# Contact Lens Complications

Nathan Efron is one of the most prolific and effective translators of research into 'clinical pearls'. In this excellent book he has encapsulated, in typical succinct prose, the key elements of the most common contact lens complications and illustrated these conditions with some of the world's best photographs and diagrams. This book is a must for any student or practitioner who wishes to detect, diagnose and understand the adverse events that can occur with contact lenses.

Brien A. Holden AOM PhD DSc BAppSc LOSc
Director, Co-operative Research Centre for Eye Research and Technology
Director, Cornea and Contact Lens Research Unit
Professor of Optometry, University of New South Wales, Sydney, Australia

Professor Efron is to be congratulated for the scale and thoroughness of his work on contact lens complications. This book will be of enormous value to all contact lens practitioners.

Roger J. Buckley MA FRCS FRCOphth
Consultant Ophthalmologist, Moorfields Eye Hospital, London
Professor of Ocular Medicine, City University, London

In reader-friendly format for those in practice and those in training, this book details diagnosis and management of contact lens complications – and is illustrated with useful tables and excellent colour photographs.

Rosemary E. Bailey FBDO (Hons) CL
Director of Contact Lens Examinations, Association of British Dispensing Opticians
Trainee Contact Lens Optician Co-ordinator, Boots Opticians Ltd, Nottingham

# CONTACT LENS COMPLICATIONS

**Nathan Efron**

*BScOptom PhD (Melbourne) DSc (UMIST)*
*MCOptom FAAO (Dip CL) FIACLE FCLSA FVCO*

Professor of Clinical Optometry
Director, Eurolens Research
Department of Optometry and Neuroscience
University of Manchester Institute of Science and Technology
Manchester
United Kingdom

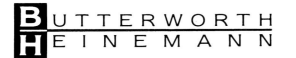

Optician

OXFORD AUCKLAND BOSTON JOHANNESBURG MELBOURNE NEW DELHI

*This book is dedicated to*
*my wife, Suzanne*
*my daughter, Zoe*
*and my son, Bruce*

Butterworth-Heinemann
Linacre House, Jordan Hill, Oxford OX2 8DP
225 Wildwood Avenue, Woburn, MA 01801-2041
A division of Reed Educational and Professional Publishing Ltd

℞ A member of the Reed Elsevier plc group

First published 1999

Reprinted 2000

**British Library Cataloguing in Publication Data**
A catalogue record for this book is available from the British Library

**Library of Congress Cataloguing in Publication Data**
A catalogue record for this book is available from the Library of Congress

ISBN 0 7506 0582 0

Typeset by David Gregson Associates, Beccles, Suffolk
Printed and bound in Spain

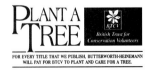

# Contents

*Preface*                                          vii
*Acknowledgements*                                  ix
*Authorship and copyright owners of figures*        xi
*Tabular summary of contact lens*
*    complications*                                 xv

## Part I
## Eyelids

### Chapter 1
### Blinking                                         3
The normal spontaneous blink                         3
Alterations to blinking caused by
    contact lenses                                   5
Complications of abnormal blinking
    with contact lenses                              5
Management of abnormal blinking
    with contact lenses                              8
Differential diagnosis of blinking
    disorders                                        8

### Chapter 2
### Ptosis                                           10
Signs and symptoms of contact lens-
    induced ptosis (CLIP)                            10
Prevalence of CLIP                                   11
Pathology of CLIP                                    11
Aetiology of CLIP                                    12
Patient management in CLIP                           13
Prognosis in CLIP                                    14
Differential diagnosis of CLIP                       14
Other contact lens-associated eyelid
    disorders                                        14

### Chapter 3
### Meibomian gland
###     dysfunction                                  18
Prevalence                                           19
Signs and symptoms                                   19
Pathology                                            20
Aetiology                                            20

Patient management                                   21
Prognosis                                            22
Differential diagnosis                               22
Other contact lens-associated
    meibomian gland disorders                        22

### Chapter 4
### Eyelash disorders                                24
External hordeolum (stye)                            24
Marginal blepharitis                                 24
Parasitic infestation of eyelashes                   25
Other contact lens-associated eyelash
    disorders                                        28

## Part II
## Conjunctiva

### Chapter 5
### Bulbar hyperaemia                                33
Definitions                                          33
Prevalence                                           34
Signs and symptoms                                   34
Pathology                                            35
Aetiology                                            35
Observation and grading                              36
Treatment                                            37
Prognosis                                            38
Differential diagnosis                               38

### Chapter 6
### Papillary conjunctivitis                         40
Prevalence                                           40
Normal tarsal conjunctiva                            41
Signs and symptoms                                   41
Pathology                                            42
Aetiology                                            43
Observation and grading                              44
Treatment                                            45
Prognosis                                            47
Differential diagnosis                               47

### Chapter 7
### Superior limbic
###     keratoconjunctivitis                         50
Prevalence                                           50
Signs and symptoms                                   51
Pathology                                            52
Aetiology                                            52
Treatment                                            55
Prognosis                                            56
Differential diagnosis                               56

## Part III
## Tear Film

### Chapter 8
### Tear film dysfunction                            61
Normal tear film                                     61
Tear film function during contact lens
    wear                                             62
Signs of tear film dysfunction during
    contact lens wear                                62
Symptoms                                             66
Pathology and aetiology                              66
Treatment                                            68
Prognosis                                            70
Differential diagnosis                               70

## Part IV
## Corneal Epithelium

### Chapter 9
### Staining                                         75
Prevalence                                           75
Signs and symptoms                                   75
Pathology                                            77
Aetiology                                            77
Observation and grading                              79
Management and treatment                             79
Prognosis                                            80
Differential diagnosis                               80

**Chapter 10**
**Microcysts** 82
Prevalence 82
Signs and symptoms 82
Pathology 84
Aetiology 84
Observation and grading 85
Management and treatment 85
Prognosis 86
Differential diagnosis 86

### Part V
## Corneal Stroma

**Chapter 11**
**Oedema** 91
Definition of oedema 91
Demise of the 'CCC' criterion 91
Prevalence 92
Signs and symptoms 92
Pathology 93
Aetiology 94
Observation and grading 95
Management and treatment 95
Prognosis 97
Differential diagnosis 97

**Chapter 12**
**Neovascularisation** 99
Prevalence 99
Signs and symptoms 100
Pathology 101
Aetiology 102
Observation and grading 103
Management and treatment 103
Prognosis 104
Differential diagnosis 105

**Chapter 13**
**Sterile infiltrative keratitis** 108
Terminology 108
Prevalence 109
Signs and symptoms 109
Pathology 111
Aetiology 111
Patient management 112
Prognosis 113
Differential diagnosis 114

**Chapter 14**
**Microbial infiltrative keratitis** 116
Incidence 117
Relative risk 117
Signs and symptoms 117
Pathology 118
Aetiology 120
Patient management 122
Prognosis 123
Differential diagnosis 123

### Part VI
## Corneal Endothelium

**Chapter 15**
**Bedewing** 129
Incidence 129
Signs and symptoms 129
Pathology 130
Aetiology 131
Patient management 131
Prognosis 132
Differential diagnosis 132

**Chapter 16**
**Blebs** 134
Prevalence 134
Signs and symptoms 135
Pathology 135
Aetiology 135
Observation and grading 136
Management and prognosis 136
Differential diagnosis 137

**Chapter 17**
**Polymegethism** 139
The normal endothelium 139
Defining endothelial changes 139
Contact lens effects 140
Prevalence 140
Signs and symptoms 141
Pathology 141
Aetiology 143
Observation and grading 143
Management 144
Prognosis 145
Differential diagnosis 145

### Part VII
## Corneal Topography

**Chapter 18**
**Corneal shape change** 149
Incidence 149
Signs and symptoms 150
Pathology 152
Aetiology 152
Patient management 154
Prognosis 155
Differential diagnosis 156
Intentional corneal moulding 157

### Part VIII
## Grading and Classification

**Chapter 19**
**Grading scales and morphs** 161
Photographic vs painted scales 162
Painted grading scales 162
Explanation of illustrations 163
Method of grading 165
Interpretation of grading 165
Grading morphs 166
Tear film classification 166
Conclusions 167

*Appendices*
Appendix A Grading scales for contact lens complications 171
Appendix B Guillon–Keeler tear film classification system 181
Appendix C Instructions for use of grading morphs on CD-ROM 187

*Index* 189

# Preface

My main motivation for writing this textbook has been to produce a 'clinician-friendly' account of ocular complications that are induced by, and associated with, contact lens wear. Previously published textbooks on the subject of contact lens complications typically have been organised with a primary focus on aetiology (causation). Although such an approach has been extremely useful in developing a broad theoretical understanding of how contact lenses interact with the anterior ocular structures, clinicians may not find this approach intuitive. In dealing with contact lens complications, clinicians first learn of the symptoms and then look for signs of pathology – typically using a slit-lamp biomicroscope in the first instance. Once the problem has been identified, deductive evidence-based reasoning begins and further investigations are undertaken in an attempt to understand and then manage the condition.

In view of the above, therefore, I offer a different approach in this textbook – one that is designed to be of practical value to clinicians. The subject matter is divided into eight parts, seven of which relate to the primary anterior ocular structures that can affect, or be affected by, contact lenses. (The eighth section is about grading scales; see below.) Within each part, various identifiable tissue pathologies or conditions are discussed by way of a systematic consideration of signs, symptoms, aetiology, pathology, management options, prognosis and differential diagnosis. This systematic approach is reflected in the tabular summary on pages xvi to xxxiii, which is designed to assist practitioners in (a) locating information on a particular complication in the main text, and (b) gaining a quick overview of a specific complication in a broader context.

I have deliberately placed heavy emphasis on the importance of understanding the various ocular complications that can occur. In particular, the development of an understanding of the aetiology and pathology of a condition is critical to formulating a link between the presenting signs and symptoms, and the development of an appropriate management plan and formulation of an accurate prognosis. Our understanding of contact lens-associated ocular complications has surged ahead over the past decade. There are still some elements of the various tissue complications that will require further research in order to develop a fuller understanding; nevertheless, there now exists an extensive knowledge base that has allowed me to construct a coherent account of the subject, which hopefully I have comprehensively captured, correctly interpreted and faithfully translated to be of immediate clinical relevance.

A critical aspect of the clinical management of an ocular complication of contact lens wear is the ability accurately to gauge and record the severity of the condition. To assist clinicians in this task, I have developed grading scales for a representative range of complications; these are presented in Appendix A of this book, together with a comprehensive account of how they can be used (Chapter 19). In addition, the grading scales have been converted to user-friendly movie morph sequences, which offer the possibility of computer-based grading. Grading morphs are included in the enclosed CD-ROM. Also presented in Appendix B is a system for classifying the various appearances of the tear film during contact lens wear.

A brief word on referencing – I have adopted the now often-used convention of citing only the first three authors of multi-authored papers, but have differed in style from most other authors by not including 'et al' after the third author where there are more than three. This is meant as no disrespect to those who 'ranked' fourth or higher; you know who you are (indeed, about 15 acknowledgements of my own scholarly contributions will not appear in this book as a result of this adopted style). Similarly, I have only listed the first page of cited works.

With ongoing improvements in contact lens materials and designs, it is my hope that contact lens tissue complications will eventually cease to occur, making this book redundant. In the mean time, I hope that this book will aid practitioners in either preventing problems from occurring, or identifying problems at an early stage so that effective management strategies can be put in place for the ultimate benefit of our patients.

*Nathan Efron*

# Acknowledgements

Although I am the sole author of this book, I am not the sole illustrator. I am very fortunate to have been given open access to four magnificent slide libraries of contact lens complications. Between 1987 and 1994, Bausch & Lomb compiled an extensive set of slides which were submissions to a photographic competition of contact lens-related topics, held as part of the European Symposium on Contact Lenses. I thank Rob Rosenbrand of Bausch & Lomb for all his efforts in putting together and carefully cataloguing this outstanding slide set.

I would like to thank the British Contact Lens Association (BCLA), the International Association of Contact Lens Educators (IACLE), and the Cornea and Contact Lens Research Unit (CCLRU), who also have given me access to their extensive slide collections. I salute the clinical excellence and skills of the many practitioners who took the photographs that are used in this book; each of whom is acknowledged in the following table.

It has been an honour and a privilege to work with the renowned medical ophthalmic artist Terry Tarrant. I have been an admirer of Terry's work ever since I was an undergraduate optometry student at the University of Melbourne in the 1970s, having studied from many of the books he illustrated. The grading illustrations he painted for this book are as good as, if not better than, any of his previous work I have seen. Thanks also to Hydron UK, who, through the kind offices of Joe Tanner, provided resources and support that allowed the production and world wide distribution of hand-held and poster-size versions of the grading scales that appear in Appendix A.

I am most grateful to Gordon Addison, who, as a final year optometry student at UMIST, created the morph movie sequences which appear on the enclosed CD-ROM. I also appreciate the assistance of Dr Philip Morgan for creating the interface for the interactive program in which the morphs are presented. I am sure that the fruits of their labours will be enjoyed by all who use the CD-ROM. Thanks also go to Dr J. P. Guillon, and Laura Haverley of Keeler, for giving permission to publish the Guillon–Keeler tear film classification system.

I am most grateful to my publisher, Caroline Makepeace, for her constant encouragement over many years, and to Caroline's hard-working team at Butterworth-Heinemann. I would like to thank Alison Ewbank, editor of the *Optician* journal, and her editorial team, who presented me with the unique opportunity of serialising my book in *Optician*, thus providing impetus for completing the book according to a demanding schedule of bi-monthly deadlines spread over three years.

I thank my wife, Suzanne, for her patience, understanding, support and constant encouragement throughout the long and relentless writing process, and my children, Zoe and Bruce, who must have wondered why their daddy was so often playing with his computer instead of with them.

And finally, I thank you the reader, for your expression of confidence in me by way of buying and/or using this book. I truly hope that my devotion and dedication to this subject has translated into an offering that will be of real clinical value, in the first instance to yourself, and ultimately to our contact lens patients, who deserve only the very best clinical care.

The publishers would like to thank Keeler Ltd, Windsor, UK and Hydron Ltd, Farnborough, UK for sponsoring this publication.

# Authorship and copyright owners of figures

Every effort has been made to trace copyright holders of illustrations, but if any have been inadvertently overlooked or if any errors occur in the list below, the publishers will be pleased to make the necessary arrangement at the first opportunity.

**Key**
BCLA = British Contact Lens Association
B&L = Bausch & Lomb
CCLRU = Cornea and Contact Lens Research Unit
IOVS = Investigative Ophthalmology and Visual Science

| Figure | Author | Copyright owner | Figure | Author | Copyright owner |
|--------|--------|-----------------|--------|--------|-----------------|
| Fig. 1.1 | Timothy Grant | B&L | Fig. 4.9 | I. DeSchepper | B&L |
| Fig. 1.2 | Nathan Efron | *Optician* | Fig. 4.10 | J. Prummel | B&L |
| Fig. 1.3 | Nathan Efron | *Optician* | Fig. 5.1 | Brien Holden | CCLRU |
| Fig. 1.4 | Donna LaHood | B&L | Fig. 5.2 | Leon Davids | B&L |
| Fig. 1.5a | Brien Holden | CCLRU | Fig. 5.3 | M.F. Pettigrew | B&L |
| Fig. 1.5b | Brien Holden | CCLRU | Fig. 5.4 | Charline Gauthier | B&L |
| Fig. 1.5c | Brien Holden | CCLRU | Fig. 5.5 | Meng Poey Soh | Meng Poey Soh |
| Fig. 1.6 | Lucia McGrogan | Lucia McGrogan | Fig. 5.6 | H.J. Rutten | B&L |
| Fig. 1.7 | Nathan Efron | *Optician* | Fig. 5.7 | Nathan Efron | *Optician* |
| Fig. 2.1 | Desmond Fonn | B&L | Fig. 5.8 | Nathan Efron | *Optician* |
| Fig. 2.2 | Nathan Efron | *Optician* | Fig. 5.9 | Nathan Efron | *Optician* |
| Fig. 2.3 | Meng Poey Soh | Meng Poey Soh | Fig. 5.10 | Hilmar Bussaker | Hilmar Bussaker |
| Fig. 2.4 | Desmond Fonn | B&L | Fig. 6.1 | Russell Lowe | B&L |
| Fig. 2.5 | Frank Pettigrew | BCLA | Fig. 6.2 | Brien Holden | CCLRU |
| Fig. 2.6 | Jan Kok | B&L | Fig. 6.3 | A. Gustafsson | A. Gustafsson |
| Fig. 2.7 | Robert Terry | CCLRU | Fig. 6.4 | Robert Terry | B&L |
| Fig. 2.8 | Sylvie Sulaiman | B&L | Fig. 6.5 *left* | C.D. Euwijk | B&L |
| Fig. 3.1 | Lyndon Jones | B&L | Fig. 6.5 *right* | C.D. Euwijk | B&L |
| Fig. 3.2 | Xavier Llobet | B&L | Fig. 6.6 | Nathan Efron | *Optician* |
| Fig. 3.3 | Lourdes Llobet | B&L | Fig. 6.7 | Nathan Efron | *Optician* |
| Fig. 3.4 | Lourdes Llobet | B&L | Fig. 6.8 *left* | Eric Papas | B&L |
| Fig. 3.5 | Arthur Back | B&L | Fig. 6.8 *right* | Eric Papas | B&L |
| Fig. 3.6 | Luigina Sorbara | B&L | Fig. 6.9 | Martina Alt | B&L |
| Fig. 3.7 | Philip Morgan | Philip Morgan | Fig. 6.10 | Lyndon Jones | BCLA |
| Fig. 4.1 | Patrick Caroline | B&L | Fig. 6.11 | Nathan Efron | *Optician* |
| Fig. 4.2 | Deborah Jones | BCLA | Fig. 6.12 *left* | Maki Shiobara | B&L |
| Fig. 4.3 | Deborah Jones | BCLA | Fig. 6.12 *right* | Brien Holden | CCLRU |
| Fig. 4.4 | Patrick Caroline | Patrick Caroline | Fig. 6.13 | V.K. Dada | B&L |
| Fig. 4.5 | Lourdes Llobet | B&L | Fig. 6.14 | Desmond Fonn | B&L |
| Fig. 4.6 | Nathan Efron | *Optician* | Fig. 7.1 | A.J. Elder Smith | BCLA |
| Fig. 4.7 | Patrick Caroline | Patrick Caroline | Fig. 7.2 | Mee Sing Chong | B&L |
| Fig. 4.8 | Patrick Caroline | Patrick Caroline | Fig. 7.3 | Nathan Efron | *Optician* |

| Figure | Author | Copyright owner | Figure | Author | Copyright owner |
|---|---|---|---|---|---|
| Fig. 7.4 | Brien Holden | CCLRU | Fig. 12.1 | Rosemary Austen | B&L |
| Fig. 7.5 | Nathan Efron | *Optician* | Fig. 12.2 | Charles McMonnies | Charles McMonnies |
| Fig. 7.6 | Nathan Efron | *Optician* | Fig. 12.3 | Desmond Fonn | BCLA |
| Fig. 7.7 | Padmaja Sankaridurg | B&L | Fig. 12.4 | Brien Holden | CCLRU |
| Fig. 8.1 | Nathan Efron | *Optician* | Fig. 12.5 | Nathan Efron | *Optician* |
| Fig. 8.2 | Nathan Efron | *Optician* | Fig. 12.6 | Patrick Caroline | B&L |
| Fig. 8.3 | Rolf Haberer | B&L | Fig. 12.7 | Nathan Efron | *Optician* |
| Fig. 8.4 | Timothy Golding | Timothy Golding | Fig. 12.8 | Patrick Caroline | B&L |
| Fig. 8.5 | Timothy Golding | Timothy Golding | Fig. 12.9 | Nathan Efron | *Optician* |
| Fig. 8.6 | Hilmar Bussaker | Hilmar Bussaker | Fig. 12.10 | Nathan Efron | *Optician* |
| Fig. 8.7 | Hilmar Bussaker | Hilmar Bussaker | Fig. 12.11 | Nathan Efron | *Optician* |
| Fig. 8.8 | Hilmar Bussaker | Hilmar Bussaker | Fig. 12.12 | Robert Grohe | Robert Grohe |
| Fig. 8.9 | Hilmar Bussaker | Hilmar Bussaker | Fig. 13.1 | Luigina Sorbara | B&L |
| Fig. 8.10 | Xavier Llobet | B&L | Fig. 13.2 | Nathan Efron | *Optician* |
| Fig. 8.11 | Arthur Back | B&L | Fig. 13.3 | Gisele Sachs | B&L |
| Fig. 8.12 | Timothy Golding | Timothy Golding | Fig. 13.4 | Nathan Efron | *Optician* |
| Fig. 8.13 | Timothy Golding | Timothy Golding | Fig. 13.5 | Deborah Jones | BCLA |
| Fig. 8.14 | Patrick Caroline | B&L | Fig. 13.6 | Nathan Efron | *Optician* |
| Fig. 8.15 | A. Aan de Kerk | B&L | Fig. 13.7 | Patrick Caroline | B&L |
| Fig. 8.16 | Arthur Back | B&L | Fig. 13.8 | Miguel Lumeras | B&L |
| Fig. 8.17 | Adrian Bruce | B&L | Fig. 13.9 | Kathy Dumbleton | B&L |
| Fig. 8.18 | Timothy Golding | Timothy Golding | Fig. 13.10 | Patrick Caroline | B&L |
| Fig. 8.19 | Timothy Golding | Timothy Golding | Fig. 14.1 | Brien Holden | CCLRU |
| Fig. 8.20 | Meng Poey Soh | Meng Poey Soh | Fig. 14.2 | Lyndon Jones | BCLA |
| Fig. 8.21 | Nathan Efron | *Optician* | Fig. 14.3 | Lyndon Jones | BCLA |
| Fig. 9.1 | Gary Orsborn | B&L | Fig. 14.4 | Donna LaHood | CCLRU |
| Fig. 9.2 | Brien Holden | CCLRU | Fig. 14.5 | Meng Poey Soh | Meng Poey Soh |
| Fig. 9.3 | Luigina Sorbara | B&L | Fig. 14.6 | Florence Mallet | B&L |
| Fig. 9.4 | Lyndon Jones | B&L | Fig. 14.7 | Suzanne Fleiszig | Suzanne Fleiszig |
| Fig. 9.5 | Arthur Back | B&L | Fig. 14.8 | Nathan Efron | *Optician* |
| Fig. 9.6 | Richard Lindsay | B&L | Fig. 14.9 | Suzanne Fleiszig | Suzanne Fleiszig |
| Fig. 9.7 | Nathan Efron | *Optician* | Fig. 14.10 | Andrew Tullo | Andrew Tullo |
| Fig. 9.8 | Donna LaHood | B&L | Fig. 14.11 | Luigina Sorbara | B&L |
| Fig. 9.9 | Deborah Jones | B&L | Fig. 14.12 | F. J. Palomar-Mascaro | B&L |
| Fig. 9.10 | Desmond Fonn | Desmond Fonn | Fig. 14.13 | Patrick Caroline | B&L |
| Fig. 9.11 | W. Vreugdenhil | B&L | Fig. 15.1 | Steve Zantos | CCLRU |
| Fig. 9.12 | Mee Sing Chong | B&L | Fig. 15.2 | Charles McMonnies | Charles McMonnies |
| Fig. 10.1 | Craig Woods | BCLA | Fig. 15.3 | Ronald Stevenson | BCLA |
| Fig. 10.2 | David Ruston | BCLA | Fig. 15.4 | Nathan Efron | *Optician* |
| Fig. 10.3 | Steve Zantos | CCLRU | Fig. 15.5 | Nathan Efron | *Optician* |
| Fig. 10.4 | Nathan Efron | *Optician* | Fig. 15.6 | Steve Zantos | CCLRU |
| Fig. 10.5 | Nathan Efron | *Optician* | Fig. 15.7 | Steve Zantos | CCLRU |
| Fig. 10.6 | Nathan Efron | *Optician* | Fig. 16.1 | Arthur Ho | CCLRU |
| Fig. 10.7 | Nathan Efron | *Optician* | Fig. 16.2 | Nathan Efron | *Optician* |
| Fig. 10.8 | Sylvie Sulaiman | B&L | Fig. 16.3 | Nathan Efron | *Optician* |
| Fig. 11.1 | Patrick Caroline | B&L | Fig. 16.4 | Nathan Efron | *Optician* |
| Fig. 11.2 *left* | Desmond Fonn | Desmond Fonn | Fig. 16.5 *left* | Steve Zantos, | CCLRU |
| Fig. 11.2 *centre* | Brien Holden | CCLRU | Fig. 16.5 *centre* | Lewis Williams | CCLRU |
| Fig. 11.2 *right* | Brien Holden | CCLRU | Fig. 16.5 *right* | Brien Holden | CCLRU |
| Fig. 11.3 | Nathan Efron | *Optician* | Fig. 16.6 | Charline Gauthier | B&L |
| Fig. 11.4 | Steve Zantos | CCLRU | Fig. 17.1 | Rolf Haberer | B&L |
| Fig. 11.5 | Nathan Efron | *Optician* | Fig. 17.2 *left* | Brien Holden | CCLRU |
| Fig. 11.6 | Nathan Efron | *Optician* | Fig. 17.2 *right* | Brien Holden | CCLRU |
| Fig. 11.7 | Nathan Efron | *Optician* | Fig. 17.3 | Brien Holden | IOVS |
| Fig. 11.8 | Patrick Caroline | B&L | Fig. 17.4 *left* | Brien Holden | CCLRU |
| Fig. 11.9 | Nathan Efron | *Optician* | Fig. 17.4 *right* | Brien Holden | CCLRU |

| Figure | Author | Copyright owner | Figure | Author | Copyright owner |
|---|---|---|---|---|---|
| Fig. 17.5 | Nathan Efron | *Optician* | Fig. 18.10 | Helen Swarbrick | B&L |
| Fig. 17.6 | Nathan Efron | *Optician* | Fig. 18.11 | Stephen Klyce | Stephen Klyce |
| Fig. 17.7 | Nathan Efron | *Optician* | Fig. 18.12 | Meredith Reyes | B&L |
| Fig. 17.8 | Nathan Efron | *Optician* | Fig. 18.13 | Ruth Cornish | B&L |
| Fig. 17.9 | Nathan Efron | *Optician* | Fig. 18.14 | Ruth Cornish | B&L |
| Fig. 17.10 | Nathan Efron | *Optician* | Fig. 19.1 | Nathan Efron | *Optician* |
| Fig. 17.11 | Nathan Efron | *Optician* | Fig. 19.2 | Nathan Efron | *Optician* |
| Fig. 17.12 | Nathan Efron | *Optician* | Fig. 19.3 | Nathan Efron | *Optician* |
| Fig. 18.1 | Russell Lowe | B&L | Fig. 19.4 | Nathan Efron | *Optician* |
| Fig. 18.2 | Stephen Klyce | Stephen Klyce | Fig. 19.5 | Nathan Efron | *Optician* |
| Fig. 18.3 | Stephen Klyce | Stephen Klyce | Fig. 19.6 | Nathan Efron | *Optician* |
| Fig. 18.4 | C. D. Euwijk | B&L | Fig. 19.7 | Nathan Efron | *Optician* |
| Fig. 18.5 | Donna LaHood | B&L | Fig. 19.8 | Nathan Efron | *Optician* |
| Fig. 18.6 | Craig Woods | B&L | Fig. 19.9 | Nathan Efron | *Optician* |
| Fig. 18.7 | Gary Orsborn | B&L | Fig. 19.10 | Nathan Efron | *Optician* |
| Fig. 18.8 | Russell Lowe | B&L | Fig. 19.11 | Nathan Efron | *Optician* |
| Fig. 18.9 | Robert Terry | B&L | | | |

# Tabular summary of contact lens complications

## I  EYELIDS

| Condition | Appearance | Signs | Symptoms |
|---|---|---|---|
| **Blinking** | 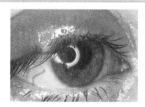 | ■ Complete blink (80%)<br>■ Incomplete blink (17%)<br>■ Twitch blink (2%)<br>■ Forced blink (1%)<br><br>p. 4 | ■ None<br><br><br><br>p. 5 |
| **Ptosis** | 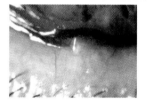 | ■ Narrowing of palpebral aperture size<br>  • no lens: 10.10 mm<br>  • soft lens: 10.24 mm<br>  • RGP lens: 9.76 mm<br>■ Large gap between upper skin fold and upper lid margin<br>■ Only seen in RGP lens wearers<br><br>p. 10 | ■ Complaints of poor cosmesis when excessive<br><br><br><br><br><br>p. 11 |
| **Meibomian gland dysfunction** | 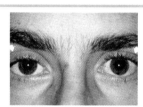 | ■ Cloudy, creamy, yellow expression<br>■ Inspissated discharge<br>■ Poorly wetting lenses<br>■ Tear meniscus frothing<br>■ No secretion if blocked<br>■ Distended or distorted meibomian glands seen in lid retroillumination<br><br>p. 19 | ■ Smeary vision<br>■ Greasy lenses<br>■ Dry eye<br>■ Lens intolerance<br><br><br><br>p. 19 |
| **External hordeolum (stye)** | 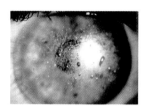 | ■ Discrete inflamed swelling of anterior lid margin<br>■ Occurs singly or as multiple small abscesses<br><br><br><br><br><br>p. 24 | ■ Mild discomfort<br>■ Extremely tender to touch<br>■ Mechanical effect of contact lenses:<br>  • soft lens presses on stye causing discomfort and increased lens movement<br>  • RGP lens fitted interpalpebrally buffets lid margin<br><br>p. 24 |
| **Staphylococcal anterior blepharitis** | 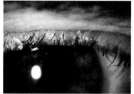 | ■ Hyperaemia<br>■ Telangiectasis<br>■ Scaling of lid margins<br>  • brittle, leaving bleeding ulcer when removed<br>■ Lashes stuck together<br>■ Lash collarette<br>■ Madarosis<br>■ Poliosis<br>■ Tylosis<br><br>p. 24 | ■ Burning<br>■ Itching<br>■ Mild photophobia<br>■ Foreign body sensation<br>■ Dry eye<br>  • worse in morning<br>■ Lens intolerance<br><br><br><br>p. 25 |

# contact lens complications

| Pathology | Aetiology | Treatment | Prognosis | Differential diagnosis |
|---|---|---|---|---|
| ■ Abnormal blinking can cause:<br>• lens surface drying<br>• deposition<br>• epithelial desiccation<br>• post-lens tear stagnation<br>• hypoxia<br>• hypercapnia<br>• 3 and 9 o'clock staining<br>• poor lens fitting | ■ Tear break-up induces blinking<br>■ Other unknown factors are involved<br>■ Oral contraceptives reduce blink rate in females | ■ Blink training<br>■ Alter lens fit<br>• less post-lens debris with RGP lenses<br>• interpalpebral RGP fit<br>• soft lenses solve 3 and 9 o'clock staining | ■ Training can improve blinking<br>■ Altering lens design can improve blinking | ■ Interruption to neural input<br>■ Interruption to muscular systems<br>■ Local eyelid pathology |
| p. 5 | p. 5 | p. 8 | p. 8 | p. 8 |
| ■ Trauma during insertion and removal due to:<br>• forced lid squeezing<br>• lateral lid stretching<br>■ Rigid lens displacement of tarsus<br>■ Blink-induced lens rubbing<br>■ Blepharospasm<br>■ Papillary conjunctivitis | ■ Lid oedema<br>■ Levator aponeurosis:<br>• disinsertion<br>• dehiscence<br>• thinning<br>• lengthening | ■ Cease lens wear for 1–3 months<br>■ Cure papillary conjunctivitis<br>■ Refit with soft lenses<br>■ Lid surgery<br>■ Scleral lens ptosis crutch<br>■ Spectacle prop<br>■ Surgical tape | ■ If oedema: good<br>■ If aponeurogenic: poor<br>■ Surgery can yield good results | ■ Soft lenses can alter palpebral aperture size<br>■ Embedded lens<br>■ Ectropion<br>■ Entropion<br>■ Lagophthalmos |
| p. 11 | p. 12 | p. 13 | p. 14 | p. 14 |
| ■ Blocked meibomian orifice<br>■ Increased keratinisation of duct walls | ■ Increased turnover of ductal epidermis<br>■ Abnormal meibomian oils<br>• more keratin proteins<br>■ Absence of lid rubbing | ■ Warm compresses<br>■ Lid scrubs<br>■ Mechanical expression<br>■ Antibiotics<br>■ Artificial tears<br>■ Surfactant lens cleaning<br>■ Improved lid hygiene | ■ Excellent if good control can be achieved | ■ External hordeolum<br>• localised swelling at lid margin<br>■ Internal hordeolum<br>• tender localised swelling<br>■ Chalazion<br>• chronic form of meibomian gland dysfunction |
| p. 20 | p. 20 | p. 21 | p. 22 | p. 22 |
| ■ Inflammation of:<br>• tissue lining lash follicle, and/or<br>• associated gland of Zeis or Moll | ■ Typically acute *Staphylococcal* infection<br>■ Often occurs in patients with staphylococcal anterior blepharitis | ■ Remove eyelash from affected follicle<br>■ Apply hot compress<br>■ May spontaneously discharge anteriorly<br>■ Cease lens wear during acute phase | ■ Self-limiting<br>■ Typical time course: 7 days | ■ External hordeolum<br>• localised swelling at lid margin<br>■ Internal hordeolum<br>• tender localised swelling<br>• not at lid margin<br>■ Chalazion<br>• chronic form of meibomian gland dysfunction<br>• not at lid margin |
| p. 24 | p. 24 | p. 24 | p. 24 | p. 24 |
| ■ *Staphylococcal* endotoxin-induced complications include:<br>• low grade conjunctivitis<br>• toxic punctate epitheliopathy | ■ *Staphylococcal* infection of eyelash follicles | ■ Antibiotic ointments<br>■ Promote lid hygiene<br>■ Steroids<br>■ Artificial tears<br>■ May need to suspend lens wear during acute treatment phase | ■ Variable: expect periods of remission and exacerbation | ■ Need to differentiate from seborrhoeic anterior blepharitis (see below) |
| p. 25 | p. 25 | p. 25 | p. 25 | p. 25 |

## I  EYELIDS (continued)

| Condition | Appearance | Signs | Symptoms |
|---|---|---|---|
| **Seborrhoeic anterior blepharitis** | 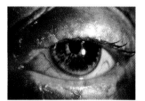 | ■ Hyperaemia<br>■ Telangiectasis<br>■ Scaling of lid margins<br>  • shiny, waxy<br>■ Lashes stuck together<br>■ Madarosis<br>■ Poliosis<br><br>p. 25 | ■ Burning<br>■ Itching<br>■ Mild photophobia<br>■ Foreign body sensation<br>■ Dry eye<br>  • worse in morning<br>■ Lens intolerance<br>■ Symptoms less severe than staphylococcal<br><br>p. 25 |
| **Mites** | 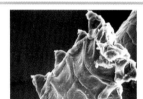 | ■ Presence of mites<br>■ Erythema of lid margins<br>■ Lid hyperplasia<br>■ Madarosis<br>■ Conjunctival injection<br>■ Lash collarette<br>■ Follicular distension<br>■ Meibomian gland blockage<br>■ Lashes easily removed<br><br>p. 25 | ■ Burning<br>■ Itching<br>■ Crusting<br>■ Swelling of lid margins<br>■ Loss of lashes<br>■ Lens intolerance<br><br>p. 26 |
| **Lice** | 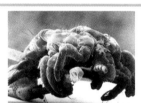 | ■ Presence of lice and nits<br>■ Erythema of lid margins<br>■ Conjunctival injection<br>■ Madarosis<br>■ Pre-auricular lymphadenopathy<br>■ Brown deposit at base of lashes<br>  • blood from host<br>  • faeces from lice<br>■ Blue spots on lid margins<br>  • secreted by lice<br><br>p. 26 | ■ Burning<br>■ Itching<br>■ Crusting<br>■ Swelling of lid margins<br>■ Lens intolerance<br><br>p. 27 |

# contact lens complications

| Pathology | Aetiology | Treatment | Prognosis | Differential diagnosis |
|---|---|---|---|---|
| ■ *Staphylococcal* endotoxin-induced complications include:<br>• low grade conjunctivitis<br>• toxic punctate epitheliopathy | ■ Disorder of glands of Zeis or Moll | ■ Promote lid hygiene<br>■ Artificial tears<br>■ May need to suspend lens wear during acute treatment phase | Variable: expect periods of remission and exacerbation | Need to differentiate from *Staphylococcal* anterior blepharitis (see above) |
| p. 25 | p. 25 | p. 25 | p. 25 | p. 25 |
| ■ *Demodex folliculorum*<br>• resides in space between follicle wall and lash<br>• eats epithelial lining of lash follicle<br>■ *Demodex brevis*<br>• resides in gland of Zeis<br>• reproduces in oily environment | ■ *Demodex folliculorum*<br>■ *Demodex brevis* | ■ Topical anaesthetic and application of toxic substances<br>■ Vigorous lid scrubbing<br>■ Viscous ointment overnight<br>■ Heavy metal ointments<br>■ Pilocarpine gel<br>■ Avoid use of facial oils | ■ Good – if patient complies with treatment | ■ Lice<br>• see below<br>■ Blepharitis<br>• see above |
| p. 26 | p. 26 | p. 27 | p. 28 | p. 27 |
| ■ Lice suck blood and serum from lid margin via stylus<br>■ Secondary inflammation along lid margins | ■ *Phthirus pubis*<br>• pubic louse<br>• 'sucking louse'<br>• 'crab louse' | ■ Mechanical removal<br>■ Cryotherapy (freezing)<br>■ Argon laser photoablation<br>■ 20% sodium fluorescein<br>■ Yellow mercuric oxide<br>■ Anticholinesterase agents<br>■ Vigorous lid scrubbing<br>■ Possibility of associated sexually transmitted disease<br>■ Heat application to clothing, bed clothing, sheets, towels etc.<br>■ Soak combs, brushes etc.<br>■ Isolate contaminated material for 2 weeks | ■ Good – if patient complies with treatment | ■ Mites<br>• see above<br>■ Blepharitis<br>• see above |
| p. 27 | p. 27 | p. 27 | p. 28 | p. 27 |

## II CONJUNCTIVA

| Condition | Appearance | Signs | Symptoms |
|---|---|---|---|
| **Bulbar hyperaemia** | 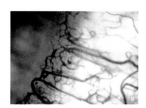 | ■ Conjunctival redness<br>■ May be regional variation (specify)<br>■ Depends on lens type:<br>  • no lens: grade 0.78<br>  • RGP lens: grade 0.96<br>  • soft lens: grade 1.54<br><br>p. 34 | ■ Often none<br>■ Itchiness<br>■ Congestion<br>■ Warm feeling<br>■ Cold feeling<br>■ Non-specific mild irritation<br><br>p. 34 |
| **Papillary conjunctivitis** | 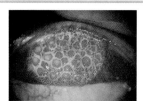 | ■ Papillae on tarsal conjunctiva<br>  • cobblestone<br>  • giant papillary<br>■ Conjunctival hyperaemia<br>■ Conjunctival oedema<br>■ Excess lens movement<br>■ Coated contact lens<br>■ Mucus discharge<br><br>p. 41 | ■ Early (grades 1 and 2)<br>  • lens awareness<br>  • mild itching<br>  • slight blur<br>■ Late (grades 3 and 4)<br>  • lens discomfort<br>  • intense itching<br>  • blur<br>  • reduced wearing time<br><br>p. 41 |
| **Superior limbic kerato-conjunctivitis** | 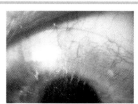 | ■ Superior limbic redness<br>■ Infiltrates<br>■ Micropannus<br>■ Corneal staining<br>■ Conjunctival staining<br>■ Hazy epithelium<br>■ Papillary hypertrophy<br>■ Corneal filaments<br>■ Corneal warpage<br><br>p. 51 | ■ Lens awareness<br>■ Burning<br>■ Itching<br>■ Photophobia<br>■ Slight vision loss<br>  • with extensive pannus<br><br>p. 51 |

# contact lens complications

| Pathology | Aetiology | Treatment | Prognosis | Differential diagnosis |
|---|---|---|---|---|
| ■ Vasodilatation due to:<br>• relaxation of smooth muscle<br>• vessel blockage | ■ Hypoxia and hypercapnia<br>■ Mechanical irritation<br>■ Immunological reaction<br>■ Infection<br>■ Inflammation<br>• acute red eye<br>■ Solution toxicity<br>■ Change in tonicity<br>■ Change in pH<br>■ Neural control | ■ Remove cause (see aetiology)<br>■ Decongestants<br>■ If >Grade 2 cease wear | ■ Excellent<br>• recovery from acute hyperaemia within 2 hours<br>• recovery from chronic hyperaemia within 2 days | ■ Cease lens wear<br>• rapid resolution implicates lens wear<br>• slow resolution suggests other cause<br>■ Hyperaemia<br>• vessels move (push)<br>■ Scleritis<br>• vessels static (push)<br>■ Haemorrhage<br>• redness between vessels |
| p. 35 | p. 35 | p. 37 | p. 38 | p. 38 |
| ■ Thickened conjunctiva<br>■ Distorted epithelial cells<br>■ Altered goblet cells<br>■ Inflammatory cells<br>• mast cells<br>• eosinophils<br>• basophils | ■ Lens deposits<br>• anterior lens surface<br>■ Mechanical irritation<br>■ Immunological reaction<br>■ Hypoxia under lid<br>■ Solution toxicity<br>• thimerosal<br>■ May be related to meibomian gland dysfunction | ■ Cease lens wear until inflammation subsides<br>■ Reduce wearing time<br>■ Improve solutions<br>■ Ocular lubricant<br>■ Mast cell stabilisers<br>■ Non-steroid anti-inflammatory agents<br>■ Change to a lens material that deposits differently<br>■ Increase frequency of lens replacement<br>■ Improve ocular hygiene | ■ Papillae can remain for weeks, months or years<br>■ Lenses can still be worn<br>■ Treat according to symptoms | ■ Follicle<br>• vessels on outside<br>■ Papilla<br>• central vascular tuft |
| p. 42 | p. 43 | p. 45 | p. 47 | p. 47 |
| ■ Cornea<br>• epitheliopathy<br>• infiltrates<br>■ Conjunctiva<br>• epithelial keratinization<br>• epithelial oedema<br>• inflammatory cells | ■ Lens deposits<br>• posterior lens surface<br>■ Mechanical irritation<br>■ Immunological reaction<br>■ Hypoxia under lid<br>■ Thimerosal<br>• hypersensitivity<br>• toxicity | ■ Cease lens wear until inflammation subsides<br>■ Reduce wearing time<br>■ Improve solutions<br>■ Ocular lubricant<br>■ Mast cell stabilisers<br>■ Non-steroid anti-inflammatory agents<br>■ Increase frequency of lens replacement<br>■ Surgery if severe | ■ After ceasing lens wear<br>• injection resolves rapidly<br>• epithelium resolves slowly<br>• can take from 3 weeks to 9 months to resolve | ■ Superficial epithelial arcuate lesion<br>• conjunctiva not involved<br>■ Bacterial conjunctivitis<br>■ Infiltrative keratitis<br>■ Theodore's superior limbic keratoconjunctivitis |
| p. 52 | p. 52 | p. 55 | p. 56 | p. 56 |

## III   TEAR FILM

| Condition | Appearance | Signs | Symptoms |
|---|---|---|---|
| **Tear film dysfunction** | 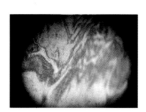 | ■ Abnormalities in:<br>  • lipid layer viewed in specular reflection<br>  • tear volume<br>  • tear structure<br>  • tear film stability<br>  • post-lens tear film<br>■ Epithelial staining | ■ Primarily 'dryness'<br>  • use a dry-eye questionnaire<br>■ Worse in females using oral contraceptives |
| | | p. 62 | p. 66 |

# contact lens complications

| Pathology | Aetiology | Treatment | Prognosis | Differential diagnosis |
|---|---|---|---|---|
| ■ Lipid deficiency or excess<br>■ Aqueous deficiency<br>■ Tear break-up<br>  • due to inter-mixing of lipid and mucus layers | ■ Lens induced changes in tear film:<br>  • tonicity<br>  • pH<br>  • composition<br>  • temperature profile<br>  • turnover<br>  • break-up | ■ Alter lens<br>■ Alter solutions<br>■ Rewetting drops<br>■ Soft lens soaking<br>■ Nutritional supplements<br>■ Control of evaporation<br>■ Reduce tear drainage<br>  • punctal plugs<br>■ Tear stimulants<br>■ Management of associated disease<br>■ Reducing or ceasing lens wear | ■ Good if problem relates to lenses/solutions<br>■ Poor if due to underlying pathology, e.g. keratoconjunctivitis sicca | ■ Aqueous tear deficiency<br>■ Lipid anomaly<br>■ Lid surfacing anomalies<br>■ Mucus deficiency<br>■ Primary epitheliopathy<br>■ Allergic dry eye |
| p. 66 | p. 66 | p. 68 | p. 70 | p. 70 |

## IV  CORNEAL EPITHELIUM

| Condition | Appearance | Signs | Symptoms |
|---|---|---|---|
| **Staining** | 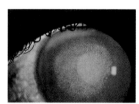 | ■ Areas of fluorescence<br>■ Can be<br>  • punctate<br>  • diffuse<br>  • coalescent<br><br>p. 75 | ■ Vision generally unaffected<br>■ Degree of discomfort depends on cause:<br>  • e.g. exposure: asymptomatic<br>  • e.g. foreign body: pain<br><br>p. 75 |
| **Microcysts** | 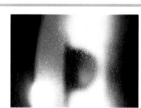 | ■ Minute scattered dots<br>■ Spherical or ovoid shape<br>■ 20 μm diameter<br>■ Reversed illumination<br><br>p. 82 | ■ Can cause slight discomfort<br>■ Can reduce vision slightly<br><br>p. 82 |

# contact lens complications

| Pathology | Aetiology | Treatment | Prognosis | Differential diagnosis |
|---|---|---|---|---|
| ■ Fluorescein<br>  • fills intercellular spaces<br>  • stains damaged cells<br>■ Rose bengal<br>  • stains dead cells<br>  • stains mucus | ■ Six categories<br>  • traumatic<br>  • exposure<br>  • metabolic<br>  • toxic<br>  • allergic<br>  • infectious | ■ Depends on cause<br>  • rinse lens<br>  • blinking instructions<br>  • fit higher Dk/L<br>  • change lens material<br>  • change solutions<br>  • kill micro-organisms | ■ Following lens removal<br>  • rapid recovery<br>  • <24 hours<br>■ While wearing lenses<br>  • slower recovery<br>  • 4–5 days | ■ Consider staining:<br>  • distribution<br>  • depth<br>  • intensity<br>  • laterality<br>  • associated history<br>  • staining patterns with<br>    different agents |
| p. 77 | p. 77 | p. 79 | p. 80 | p. 80 |
| ■ Intraepithelial sheets<br>■ Disorganised cell growth<br>■ Pockets of dead cells<br>■ Slowly pushed to surface | ■ Possible factors<br>  • prolonged hypoxia<br>  • mechanical irritation<br>  • reduced oxygen uptake<br>  • reduced mitosis<br>  • typically extended wear<br>    (EW) | ■ <30 microcysts (EW)<br>  • no action<br>  • monitor carefully<br>■ >30 microcysts (EW)<br>  • cease wear (1 month)<br>  • reduce wearing time<br>  • change to daily wear<br>  • increase lens Dk/L | ■ After ceasing wear<br>  • increase (7 days)<br>  • then decrease<br>■ Recovery in 2 months | ■ Tear film debris<br>  • move on blink<br>■ Vacuoles<br>  • unreversed optics<br>■ Bedewing<br>  • endothelial<br>■ Dimple veiling<br>  • very large<br>■ Mucus balls<br>  • unreversed optics |
| p. 84 | p. 84 | p. 85 | p. 86 | p. 86 |

## V CORNEAL STROMA

| Condition | Appearance | Signs | Symptoms |
|---|---|---|---|
| **Oedema** | | ■ <2%: undetectable<br> • 'safe'<br>■ >5%: vertical striae<br> • caution<br>■ >8%: posterior folds<br> • danger<br>■ >15%: loss of corneal transparency<br> • pathological<br><br>p. 92 | ■ <10% oedema<br> • none<br>■ >10% oedema<br> • discomfort<br><br><br><br><br><br>p. 92 |
| **Thinning** | | ■ Only detected using pachometry after oedema has resolved<br><br>p. 93 | ■ None<br><br>p. 93 |
| **Neo-vascularisation** | | ■ Superficial vessels<br> • from conjunctiva<br>■ Deep stromal vessels<br> • rare<br> • appear to end abruptly at limbus<br>■ 'Normal' responses:<br> • no lens: 0.2 mm<br> • DW hard: 0.4 mm<br> • DW soft: 0.6 mm<br> • EW soft: 1.4 mm<br><br>p. 100 | ■ No discomfort<br>■ VA loss if extreme<br><br><br><br><br><br><br><br><br>p. 100 |
| **Sterile infiltrative keratitis** | | ■ Typically uniocular<br>■ Culture-negative<br>■ May be non-ulcerative, e.g. contact-lens induced acute red eye<br> • haziness in stroma<br>■ May be ulcerative, e.g. culture-negative peripheral ulcer<br> • haziness in stroma<br> • overlying epithelial defect<br><br>p. 109 | ■ Extremely variable<br> • asymptomatic, or<br> • mild discomfort, or<br> • pain<br><br><br><br><br><br>p. 109 |

# contact lens complications

| Pathology | Aetiology | Treatment | Prognosis | Differential diagnosis |
|---|---|---|---|---|
| ■ Oedema<br>　• increased fluid<br>■ Striae<br>　• separated collagen fibrils<br>■ Folds<br>　• physical buckling | ■ Primarily hypoxia (50%)<br>　• lactate theory<br>■ Other factors (50%):<br>　• tear hypotonicity<br>　• hypercapnia<br>　• increased temperature<br>　• increased humidity<br>　• mechanical | ■ Alleviate hypoxia<br>　• increase material Dk<br>　• reduce lens thickness<br>　• increase lens movement<br>　• increase edge lift<br>■ Alleviate hypercapnia (as per hypoxia) | ■ Acute oedema<br>　• resolves in 2.5 hours<br>■ Chronic oedema<br>　• resolves in 7 days<br>■ Chronic oedema thins stroma (see below) | ■ Striae<br>　• nerve fibres<br>　• ghost vessels<br>■ Folds<br>　• seen in diabetes<br>■ Haze<br>　• scarring<br>　• epithelial oedema |
| p. 93 | p. 94 | p. 95 | p. 97 | p. 97 |
| ■ Reduced stromal mass | ■ Chronic oedema<br>■ Keratocyte dysfunction due to:<br>　• hypoxia<br>　• tissue acidosis<br>■ Dissolution of mucopolysaccharide ground substance | ■ Alleviate chronic hypoxia<br>　• increase material Dk<br>　• reduce lens thickness<br>　• increase lens movement<br>　• increase edge lift<br>■ Alleviate chronic hypercapnia (as per hypoxia) | ■ Unknown time course<br>　• thought to be permanent<br>■ Of physiological interest only<br>　• rate of thinning is very slow | ■ Keratoconus<br>　• central corneal thinning |
| p. 93 | p. 94 | p. 95 | p. 93 | p. 97 |
| ■ Sprouting or budding<br>■ Solid cord of vascular endothelial cells at growing tip<br>■ Thin vessel wall<br>■ Pericytes<br>■ Cell migration<br>■ Surrounding inflammatory cells<br>■ Disruption of stromal lamellae | ■ Stromal softening<br>　• hypoxia-induced oedema<br>■ Triggering agent<br>　• epithelial damage<br>　• solution toxicity<br>　• infection | ■ If severe<br>　• cease lens wear permanently<br>■ If mild<br>　• improve care system<br>　• increase Dk/L<br>　• reduce wearing time<br>　• monitor carefully | ■ On ceasing lens wear<br>　• vessels empty rapidly<br>　• ghost vessels remain<br>　• years to resolve<br>■ On reintroducing lens<br>　• ghost vessels rapidly refill | ■ Nerve fibres<br>　• any orientation<br>　• 'solid'<br>■ Striae<br>　• always vertical<br>　• white, whispy<br>■ Ghost vessels<br>　• start at limbus<br>　• relatively thick |
| p. 101 | p. 102 | p. 103 | p.104 | p. 105 |
| ■ Infiltrates could comprise of:<br>　• inflammatory cells (polymorphonuclear leucocytes)<br>　• bacterial endotoxins<br>　• serum<br>　• proteins<br>■ Bowman's layer is usually intact | ■ Bacterial contamination<br>■ Eye closure<br>■ Tight lens<br>■ Hypoxia<br>■ Mechanical trauma<br>■ Lens deposits<br>■ Solution toxicity | ■ Cold compresses<br>■ Fit disposable lenses<br>■ Alleviate trauma<br>■ Improve care system<br>■ Improve hygiene<br>■ Loosen lens fit<br>■ Change to daily wear<br>■ Fit RGP lenses<br>■ Fit low water lenses<br>■ Improve Dk/L | ■ Excellent<br>　• symptoms resolve within 48 hours<br>　• infiltrates resolve within 3 months | ■ Epidemic keratoconjunctivitis<br>　• typically bilateral<br>■ Stromal opacities<br>■ Stromal scars<br>■ Sterile vs infectious ulcer |
| p. 111 | p. 111 | p. 112 | p. 113 | p. 114 |

## V   CORNEAL  STROMA (continued)

| Condition | Appearance | Signs | Symptoms |
|---|---|---|---|
| **Microbial infiltrative keratitis** | 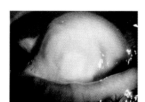 | ■ Typically uniocular<br>■ Conjunctival hyperaemia<br>■ Lid swelling<br>■ Lacrimation<br>■ Photophobia<br>■ Discharge<br>■ Loss of vision<br>■ Culture-positive<br>■ May be non-ulcerative, e.g. epidemic keratoconjunctivitis<br>  • haziness in stroma<br>■ May be ulcerative, e.g. *Pseudomonas aeruginosa*<br>  • haziness in stroma<br>  • overlying epithelial defect | ■ Initial foreign body sensation<br>■ Worsening pain |

p. 117                                            p. 117

# contact lens complications

| Pathology | Aetiology | Treatment | Prognosis | Differential diagnosis |
|---|---|---|---|---|
| ■ Infiltrates could comprise of:<br>  • the offending micro-organisms<br>  • inflammatory cells (polymorphonuclear leucocytes)<br>  • bacterial endotoxins<br>  • serum<br>  • proteins<br>■ Bowman's layer is usually compromised<br>■ Stromal destruction beneath epithelial defect | ■ Microbial infection<br>  • bacteria: e.g. *Pseudomonas aeruginosa*<br>  • amoeba: e.g. *Acanthamoeba* species<br>■ Exacerbated by other factors (see aetiology of sterile infiltrative keratitis above) | ■ Advise of risks<br>  • sleeping in lenses<br>  • diabetes<br>■ Antibiotics<br>■ Mydriatics<br>■ Non-steroidal anti-inflammatory agents<br>■ Analgesics<br>■ Tissue adhesives<br>■ Debridement<br>■ Alleviate trauma<br>■ Improve care system<br>■ Improve Dk/L<br>■ Improve hygiene<br>■ Avoid tap water<br>■ Revert to daily wear<br>■ Fit RGP lenses | ■ Depends on speed of treatment<br>  • excellent if rapid action is taken<br>■ *Pseudomonas*<br>  • condition usually worsens during initial 24 hours, then improves<br>■ *Acanthamoeba*<br>  • slow recovery<br>  • small scar remains | ■ Sterile vs infectious ulcer<br>■ *Pseudomonas* vs *Acanthamoeba*<br>■ *Acanthamoeba* vs herpetic keratitis |
| p. 118 | p. 120 | p. 122 | p. 123 | p. 123 |

## VI   CORNEAL ENDOTHELIUM

| Condition | Appearance | Signs | Symptoms |
|---|---|---|---|
| **Bedewing** | | ■ Cluster of particles<br>■ 20–50 in number<br>■ Inferior cornea, near lower pupil margin<br>■ Display reversed illumination<br><br>p. 129 | ■ Intolerance to lenses<br>■ Stinging sensation<br>■ Reduced vision<br><br><br>p. 129 |
| **Blebs** | | ■ Black non-reflecting areas<br>■ Apparent separation of cells<br><br>p. 135 | ■ None<br><br><br>p. 135 |
| **Polymegethism** | | ■ Large variation in endothelial cell size<br>■ Small : large cell ratio<br>　• normal: 1 : 5<br>　• polymegethism: 1 : 20<br><br>p. 141 | ■ Corneal exhaustion syndrome<br>　• reduced wearing time<br>　• discomfort<br><br><br>p. 141 |

# contact lens complications

| Pathology | Aetiology | Treatment | Prognosis | Differential diagnosis |
|---|---|---|---|---|
| ■ Inflammatory cells<br>　• on endothelial surface<br>　• may become 'entrapped' within endothelium | ■ Hypoxia<br>■ Inflammatory mediators<br>　• prostaglandins?<br>■ Inflammation of anterior uvea? | ■ Reduce wearing time<br>■ Check for concurrent pathology<br>■ Check for raised intraocular pressure | ■ Symptoms disappear in 3–5 days<br>■ Bedewing disappears in 3–5 months<br>■ Prolonged intolerance to lens wear | ■ Microcysts<br>　• epithelial<br>■ Guttata<br>　• large dark spots<br>■ Bedewing<br>　• on endothelium |
| p. 130 | p. 131 | p. 131 | p. 132 | p. 132 |
| ■ Oedema of cell nucleus<br>■ Intracellular vacuoles<br>■ Extracellular vacuoles<br>■ Posterior surface bulging | ■ Acidic pH shift at endothelium due to<br>　• hypercapnia: carbonic acid<br>　• hypoxia: lactic acid<br>■ Acute response | ■ Not necessary | ■ After inserting lens<br>　• peak response in 10 min<br>　• low level blebs continue<br>■ After removing lens<br>　• disappear in 2 min | ■ Guttata<br>　• permanent<br>■ Bedewing<br>　• lasts months<br>■ Blebs<br>　• last minutes |
| p. 135 | p. 135 | p. 136 | p. 136 | p. 137 |
| ■ Altered lateral cell walls<br>■ Straightening of interdigitations<br>■ Cell volume unchanged<br>■ Cell organelles normal<br>■ Poor oedema recovery | ■ Acidic pH shift at endothelium due to<br>　• hypercapnia: carbonic acid<br>　• hypoxia: lactic acid<br>■ Chronic response | ■ General strategy<br>　• alleviate acidosis<br>　• better materials<br>■ Corneal exhaustion syndrome<br>　• reduce wearing time<br>　• fit higher Dk/L lens | ■ Possible long term recovery (many years) after ceasing lens wear | ■ Pleomorphism<br>　• variation in shape<br>■ Polymegethism<br>　• variation in size |
| p. 141 | p. 143 | p. 144 | p. 145 | p. 145 |

## VII   CORNEAL TOPOGRAPHY

| Condition | Appearance | Signs | Symptoms |
|---|---|---|---|
| **Epithelial wrinkling** | 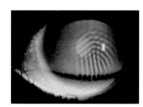 | ■ Multiple furrows<br>■ Thin medium-water lenses<br>■ Linear wave staining<br>■ Distorted 'K' mires<br><br>p. 151 | ■ Very painful<br>■ Extreme VA loss<br>  • can drop to <6/60 within minutes of lens insertion<br><br>p. 151 |
| **Corneal warpage** | 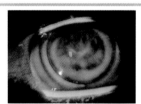 | ■ Can manifest as change in corneal:<br>  • curvature (overall)<br>  • symmetry<br>  • regularity<br>■ Corneal indentation<br>  • may be associated with corneal binding<br><br>p. 150 | ■ Spectacle blur<br>■ Haze<br>  • if associated with excess oedema<br><br>p. 150 |

# contact lens complications

| Pathology | Aetiology | Treatment | Prognosis | Differential diagnosis |
|---|---|---|---|---|
| ■ Possible changes<br> • epithelial folding<br> • local drying | ■ Possible factors<br> • mechanical pressure<br> • 'poor' lens design<br> • elastic lens properties | ■ Remove lens immediately<br>■ Refit different soft lens<br>■ Refit with RGP | ■ Discomfort for 24 hr<br>■ Lens recovery time is directly related to lens wear time | ■ Fischer–Schweitzer mosaic<br> • eye rubbing effect<br>■ Wrinkling<br> • more defined |
| p. 152 | p. 154 | p. 155 | p. 156 | p. 156 |
| ■ Surface Asymmetry Index<br> • more likely with RGP lenses<br> • decentred lens flattens cornea<br>■ Surface Irregularity Index<br> • distortion may be symmetrical<br> • more likely with RGP lenses<br>■ Corneal indentation – pressure from lens edge | ■ Oedema<br> • increased fluid<br>■ Physical moulding<br> • pressure from RGP lenses<br> • supplementary pressure from eyelids<br>■ Associated pathology, e.g. keratoconus | ■ Alleviate RGP bearing<br>■ Alleviate hypoxia<br>■ Corneal indentation<br> • patient-dependent, i.e. likely to recur again in same patient<br>■ Keratoplasty for keratoconus | ■ RGP warpage<br> • full recovery in 5–8 months<br>■ RGP binding<br> • full recovery in 24 hours<br>■ Soft lens warpage<br> • resolves in 7 days | ■ Keratoconus<br> • other signs present such as stromal thinning, Vogt's striae, Fleischer's ring etc. |
| p. 152 | p. 152 | p. 154 | p. 155 | p. 156 |

# Part I
# **Eyelids**

# 1
# Blinking

The normal spontaneous blink
Alterations to blinking caused by contact lenses
Complications of abnormal blinking with contact lenses
Management of abnormal blinking with contact lenses
Differential diagnosis of blinking disorders

Blinking is a short duration high-speed closure movement of the eyelids that has both reflex and spontaneous origins.[1] Reflex blinking can be elicited by a variety of external stimuli, such as strong lights, approaching objects, loud noises, and corneal, conjunctival or ciliary touch.

Contact lenses will elicit reflex blinking during lens insertion, removal and other instances of manual manipulation. Also, as a result of a reflex blink, contact lenses may mislocate or become dislodged from the eye. Apart from these phenomena, there is no reason to suppose that contact lens wear alters the essential nature of the reflex blink. For this reason, this chapter will concentrate on spontaneous blinking activity associated with contact lens wear, and the term 'blink' should generally be taken to read 'spontaneous blink'.

Blinking serves a number of useful functions, both with and without contact lenses. Although eye care practitioners have long subscribed to the notion that their contact lens patients should execute full and regular blinks during lens wear, this topic has received little attention in the literature.

This chapter will review characteristics of the normal blink and examine how contact lens wear can affect, and be affected by, blinking behaviour. Complications that arise from poor blinking behaviour with contact lenses (such as lens surface drying as shown in Figure 1.1) will be reviewed, along with the question of clinical management of dysfunctional blinking.

## The normal spontaneous blink

### Mechanism of blinking
Eyelid closure during blinking is effected by the orbicularis oculi muscle, which is in-nervated by the seventh cranial nerve. The act of blinking is accomplished primarily by the upper lid. The lower lid remains virtually stationary. Closure is characterised by a progressive narrowing of the palpebral fissure, in a zipper-like fashion, from the outer to inner canthus. This moving wave of closure serves to force tears in the interpalpebral fissure towards the lacrimal puncta, thus aiding tear drainage.[2]

Spontaneous blinking occurs in all terrestrial vertebrates possessing eyelids, although the rate of blinking varies considerably between species. Large predatory cats execute less than one blink per minute, whereas some small species of monkey have blink rates as high as 45 times per minute. Infants have a low spontaneous blink rate.[1]

Spontaneous blinking occurs in patients who have total congenital blindness, indicating that it is a phenomenon that is not learned and is not dependent on visual input.[1] The rate of spontaneous blinking may alter in response to changes in the level of visual activity and in different emotional states. General environmental changes, such as the level of dryness or wind flow, may also alter spontaneous blink rate. The frequency and completeness of blink is reduced during intense concen-

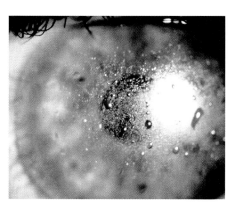

**Figure 1.1**
*Non-wetting surface of a silicone elastomer lens*

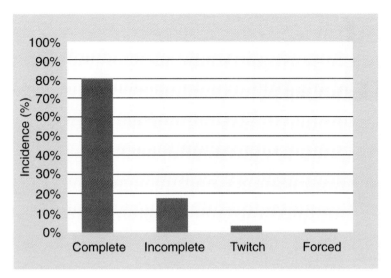

**Figure 1.2**
*Frequency of occurrence of various blink types*

the momentary interruption to visual input does not produce a conscious interruption to visual perception.

Various authors have suggested that there is a gender difference in blink rate. Adler proposes that males blink more frequently than females, whereas Tsubota *et al*[7] have suggested the opposite; neither validated their claims statistically. Yolton *et al*[8] recently shed light on this issue by measuring the spontaneous blink rate in males, females not using oral contraceptives, and females using oral contraceptives. The blink rates observed in these three groups were 14.5, 14.9 and 19.6 blinks/min, respectively. This finding indicates that there is no intrinsic gender difference in blink rate, but the use of oral contraceptives induces a significantly greater blink rate, for reasons which are unclear.

**Purpose of blinking**
Spontaneous blinking in non-lens wearers serves the following functions:

- Maintenance of an intact pre-corneal tear film by constantly spreading tear film evenly across the corneal surface.
- Removal of intrinsic and extrinsic particulate matter by forcing such debris into the lower lacrimal river.
- Facilitation of tear exchange by constantly swiping tears towards the puncta located at the inner canthus.

The importance of the first of the functions listed above (maintenance of an intact pre-corneal tear film) has been illustrated in a number of studies that have examined blinking behaviour in patients suffering from symptoms of dry eye.

Prause and Norn[10] advanced the theory that spontaneous blinking is, in part, a stimulus to the rupture of the pre-corneal tear film. They tested this hypothesis by measuring tear break-up time (TBUT) and the inter-blink period (IBP) in a group of normal and dry-eye patients. In both groups, there was a statistically significant positive correlation between these two parameters; that is, the more rapidly tear film breaks up, the more frequently the patient blinks. The above finding was subsequently confirmed by Yap[11] in a group of normal subjects, although two other research groups found no such association.[8,12]

Prause and Norn[10] also demonstrated that, in general, the IBP was slightly less

tration, such as when reading[2] or working on a visual display unit.

**Types and patterns of blinking**
Researchers must employ devious methods to monitor types and patterns of spontaneous blinking because of the methodological problem that subjects will alter their blinking activity if they are aware that this is being measured.[2] Typically, subjects in such circumstances will execute an increased proportion of voluntary forced blinks and a greater blink frequency. For this reason, hidden observers or video cameras are employed to record blinkng activity while the subject, for example, is engaged in an interview about an unrelated matter or observes a silent movie.

Zaman and Doughty[3] have highlighted other potential methodological pitfalls. For example, simple averaging of blink rates may not always be appropriate because of the high chance of non-Gaussian distribution of data. These authors conclude that eye-blink monitoring over at least 3 minutes is required for valid data analysis. Fortunately, almost all blink researchers have used times in excess of this.

According to Abelson and Holly,[4] blinking can be classified into four basic types:

- *Complete blink* – the upper eyelid covers more than 67 per cent of the cornea.
- *Incomplete blink* – the upper eyelid covers less than 67 per cent of the cornea.
- *Twitch blink* – a small movement of the upper eyelid.

- *Forced blink* – lower lid raises to complete eye closure.

The percentage of all blinks that can be characterised by each of these four blink types, as determined by Abelson and Holly,[4] is illustrated in Figure 1.2. Subsequent research has confirmed these findings.[5,6]

Tsubota *et al.*[7] developed a computer-interfaced 'blink analyser' to accurately measure the time course and pattern of blinking in 64 normal volunteers. They found that the average time taken to execute one complete blink (which they defined as the upper lid covering more than 85 per cent of the cornea) was $0.20 \pm 0.04$ sec, and that the average inter-blink period was $4.0 \pm 2.0$ sec. Taking one complete blink cycle as the sum of the blink time and inter-blink period $(0.2 + 4.0 = 4.2$ sec) gives an average blink frequency of 14.3 blinks per minute (60/4.2). This result is consistent with previous estimates of the spontaneous blink rate in humans.[5,8]

The small interruption to visual input during a blink is thought to be of practical significance only in occupations or tasks requiring constant monitoring of rapidly changing visual images. (Paradoxically, blinking is problematic for researchers monitoring blinking activity of experimental subjects, either directly or via video replays; in the latter case, viewing in slow motion solves this problem.) Volkmann *et al*[9] proposed that there is a suppression of the visual pathway associated with blinks so that than TBUT, suggesting that the patient adopts a blink rate that will prevent tear break-up. Using quantitative videographic analysis, Tsubota et al[7] found that the IBP in dry-eye patients was $1.5 \pm 0.9$ sec, compared with $4.0 \pm 2.0$ sec in normal subjects.

Indirect evidence of the link between TBUT and IBP comes from the work of Tsubota and Nakamori,[13] who measured the tear evaporation rate from the ocular surface (TEROS) in 17 normal volunteers and found an increase in blink rate with increasing TEROS. This result is consistent with previous demonstrations of the positive correlation between IBP and TBUT because tear break-up associated with more rapid blinking would be expected to result in higher rates of tear evaporation.

Although the weight of evidence suggests that blink rate is in part dependent on the integrity of the tear film, other factors must also be involved. This fact was demonstrated by Collins et al[14] who found that blinking continued following instillation of a corneal topical anaesthetic in a group of normal subjects. The blink rate did, however, drop from 24.8 to 17.2 blinks/min. If discomfort due to tear break-up was the sole determinant of blink rate, blinking would have stopped in eyes with anaesthetised corneas.

## Alterations to blinking caused by contact lenses

### Blink rate
Hill and Carney[15] demonstrated, in a group of seven subjects, that blink rate increased from 15.5 blinks/min to 23.2 blinks/min after being fitted with polymethyl methacrylate (PMMA) contact lenses.

A similar result was reported by York et al[16] although Brown et al[17] did not confirm this result. It appears, however, that PMMA lens-induced alterations to blink rate may be more related to reflex blinking than to spontaneous blinking; that is, the increased blink rate may be a result of continual irritation caused by the contact lens edge buffeting against the lid margin.

In another group of seven subjects, Hill and Carney[18] demonstrated that blink rate increased from 12.1 blinks/min to 20.3 blinks/min after being fitted with soft contact lenses (presumably hydroxyethyl methacrylate [HEMA]). The reason for this is less clear, as soft lenses would be expected to be more comfortable and to induce less

reflex blinking activity, although it should be noted that the earlier study of Brown et al[16] found that blink rate was essentially unaffected by soft lens wear.

Although blink rate may be altered during contact lens wear, another consideration is whether or not any alteration to blinking activity is permanent. Yolton et al[8] reported that the blink rate ($16.2 \pm 8.9$ blinks/min) in a cohort of habitual contact lens wearers (the lens type was not specified) who had ceased contact lens wear at least 24 hours before blinking assessment was identical to that of a matched control group who had never worn contact lenses ($16.2 \pm 9.5$ blinks/min). This suggests that contact lens-induced alterations to blink rate are evident only during lens wear.

### Blink type
Carney and Hill[15,18] have examined the effects of hard and soft lens wear on the pattern of blinking. A decrease in the frequency of occurrence of long-duration IBPs was observed in association with rigid lens wear, but not soft lens wear. Neither rigid nor soft lens wear altered the proportion of complete, incomplete, twitch and forced blinks.

## Complications of abnormal blinking with contact lenses

### Lens surface drying and deposition
The tear film on the front surface of both rigid and soft lenses has a different structure compared to the pre-ocular tear film (POTF), with the lipid layer being thinner or absent, and the aqueous layer being of variable thickness, depending on the lens material and design.[19,20] Similarly, the tear film on the front surface of both rigid and soft lenses is less stable than that of the POTF.

Whereas the POTF in normal human subjects has a TBUT of at least 15 seconds,[21] the pre-lens tear film (PLTF) has a TBUT of between 3 and 10 seconds for soft lenses[22] and between 4 and 6 seconds for rigid lenses.[20] Bearing in mind that the mean IBP in humans is $4.0 \pm 2.0$ sec, and that contact lens wear has little effect on the IBP, it is clear that in some patients the IBP will exceed the PLTF TBUT, leading to intermittent lens surface drying.

A case of severe drying of the surface of a silicone elastomer lens (which is naturally hydrophobic) is depicted in Figure 1.1. In

view of the rapid TBUT of such a lens, an unsustainable and cosmetically unacceptable inter-blink frequency of approximately 2 seconds would be required to prevent the lens surface from drying.

It is generally recognised that a full and continuous tear film on the lens surface is important in maintaining a clean surface with minimum deposition. The greater the discrepancy between the IBP and the PLTF TBUT, and the longer it is maintained, the greater will be the possibility for both extrinsic and intrinsic material to adhere to the lens surface.

It would also seem theoretically plausible that a discrepancy between the IBP and the PLTF TBUT of soft lenses could result in a greater degree of lens dehydration, because water from the lens could evaporate directly into the atmosphere from a dry lens surface. This theory was tested by Young and Efron,[22] but no association could be demonstrated between PLTF TBUT and lens dehydration.

In general, therefore, lens surface characteristics can be optimised by ensuring that the IBP is shorter than the PLTF TBUT.

### Epithelial desiccation
Severe desiccation staining of the corneal epithelium is known to occur as a result of fitting extremely thin, high-water content soft contact lenses.[23] This phenomenon relates primarily to the fitting of lenses of inappropriate design. However, Guillon et al[24] have demonstrated that epithelial desiccation can occur with good-fitting high-water content lenses of adequate thickness. They attributed this phenomenon to a breakup of the tear film at the inferior tear prism margin. This complication is theoretically avoidable if the blink rate is sufficient to prevent such PLTF break up.

### Post-lens tear stagnation
The anterior ocular surface is host to a plethora of organic material, such as desquamated superficial epithelial and conjunctival cells, mucus, proteins, lipids, micro-organisms and inflammatory cells. Environmental antigens such as iron particles, dust, pollen, smoke, smog, and other atmospheric pollutants and particulate matter can also easily enter the tear film. The material listed above rarely poses a problem because it is constantly being washed away, primarily as a result of blinking. However, when such material gets behind the lens, problems can arise if the

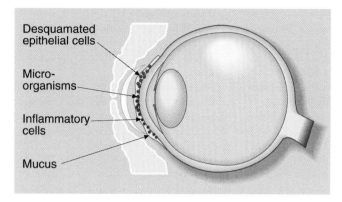

**Figure 1.3**
*Various types of debris trapped beneath a soft lens*

post-lens tear film is allowed to stagnate (Figure 1.3).

Infrequent and/or incomplete blinking during contact lens wear can theoretically be problematic because the residency time of ocular pollutants in the post-lens tear film is increased, thus heightening the potential for traumatic, toxic, allergic or infectious insult to the cornea. Blinking serves to flush such debris out from beneath the lens, to be replaced by 'fresh' tears containing a new set of pollutants. As long as there is this constant turnover of tears beneath the lens, which is referred to as 'tear exchange', high pollutant resident times can be avoided.

Daily wear of rigid contact lenses is known to be associated with a tear exchange of between 10 and 17 per cent with each blink.[25] This contrasts with a tear exchange of only about 1 per cent with each blink during soft lens wear.[26] These research findings, and accumulated clinical experience, have led practitioners to be aware of the importance of fitting soft lenses so that there is adequate movement of contact lenses (in particular soft lenses) with each blink. Failure to ensure adequate lens movement may allow the stagnating post-lens tear film debris to induce an adverse reaction via a variety of different mechanisms, leading to lens discomfort.

Problems relating to post-lens tear film tear stagnation are uncommon in daily wear because an awake, conscious patient can manipulate or remove an uncomfortable lens, thus minimising any ocular trauma. Also, the lens will be removed each day, allowing any sub-clinical insult that may have been developing to recover.

Post-lens tear stagnation is, however, of real concern in patients who sleep in lenses,

and the problems manifest differently for rigid and soft lenses. In the case of rigid lenses, the aqueous phase is depleted overnight leaving a mucus-rich post-lens tear film which tends to create adhesion between the lens and cornea (Figure 1.4).[27] Blinking on awakening in patients who have slept in rigid lenses is critical because the blinking action will tend to mechanically dislodge the adherent lens so that a normal post-lens tear film can be re-established.

In the absence of blinking during overnight lens wear, material that was present in the post-lens tear film immediately before going to sleep, in addition to desquamated epithelial cells and inflammatory cells that will have accumulated throughout the night, will be present beneath the lens on waking.[28] Various forms of toxic, infectious, inflammatory or immunologic reactions may be initiated. If the patient continues to wear the lenses during waking

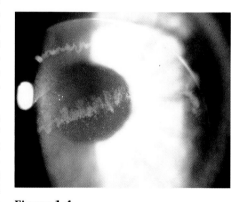

**Figure 1.4**
*Mucus at the centre and periphery of the cornea in the tear film beneath a rigid lens that has been worn overnight*

hours, the rate of tear exchange, especially with soft lenses, may be insufficient to effect a rapid clearance of the post-lens tear film, allowing any adverse reactions that have been initiated to continue.

A model can be constructed to illustrate the sequelae of events that lead to corneal ulceration, in a patient who sleeps in soft contact lenses, as a result of inadequate blink-assisted clearance of debris from the post-lens tear film on waking (Figure 1.5). Desquamated epithelial cells are trapped beneath a soft lens. These cells undergo lysis and irritate the underlying corneal epithelium, causing corneal staining. The epithelium is unable to repair itself in the toxic post-lens tear film environment, and a sterile ulcer results.

Factors governing the removal of debris from the post-lens tear film have been investigated by McGrogan *et al*[29] who inserted soft lenses containing polystyrene microspheres of various sizes and monitored the rate of removal of these microspheres from the post-lens tear firm during blinking (Figure 1.6). The key determinant of microsphere removal was the size of the microspheres; larger microspheres were less easily dislodged from beneath the lens than smaller microspheres. Lens modulus and lens fit had little effect on microsphere clearance.

**Hypoxia and hypercapnia**
The normal cornea is constantly drawing oxygen from the atmosphere to sustain its high levels of metabolic activity. At the same time, carbon dioxide – an unwanted by-product of corneal metabolism – is released into the atmosphere from the corneal surface. Contact lenses form a potential barrier to corneal oxygenation and carbon dioxide efflux, resulting in reduced oxygenation (hypoxia) and increased levels of carbon dioxide (hypercapnia); complications arising from lens-induced hypoxia and hypercapnia have been widely discussed and will not be recounted here; suffice to say that a key goal of contact lens fitting is to minimise hypoxia and hypercapnia.

All contact lenses fitted today (aside from PMMA) have some degree of gas transmissibility that allows oxygen to flow through the lens into the cornea and carbon dioxide to flow out of the lens into the atmosphere. This necessary gaseous exchange can be further enhanced by tear exchange, whereby the oxygen-depleted and carbon dioxide-rich tear film beneath the lens is

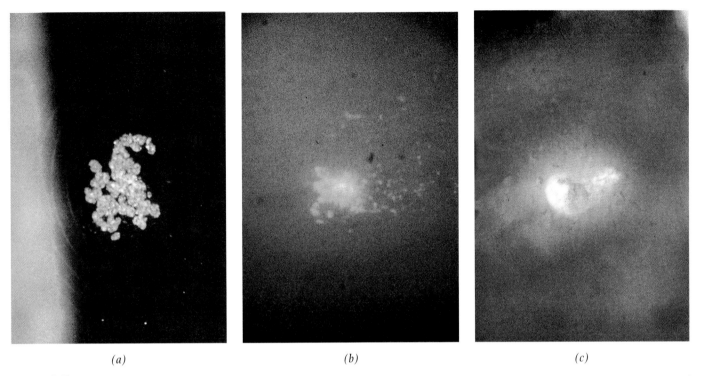

**Figure 1.5**
*Complications due to stagnating debris in the post-lens tear film. (a) Epithelial cells are trapped by the lens. (b) Cell lysis leads to epithelial disruption and staining. (c) A small sterile corneal ulcer forms*

partially replaced by freshly oxygenated and carbon dioxide-free tears from outside the lens. The higher the gas permeability of the lens fitted, the lower will be the reliance on tear exchange for the alleviation of hypoxia and hypercapnia.

The effect of blinking on corneal hypoxia and hypercapnia beneath rigid and soft

lenses has been studied extensively.[30,31] It has been demonstrated that blinking can partially alleviate corneal hypoxia and hypercapnia in both soft and rigid lenses.

Blinking also plays an important role in re-distributing oxygenated tears evenly across the corneal surface beneath soft lenses, via a process known as 'tear mixing'.[32]

This function is particularly important during the wearing of lenses of non-uniform thickness. For example, in the absence of effective tear mixing with a minus-powered lens (thicker in the lens periphery than the centre), the corneal periphery will suffer from greater levels of hypoxia than the central cornea, which can potentially result in pathology of the peripheral cornea and limbus. In this example, effective tear mixing would allow highly oxygenated tears beneath the centre of the lens to become interspersed with oxygen-deprived tears beneath the lens periphery, resulting in an 'averaging' of available oxygen and lessening peripheral hypoxia.

**Figure 1.6**
*Polystyrene microspheres visible as single spheres and small 'tracks' (the latter as a result of a slow photographic shutter speed). The microspheres have a diameter of 10 μm (yellow) and 6 μm (pink)*

### Three and nine o'clock staining
Three and nine o'clock staining is a common problem with rigid lenses which is

thought to be due to a lens-induced disturbance of the normal blink movement of the upper lid over the lens and cornea. A rigid lens will tend to bridge the upper lid away from the cornea so that, during the downward movement of the upper lid in the course of a blink, the lid is unable to re-wet the 'bridged' regions of the cornea at the 3 and 9 o'clock locations. This leads to local drying and consequent staining of these 'bridged' corneal locations.

**Poor lens design and fitting**

With respect to the eyelids, rigid lenses can be fitted according to two basic philosophies – the intrapalpebral fit and the lid attachment fit. The intrapalpebral fit entails fitting a lens, typically of small diameter, so that it rests on the cornea between the upper and lower lid margins during primary gaze. The upper lid rides over the lens during the blink, resulting in lens movement (essential for tear exchange) and lens re-positioning (essential for proper lens alignment with the optical axis of the eye).

Faults in lens design and fitting can interfere with proper blink-mediated lid–lens interaction. For example, an edge stand-off that is too great (due to excessive peripheral lens curvature or edge lift) could lead to discomfort during the blink because of the constant buffeting of the lens edge against the lid margin. The lid may even gain leverage beneath the lens edge causing the lens to be dislodged from the eye.

With a lid attachment fit, the upper lid lies over the lens periphery into which may be designed a negative lens carrier. The purpose of this type of fit is to aid central lens positioning. The lens will typically move synchronously with each blink. A poorly designed lens carrier, or the use of a lens of inappropriate diameter, may result in loss of synchronised movement of the lid and lens, leading to lens mislocation, discomfort and intermittent blur.

**Management of abnormal blinking with contact lenses**

Practitioners have two options when faced with a clinical problem relating to non-pathologic disorders of spontaneous blinking activity such as infrequent or incomplete blinking. These options are either to train the patient to modify their blinking activity or make no attempt to modify blink-

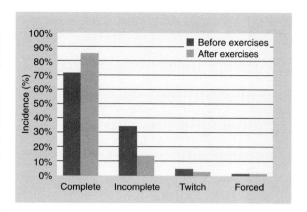

**Figure 1.7**
*Percentage distribution of the various types of blink before and after blink training (adapted from Collins et al[6])*

ing activity but instead alter the lens type or lens fit.

Early anecdotal reports proposed a variety of strategies for enhancing blinking activity. These included simple instructions and reminders,[33] and the use of a small buzzer that sounded every 10 seconds, which acted as a prompt to execute a full blink.[34] Although it was realised that such strategies were only stimulating reflex rather than spontaneous blinks, the underlying assumption was that spontaneous blinking activity could be learned via training using reflex stimulation techniques.

Collins *et al*[6] tested the hypothesis that blinking could be trained by subjecting a group of unsuspecting contact lens-wearers to blink exercises (the volunteers were told that the purpose of the exercises was to improve vision). The exercise consisted of placing the index finger of each hand just lateral to the outer canthus to hold the lids taut while performing 10 complete forced blinks. This exercise was repeated three times daily for two weeks. Blinking exercises resulted in an increased frequency of complete blinks and a decreased frequency of incomplete and twitch blinks (Figure 1.7).

If blink training is thought to be impractical or inefficacious, the only alternative management strategy to alleviate blink-related contact lens problems is to alter the lens type, design or fit. By way of example, the following strategies are advocated:

- Changing from soft to rigid lenses will tend to solve blink-associated problems relating to debris removal, hypoxia and hypercapnia

- Changing a rigid lens to a multicurve design (from, say, an aspheric design) will tend to solve blink-associated problems relating to debris removal, hypoxia and hypercapnia
- Changing a rigid lens to an intrapalpebral fit (from, say, a lid-attachment fit) will tend to solve blink-associated problems relating to debris removal, hypoxia and hypercapnia
- Changing from rigid to soft lenses will tend to solve blink-associated problems relating to lens surface drying and 3 and 9 o'clock staining.

**Differential diagnosis of blinking disorders**

Practitioners should always be alert to the possibility that apparent anomalies in the type or pattern of blinking activity in a contact lens wearer may be attributable to unrelated disease states. Interruptions to the neural input and/or muscular systems of the eyelids can adversely affect normal spontaneous blinking activity. For example, patients with Parkinson's disease exhibit a low blink rate.

Increased mechanical resistance to eyelid movement, as in Graves' disease, can also reduce blink frequency. Local pathology of the eyelids, such as ptosis, chalazia and carcinomas, can alter eyelid function and movement, and hence interfere with normal blinking activity. It is therefore essential to rule out the possibility of unrelated pathology before ascribing blinking dysfunction to contact lens wear.

# REFERENCES

1 Hart WM (1992) The eyelids. In: *Adler's Physiology of the Eye* (ed. WM Hart), 9th edn. Mosby Year Book, St Louis.

2 Doane MG (1980) Interaction of the eyelids and tears in corneal wetting and the dynamics of normal human eyeblinks. *Am J Ophthalmol* **89**: 507.

3 Zaman ML, Doughty MJ (1997) Some methodological issues in the assessment of the spontaneous eyeblink frequency in man. *Ophthal Physiol Opt* **17**: 421.

4 Abelson MB, Holly FJ (1977) A tentative mechanism for inferior punctate keratopathy. *Am J Ophthalmol* **83**: 866.

5 Carney LG, Hill RM (1982) The nature of normal blinking patterns. *Acta Ophthalmol* **60**: 427.

6 Collins M, Heron H, Larson R (1987) Blinking patterns in soft contact lens wearers can be altered with training. *Am J Optom Physiol Opt* **64**: 100.

7 Tsubota K, Hata S, Okusawa Y (1996) Quantitative videographic analysis of blinking in normal subjects and patients with dry eye. *Arch Ophthalmol* **114**: 715.

8 Yolton DP, Yolton RL, Lopez R (1994) The effect of gender and birth control pill use on spontaneous blink rates. *J Am Optom Assoc* **65**: 763.

9 Volkmann F, Riggs, Moore R (1980) Eyeblinks and visual suppression. *Science* **207**: 900.

10 Prause JU, Norn M (1987) Relation between blink frequency and break-up time? *Acta Ophthalmol* **65**: 19.

11 Yap M (1991) Tear break-up time is related to blink frequency. *Acta Ophthalmol* **69**: 92.

12 Bhatia RPS, Singh RK (1993) Tear film break-up time in contact lens wearers. *Ann Ophthalmol* **25**: 334.

13 Tsubota K, Nakamori K (1995) Effects of ocular surface area and blink rate on tear dynamics. *Arch Ophthalmol* **113**: 155.

14 Collins M, Seeto R, Campbell L (1989) Blinking and corneal sensitivity. *Acta Ophthalmol* **67**: 525.

15 Hill RM, Carney LG (1984) The effects of hard lens wear on blinking behaviour. *Int Contact Lens Clin* **11**: 242.

16 York M, Ong J, Robbins JC (1971) Variation in blink rate associated with contact lens wear and task difficulty. *Am J Optom Arch Am Acad Optom* **48**: 461.

17 Brown M, Chinn S, Fatt I (1973) The effect of soft and hard contact lenses on blink rate, amplitude and length. *J Am Optom Assoc* **44**: 254.

18 Carney LG, Hill RM (1984) Variation in blinking behaviour during soft lens wear. *Int Contact Lens Clin* **11**: 250.

19 Guillon JP, Guillon M (1988) The status of the pre soft lens tear film during overnight wear. *Am J Optom Physiol Opt* **65**: 40.

20 Guillon JP, Guillon M (1988) Pre-lens tear film characteristics of high Dk rigid gas permeable lenses. *Am J Optom Physiol Opt* **65**: 73.

21 Holly FJ, Lemp MA (1977) Tear physiology and dry eyes. *Surv Ophthalmol* **22**: 69.

22 Young G, Efron N (1991) Characteristics of the pre-lens tear film during hydrogel contact lens wear. *Ophthal Physiol Opt* **11**: 53.

23 Holden BA, Sweeney DF, Seger RG (1986) Epithelial erosions caused by thin high water contact lenses. *Clin Exp Optom* **69**: 103.

24 Guillon JP, Guillon M, Malgouyres S (1990) Corneal desiccation staining with hydrogel lenses: tear film and contact lens factors. *Ophthal Physiol Opt* **10**: 343.

25 Cuklanz HD, Hill RM (1969) Oxygen requirements of corneal contact lens systems. *Am J Optom Arch Am Acad Optom* **46**: 228.

26 Polse KA (1979) Tear flow under hydrogel contact lenses. *Invest Ophthalmol Vis Sci* **18**: 409.

27 Swarbrick HA, Holden BA (1987) Rigid gas permeable lens binding: significance and contributing factors. *Am J Optom* **64**: 815.

28 Wilson G, O'Leary DJ, Holden BA (1989) Cell content of tears following overnight wear of a contact lens. *Curr Eye Res* **8**: 329.

29 McGrogan L, Guillon M, Dilly N (1997) Post-lens particle exchange under hydrogel contact lenses – effect of contact lens characteristics. *Optom Vis Sci* **74**: 73.

30 Efron N, Carney LG (1981) Models of oxygen performance for the static, dynamic and closed lid wear of hydrogel contact lenses. *Aust J Optom* **64**: 223.

31 Efron N, Ang JHB (1990) Corneal hypoxia and hypercapnia during contact lens wear. *Optom Vis Sci* **67**: 512.

32 Efron N, Fitzgerald JP (1996) Distribution of oxygen across the surface of the human cornea during soft contact lens wear. *Optom Vis Sci* **73**: 659.

33 Korb D, Korb JE (1974) Fitting to achieve normal blinking and lid action. *Int Contact Lens Clin* **1**: 57.

34 Jenkins MS, Rehkopf PG, Brown SI (1978) A simple device to improve blinking. *Am J Ophthalmol* **85**: 869.

# 2
# Ptosis

Signs and symptoms of contact lens-induced ptosis (CLIP)
Prevalence of CLIP
Pathology of CLIP
Aetiology of CLIP
Patient management in CLIP
Prognosis in CLIP
Differential diagnosis of CLIP
Other contact lens-associated eyelid disorders

Contact lens practitioners routinely examine the tarsal conjunctiva and lid margins of their patients, but little attention is generally given to the overall integrity of the eyelids. Eyelid dysfunction, whether caused by contact lens wear or other factors, can pose a problem for contact lens wearers because this could interfere with some of the important roles played by the eyelids.

This chapter will concentrate on a condition that has received scant attention in the literature over the past decade – contact lens-induced ptosis (CLIP). Ptosis is defined as 'prolapse, abnormal depression, or falling down of an organ or part; applied especially to drooping of the upper eyelid'.[1] Because ptosis is not confined to the eyelids, some authors prefer to use the more exact term 'blepharoptosis'.

An assortment of other eyelid disorders that may be of relevance to contact lens wear will also be considered.

CLIP is perhaps the only complication of contact lens wear for which surgical intervention is contemplated and occasionally executed (notwithstanding infectious keratitis associated with corneal ulceration which sometimes requires hospitalisation

and can result in keratoplasty). It is for this reason that clinicians should have an appreciation of the typical manifestation of this condition, its likely causation, and indications for surgery and other management options.

## Signs and symptoms of contact lens-induced ptosis (CLIP)

### Signs
The classical appearance of ptosis is of a

narrowing of the palpebral fissure and a relatively large gap between the upper lid margin and the skin fold at the top of the eyelid (Figure 2.1). In a normal patient in the absence of ptosis, the skin fold at the top of the eyelid is only slightly higher than the upper eyelid margin. In some patients, these anatomical features can become virtually co-aligned towards the outer canthus.

Because contact lenses are typically worn in both eyes, any contact lens-

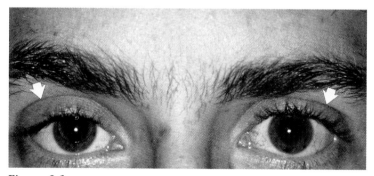

**Figure 2.1**
*Unilateral right eye ptosis induced by rigid lens extended wear approximately four weeks after initiating wear. The left eye was wearing a soft lens as part of a research experiment. The skin folds, which are used as the reference point for assessing the degree of ptosis, are indicated by the arrows*

induced narrowing of the palpebral apertures will be bilateral. It is therefore only possible to detect such changes if either (a) palpebral aperture height is measured accurately on many occasions over time (to detect a trend), or (b) one eye is affected more than the other. The latter situation can arise if a lens is only worn in one eye or if each eye is fitted with a different lens type.

Fonn and Holden[2,3] conducted a longitudinal trial designed to compare the ocular response with rigid vs hydrogel contact lenses worn on an extended wear basis. The experimental protocol called for an interocular comparison; that is, a rigid lens was worn in one eye and a hydrogel lens was worn in the other. It was observed that the palpebral aperture of the eye wearing the rigid lens was noticeably narrower than that in the eye fitted with the soft lens in 77 per cent of the 40 subjects who participated in the trial[3] (see Figure 2.1).

**Measurement of CLIP**
Subsequent studies have quantified the extent of palpebral aperture closure resulting from various modalities of contact lens wear. Fonn *et al*[4] measured the palpebral aperture size (PAS) to be $10.10 \pm 1.11$ mm in non-wearers, $10.24 \pm 0.94$ mm in soft lens wearers and $9.76 \pm 0.99$ mm in rigid lens wearers. The difference in PAS between the rigid lens wearers vs soft lens wearers (0.48 mm), and between the rigid lens wearers vs non-lens wearers (0.34 mm), was statistically significant, but there was no significant difference in PAS between soft lens wearers vs non-wearers (0.14 mm). The rigid lens wearers had been wearing lenses for $11.6 \pm 8.4$ years and the soft lens wearers for $8.2 \pm 5.5$ years. No gender difference in the development of CLIP was noted.

A similar study to that described above, by van den Bosch and Lemij,[5] found that the upper lid had lowered by 0.5 mm in a group of patients wearing rigid lenses for an average of 16.3 years. The reason for a greater amount of ptosis in this study (versus that of Fonn *et al*[4]) may be attributed to the greater lens wearing experience of the subjects examined (16.3 vs 11.6 years), although Fonn *et al*[4] noted no such relationship within his own subject group. The position of the lower lid was unaltered by rigid lens wear.[5]

**Time course of onset**
Fonn and Holden[3] monitored the time

course of onset of CLIP in 17 subjects who wore a soft lens in one eye and a rigid lens in the other. In the eye wearing the rigid lens, maximum ptosis (12 per cent closure) was observed 4–6 weeks after commencing lens wear; this was followed by a relative lessening of the ptosis to a point where the PAS was 3 per cent smaller compared with baseline after 13 weeks (Figure 2.2). The PAS remained fairly stable in the eye wearing the soft lens for the first 7 weeks, but then began to increase to be 7 per cent wider compared with baseline after 13 weeks. (Apparent widening of the palpebral aperture as a result of soft lens wear is discussed later in this chapter.)

In the longer term, the pattern of onset can be variable. In one study,[5] all but two of 17 patients presenting to a clinic complaining of CLIP reported that the condition had developed gradually over the past 12–24 months; most of these patients could illustrate this with photographs.[5] The other two patients in this study noted that the ptosis had existed for 6 and 16 years respectively, and had gradually become worse.

**Symptoms**
Based on their observation of 17 patients presenting to a clinic complaining of advanced CLIP, van den Bosch and Lemij[5] demonstrate that this is a condition that will be generally noticed by patients. No associated signs or symptoms were noted in any of these patients.

It is also interesting that, in prospective

studies of palpebral aperture height in asymptomatic contact lens wearers,[4,5] none of the patients deemed to be suffering from CLIP were aware that they had this condition.

**Prevalence of CLIP**

Ptosis is defined by van den Bosch and Lemij[5] as a situation whereby the distance between the centre of the pupil and the lower margin of the upper lid is less than 2.8 mm. Using this criterion, these authors determined that the prevalence of ptosis in a consecutively presenting group of 46 rigid contact lens wearers was 11 per cent, versus 1 per cent in a control group of non-lens wearers. More recently, Jupiter and Karesh[6] reported the prevalence of ptosis in a population of rigid lens wearers to be 4.7 per cent.

**Pathology of CLIP**

There is general agreement that the pathological basis of CLIP is either: (a) oedema leading to lid swelling, or (b) disinsertion, dehiscence (splitting), thinning or lengthening of the levator aponeurosis.[5] The relatively large gap between the upper lid margin and the skin fold at the top of the eyelid described earlier (also referred to as a 'high skin crease') develops because the posterior fibres of the levator aponeurosis on the tarsal plate disinsert, split or

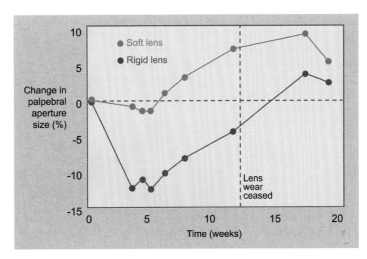

**Figure 2.2**
*Changes in palpebral aperture size (per cent) over 13 weeks of extended wear of an RGP lens in one eye and a soft lens in the other eye, and 7 weeks' recovery (adapted from Fonn and Holden[3])*

lengthen, while the anterior insertion of the levator aponeurosis into the orbicularis muscle and skin remains intact.[5] Thinning of the eyelid can also be observed.

## Aetiology of CLIP

A number of mechanisms have been advanced as possible causes of CLIP. These can broadly be categorised into aponeurogenic (i.e. involving some form of dysfunction of the aponeurosis) and non-aponeurogenic causes. Aponeurogenic causes of ptosis include the following:

### Forced lid squeezing
The unnatural 'forced blink' rigid lens removal technique places simultaneous, although antagonistic forces on the orbicularis and levator muscles. Specifically, because rigid lens wearers are instructed to open their eyes widely while executing a powerful blink, both the levator and orbicularis muscles are attempting to contract at the sime time. The opposed actions of these two muscles might cause increased traction on the levator aponeurosis, leading to disinsertion or dehiscence.[7]

### Lateral eyelid stretching
To effect rigid lens removal, patients are often instructed to pull firmly on the outer canthus to create increased tension in the eyelids so that a greater leverage force is created to enable the lens to be blinked out of the eye. Although this action may lead (if anything) to a disinsertion or dehiscence of the lateral canthal ligament or the medial canthal tendon, it should not by itself lead to a disinsertion or dehiscence from the levator aponeurosis.[5] However, in combination with the antagonistic contraction of the orbicularis and levator muscles during forced blink removal described above, stretching or thinning of the levator aponeurosis cannot be discounted.

Consideration of the above two aetiological factors – forced lid squeezing and lateral eyelid stretching – lead to the disturbing conclusion that actions undertaken by practitioners and patients may be responsible for CLIP in some cases.

This conclusion is supported by the report of five cases of CLIP by Epstein and Putterman,[7] who observed that two of these cases developed directly after the patients were fitted with rigid lenses. The

ptosis in these two patients did not resolve following cessation of lens wear.

### Rigid lens displacement of tarsus
During repeated attempts to remove a rigid lens, the lid will occasionally be pulled across the lens, which will in turn exert pressure on the palpebral conjunctiva. This unnatural pressure against the palpebral conjunctiva, effectively in an anterior direction against the posterior surface of the lid, could be directed against the levator aponeurosis, especially if the lens has migrated a little superiorly. This in turn could lead to disinsertion, dehiscence and/ or thinning of the aponeurosis.[5]

### Blink-induced lens rubbing
It has been argued by van den Bosch and Lemij[5] that every blink made during the regular wearing of a rigid lens causes the lens to rub against the eyelid structures, albeit less forcefully than during lens insertion and removal. This chronic rubbing and displacement of the lid away from the globe by the lens may cause a gradual thinning and stretching of the levator aponeurosis. Thus, the way in which the lens is fitted, and the size, thickness and positioning of the lens, may have a bearing on CLIP.

Non-aponeurogenic causes of CLIP include the following:

### Oedema
Constant physical irritation of any tissue in the body can result in a mild, sub-clinical inflammatory status and subsequent oedema.[2–4] Thus, constant rubbing of a rigid lens against the tarsal conjunctiva is a possible cause of the ptosis. Specifically, oedema could lead to ptosis due to a physical enlargement of the eyelid in all dimensions (including a downward displace-

ment) as the lid absorbs increased levels of fluid. The increased mass of the oedematous upper lid, combined with the effects of gravity, may cause a lowering of the lid (Figure 2.3).

Rigid lens-induced ptosis in the right eye of a patient who wore a soft lens in the left eye (as part of a research study) is shown in Figure 2.3. The region above and below the upper skin fold of the right eye appears slightly oedematous, which would suggest that oedema due to mechanical lens rubbing caused the ptosis in this eye.

### Blepharospasm
Involuntary narrowing of the palpebral aperture to stabilise rigid lenses, which are intrinsically uncomfortable, is another possible explanation of CLIP. In the long term, chronic involuntary blepharospasm may strain the levator muscle or cause, in turn, a higher tonus of the levator muscle. However, van den Bosch and Lemij[5] discount this mechanism as an important aetiological factor in CLIP because the lower lid – which would be expected to adopt a slightly higher position as a result of blepharospasm – is unaffected by rigid lens wear.

### Papillary conjunctivitis
Severe (grade 4) contact lens-induced papillary conjunctivitis can be associated with excessive inflammation and oedema of the eyelids, which can cause lid swelling and drooping.[8] Since papillary conjunctivitis typically manifests bilaterally, a bilateral CLIP results. This will be more prevalent in soft lens wearers. Papillary conjunctivitis also occurs in association with rigid lens wear, but it is rarely more severe than grade 2.

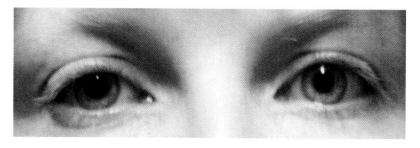

**Figure 2.3**
*Apparent rigid lens-induced lid oedema in the region above and below the upper skin fold of the right eye, leading to ptosis. The left eye was wearing a soft lens as part of a research trial*

# Patient management in CLIP

A key diagnostic criterion in deciding on appropriate action to alleviate CLIP is to determine whether the CLIP has been caused by:

- disinsertion, dehiscence or thinning of the aponeurosis
- oedema or involuntary blepharospasm
- contact lens–induced papillary conjunctivitis.

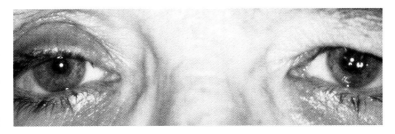

**Figure 2.4**
*Ptosis in the right eye due to rigid lens wear in that eye. The left eye was emmetropic and did not require a contact lens*

To differentiate between these possible causes, patients demonstrating CLIP should be required to cease lens wear for at least one month (to detect any trends towards recovery) and perhaps as long as 3 months (to demonstrate complete resolution).

If the CLIP partially or completely resolves after ceasing lens wear for one month, then the cause was lid oedema and/or involuntary blepharospasm. The decision as to whether action needs to be taken is based largely on cosmetic considerations, although a severe ptosis can also interfere with vision if the lid wholly or partially covers the pupil. If the extent of ptosis is cosmetically unsightly, or it is more prominent in one eye, leading to a noticeable asymmetry in palpebral aperture size, the patient may need to be refitted with soft lenses (which do not induce ptosis). The eyelids should also be inverted to determine whether papillary conjunctivitis is involved, and if so, appropriate action should be taken to alleviate the condition.

If the ptosis persists after resolution of the papillary conjunctivitis, it is likely the aponeurosis has also been damaged by lens wear.

maining alternatives being soft contact lenses, spectacles or refractive surgery.

A fascinating report by Levy and Stamper[9] reinforces the importance of observing the eyes after a prolonged period of cessation of lens wear to exclude non-aponeurogenic causes of CLIP. They reported the case of a rigid lens wearer who received extracapsular cataract surgery in the right eye. Following surgery, the right eye was emmetropic and the patient continued to wear a rigid lens in the left eye. However, as a result of the surgery, the right eyelid was oedematous and the palpebral aperture of that eye was the same as the left eye, which was also reduced due to the pre-existence of CLIP. Eight weeks after surgery, the patient presented with an apparent ptosis of the lens-wearing (left) eye. The palpebral aperture size was 12 mm in the right eye and 8 mm in the left eye.

Lid surgery was contemplated, but as a precaution the surgeon advised cessation of lens wear for a period to determine if the lens was the cause. The difference in palpebral aperture size halved within one month and disappeared after 3 months, so surgery was not performed.

Figure 2.4 illustrates the above point; it depicts the case of a patient who was fitted with an intraocular lens to the left eye. The ametropic right eye was fitted with a rigid lens and displays an obvious ptosis.

**Non-surgical management**
Management strategies are available for patients with severe CLIP who do not wish to undergo lid surgery. The patient may be fitted with a 'ptosis crutch', 'ptosis prop' or 'ptosis lugs'.[10] This is a scleral lens which has either a cemented ledge or lugs fixed to the front surface, and/or a shelf cut into the front surface of the lens. In both cases, the lower border of the upper lid rests on the ledge or shelf, thus keeping the eyelid open to the desired extent.

Figure 2.5 depicts the case of a blind eye with inoperable ptosis which was fitted with an impression scleral prosthetic moulded shell with a superior shelf and ptosis crutch lugs. In this photograph, the lid appears to be supported more by the left lug, and the shelf (the white line connecting the two lugs) appears to be displaced from the upper lid margin. This appliance has been successfully worn for 10 years.

## Surgical correction

If the CLIP does not resolve after ceasing lens wear for one month, then the cause is most likely damage to the aponeurosis. Surgical correction is the preferred option in such cases. The typical procedure is to reinsert the levator aponeurosis on the anterior surface of the tarsal plate and reconstruct the skin crease under local or general anaesthesia. This procedure was carried out successfully by van den Bosch and Lemij[5] in 10 patients who had developed ptosis as a result of rigid lens wear. Following surgery, patients should not be refitted with rigid contact lenses – the obvious re-

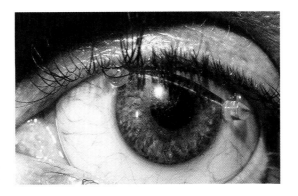

**Figure 2.5**
*Scleral lens with ptosis lugs and shelf*

This approach in a patient with CLIP constitutes something of a paradox, because the patient is being fitted with a scleral lens. Such a lens can be considered to be an extreme form of rigid lens – which was the likely cause of the problem in the first place. That is, the scleral lens with ptosis crutch may be perpetuating or even exacerbating the very problem it is supposedly curing.

Other options for non-surgical correction of CLIP Include:

- instructing patients to periodically raise the ptotic lid with their finger and relying on residual tone to keep the lid open for a period of time thereafter
- employing a spectacle frame-mounted lid prop
- attaching one end of a small piece of surgical tape to the eyelid just above the lashes and the other end to the smooth skin below the eyebrow.

This discussion of management options has concentrated on CLIP. Of course, other possible causes of ptosis must also be considered – these are discussed under 'differential diagnosis'.

## Prognosis in CLIP

The prognosis for recovery from aponeurogenic CLIP is poor; the condition can only be reversed by surgical correction or other management options as described above.

The prognosis for recovery from non-aponeurogenic CLIP is good. If the cause of ptosis is papillary conjunctivitis, the time course of resolution of the ptosis will parallel the time course of recovery of the papillary conjunctivitis. A noticeable diminution of ptosis associated with a reduction of the severity of papillary conjunctivitis from grade four to grade one or two would take 4–8 weeks.

According to Fonn and Holden,[3] complete resolution of non-aponeurogenic ptosis will occur within 6 weeks, although in severe cases resolution may take as long as 3 months.[9]

## Differential diagnosis of CLIP

If a contact lens wearer presents with ptosis, other possible causes of this condition must be considered so that the appro-priate course of management can be adopted.

### Aponeurogenic ptosis

Any ptosis caused by disinsertion, dehiscence, thinning or lengthening of the levator aponeurosis can be referred to as aponeurogenic ptosis, of which there are two categories based on aetiology – traumatic or involutional.

Surgery is the most common cause of traumatic aponeurogenic ptosis; specifically, damage to the levator aponeurosis can be caused by traction on the eyelids during surgery or clumsy attempts by the patient to remove a patch over the eye following surgery.

Trauma induced by forceful rigid lens removal and the chronic presence of a rigid lens are other possible causes of traumatic aponeurogenic ptosis.

Involutional aponeurogenic ptosis describes the process of damage to the levator aponeurosis due to ageing. Ocular inflammation and the use of steroids can exacerbate this condition.[5]

The age profile of patients presenting with contact lens-induced aponeurogenic ptosis was compared by van den Bosch and Lemij[5] with that of patients presenting to the same clinic with involutional aponeurogenic ptosis. The age range was 18 to 56 years (mean 38.5) in the former group and 48 to 88 years (mean 69) in the latter group. Thus, patient age provides an important clue as to the cause of aponeurogenic ptosis.

### Non-aponeurogenic ptosis

Non-aponeurogenic causes of ptosis include:

- Neurogenic disease such as pathway interruption or palsy of the third cranial nerve supplying the levator, Horner's syndrome or Marcus Gunn sign
- Myogenic disease, which may be congenital or acquired – examples of the latter being muscular dystrophy or myasthenia gravis
- Oedema following lid surgery
- Oedema due to traumatic eye injury
- Oedema resulting from prolonged rigid contact lens wear (as described in detail in this chapter)
- Contact lens imbedded in upper eyelid (see below)
- Chalazion
- Tumour

- Dermatochalasis
- Blepharospasm, possibly caused by photophobia secondary to other ocular diseases
- Vernal and giant papillary conjunctivitis
- Forms of nervous disposition leading to idiosyncratic partial eye closure.

## Other contact lens-associated eyelid disorders

### Soft lens-induced increase in palpebral aperture size

Mutti and Seger[11] noted in two unilateral soft lens wearers a relative ptosis of 19 per cent in the contralateral non-lens wearing eye. As these authors had no baseline data, they were unsure whether this appearance was due to a widening of the lens-wearing eye or a narrowing of the non-lens wearing eye. Fonn and Holden[3] observed an 8 per cent widening of the PAS in eyes wearing soft lenses, but failed to validate their data statistically. Fonn et al[4] noted that the PAS of soft lens wearers was 1.4 per cent greater than that of controls, but statistical analysis failed to reveal a significant difference.

Although soft lens–induced widening of PAS can only be considered as an anecdotal observation at the present time, it is interesting to speculate as to a possible cause. Mutti and Seger[11] have tentatively attributed this phenomenon to neural feedback from stimulation of the lid by the lens edge and/or lens mass, resulting in increased reflex tonus of the levator or Mueller's muscle, causing a slight raising of the eyelid.

### Embedded lens

Cases of a rigid lens becoming 'lost' and in some cases embedded in the upper palpebral conjunctiva were reported as early as 1963.[12,13] Since then, numerous accounts of similar occurrences have been published.[14–21] In the majority of these cases, the patient presented complaining of an otherwise 'quiet' lump in the upper lid, which can be misdiagnosed as a chalazion.[14–6] Jahn[14] reports the case of a 41-year-old female patient who had lost a rigid lens 12 months before noticing a lump in her left eye. She failed to associate the previously lost lens with the lid lump. The condition was diagnosed as chalazion and to the surgeon's surprise, a lens was extracted from the lump during surgical treatment of the 'chalazion'.

In two cases[17,18] the embedded lens was

inverted; that is, the convex surface of the lens faced the globe. Jones and Hassan[17] suggest that this inversion leads to greater mechanical irritation (compared with a non-inverted lens) and is a predominant factor in reducing the time taken for distressing symptoms to occur. They also suggest[17] that if the lens does not invert, deeper migration into a pretarsal or even orbital location[19] is more likely. Excessive lid swelling as a result of an embedded lens can also give the appearance of ptosis in the affected eye.[20]

Perhaps the most astonishing case of 'lost lenses' re-appearing later in the upper lid, is that reported by Kelly.[21] A female patient reported that she had lost a lens and thought that it was still in her eye. A mucus-coated pellet was removed from beneath the upper eyelid, leaving a well-defined depression on the upper globe. On further questioning, the patient reported having lost and re-ordered a number of lenses over the past three months, and having reported to other clinicians that she thought a lens was in her eye (with nothing being found). The mucus-coated pellet was found to consist of eight PMMA lenses and one rigid gas-permeable lens. The lessons to be learned from such a case are self-evident.

## Ectropion

Ectropion is an outward turning of the eyelid from the globe, and is frequently associated with epiphora and chronic conjunctivitis. Four types of ectropion can be defined:

- *Involutional* – senile change.
- *Cicatricial* – caused by scarring and contracture of skin and underlying tissue which pulls the eyelid away from the globe.
- *Congenital* – rare and typically associated with blepharophimosis syndrome.
- *Paralytic* – typically caused by a facial nerve palsy.[22]

The implication of ectropion in contact lens wearers is that the lower lid cannot be relied upon to help position the lens; that is, both rigid and soft lenses may mislocate inferiorly in an ectropic eye. An ectropic eyelid will have a reduced effectiveness in cases where the lower lid is required for lid-assisted lens translation (e.g. alternating vision bifocals) or location (e.g. truncated toric lens). In addition, an eye with an ectropic eyelid may tend to be relatively dry due to an excessive rate of loss of tears.

## Entropion

Entropion is an inversion of the eyelid towards the globe, and usually causes discomfort due to rubbing of the eyelashes against the cornea. This latter phenomenon is known as pseudotrichiasis and should not be confused with 'true' trichiasis which describes an actual ingrowth of the lashes from an otherwise normal lid margin.

Four types of entropion can be defined:

- *Involutional* – senile change.
- *Cicatricial* – caused by scarring and contracture of the palpebral conjunctiva which pulls the eyelid towards the globe. This condition can be caused by cicatricial pemphigoid, Stevens–Johnson syndrome, trachoma and chemical burns, and can involve the upper and lower lids.
- *Congenital* – rare, but can be dealt with surgically.
- *Acute spastic* – due to spasm of the orbicularis arising from ocular irritation; this condition typically resolves with removal of the irritation.[22]

An important implication of entropion in contact lens wearers is that the lower lid may interfere with correct lens positioning. An entropic eyelid with associated pseudotrichiasis can lead to corneal irritation; as an interim measure, soft contact lenses can be fitted to protect the cornea.

A pseudo-entropion can arise as a result of pressure on the eyelids from external forces. An example of such a case is shown in Figure 2.6; the lower lid has been temporarily folded inwards due to the fitting of a scleral lens of insufficient diameter.

## Lagophthalmos

Lagophthalmos refers to incomplete eyelid closure, and can be caused by a number of factors such as facial nerve lesions, orbicularis weakness, ectropion or mechanical displacement due to tumours. This condition can lead to corneal exposure and consequent keratitis. A soft lens will provide protection, although lenses tend to fall out of the eye. In such cases, partial tarsorrhaphy or temporary taping together of the eyelids is indicated.

Rigid lenses are problematic because they do not completely cover the cornea. This can lead to corneal desiccation outside the lens edge, typically in the 3 and 9 o'clock position.[22] Nocturnal lagophthalmos (partial eye opening during sleep) is an anatomical variant in the normal human population, occurring in 23 per cent of the population.[23] Excessive 3 and 9 o'clock staining in some patients who sleep in rigid lenses could be explained by the presence of nocturnal lagophthalmos.

## Rigid lens 'bridging'

Contact lenses act to displace the eyelids away from the globe. This action has been implicated in the aetiology of traumatic aponeurogenic ptosis in rigid lens wear because of the greater displacement caused by such lenses. Rigid lenses also cause a 'bridging' of the tarsal conjunctiva away from the corneal surface at the lens edge, which is thought to be of aetiological significance in the development of 3 and 9 o'clock corneal staining. The areas of

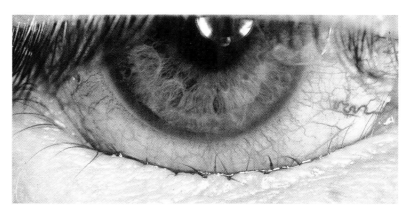

**Figure 2.6**
*Pseudo-entropion due to the fitting of a scleral lens of insufficient diameter*

cornea adjacent to the lens edge, especially at 3 and 9 o'clock, are prone to dry out because these regions are not being re-wetted by the passage of the eyelid against the eyeball.

### Lids as a lens-positioning tool

The eyelids are used to stabilise, position and translocate contact lenses to achieve various fitting and optical objectives. A detailed analysis of these strategies is beyond the scope of this chapter, but they are listed below to provide a clue to solving contact lens-related eyelid problems that may have a bearing on lens performance.

Specifically, the eyelids are employed to:

- Move the lens with each blink so as to effect an exchange of tear fluid, and a removal of particulate matter, from beneath the lens.
- Continually re-wet the front surface of the lens with each blink.
- Position truncated rigid and soft toric lenses.
- Squeeze the 'thin zones' of toric lenses against the globe to provide correct lens orientation.
- Position rigid lenses by way of 'lid attachment' or 'interpalpebral' fitting philosophies.
- Translate alternating vision bifocals across the cornea so as to align the appropriate portion of the lens over the pupil.

Deformities or swelling of the eyelids – such as scarring of the lid margins (Figure 2.7) or swelling of the palpebral conjunctiva

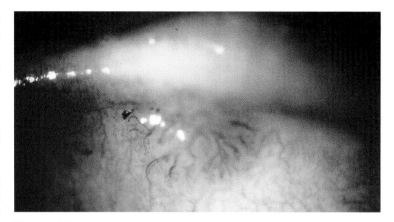

**Figure 2.8**
*Mass of vascularised oedematous tissue adjacent to the lid margin of a soft lens wearer, which could lead to lens mislocation*

(Figure 2.8) – can interfere with lid-mediated positioning of contact lenses.

### Absence of eyelid

The destruction of an eyelid due to a tumour or other disease is a potentially blinding situation. It is perhaps fitting to conclude this chapter with a reminder that the first contact lens ever fitted was in Germany by Dr Sämisch to one eye of a patient whose lower eyelid was destroyed as a result of carcinoma and whose upper lid was partially missing with the remaining portion thickened and entropic.[24] (Contact lens historians point out that, technically, a contact 'shell' was fitted, rather than a 'lens', because it had no power).[25] The other eye was totally blind. The patient obtained useful vision with the aid of this prosthetic device, which was worn continually for over 20 years until he died.

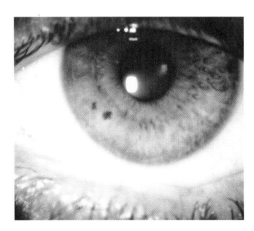

**Figure 2.7**
*Distortion of the lower lid margin due to scarring of the inferior palpebral conjunctiva, which may adversely affect lens positioning*

## REFERENCES

1 Osol A ed. (1973) *Blakiston's Pocket Medical Dictionary*. McGraw-Hill, New York.
2 Fonn D, Holden BA (1986) Extended wear of hard gas-permeable contact lenses can induce ptosis. *Contact Lens Assoc Ophthalmol J* **12**: 93.
3 Fonn D, Holden BA (1988) Rigid gas-permeable vs hydrogel contact lenses for extended wear. *Am J Optom Physiol Opt* **65**: 536.
4 Fonn D, Pritchard N, Garnett B (1996) Palpebral aperture sizes of rigid and soft contact lens wearers compared with non-wearers. *Optom Vis Sci* **73**: 211.
5 Van den Bosch WA, Lemij HG (1992) Blepharoptosis induced by prolonged hard contact lens wear. *Ophthalmology* **99**: 1759.
6 Jupiter DG, Karesh J (1997) Ptosis associated with hard/rigid gas-permeable contact lens wear. *Optom Vis Sci* **74**(s): 91.
7 Epstein G, Putterman AM (1981) Acquired blepharoptosis secondary to contact lens wear. *Am J Ophthalmol* **91**: 634.
8 Sheldon L, Biedner B, Geltman C (1979) Giant papillary conjunctivitis and ptosis in a contact lens wearer. *J Pediatr Ophthalmol Strab* **16**: 136.
9 Levy B, Stamper RL (1992) Acute ptosis secondary to contact lens wear. *Optom Vis Sci* **69**: 565.
10 Trodd TC (1971) Ptosis props in ocular myopathy. *Contact Lens* **3**: 3.
11 Mutti DO, Seger RG (1988) Eyelid asymmetry in unilateral hydrogel contact lens wear. *Int Contact Lens Clin* **15**: 252.
12 Green WR (1963) An embedded ('lost') contact lens. *Arch Ophthalmol* **69**: 23.
13 Long JC (1963) Retention of contact lens in upper fornix. *Am J Ophthalmol* **56**: 309.
14 Jahn D (1992) 'Pseudochalazion' due to a 'lost' contact lens. *Contactologia* **14**: 96.
15 Richter S, Sherman J, Horn D (1979) An embedded contact lens in the upper lid masquerading as a mass. *J Am Optom Assoc* **50**: 372.
16 Jones D, Livesey S, Wilkins P (1987) Hard contact lens migration into the upper lid: an unexpected lump. *Br J Ophthalmol* **71**: 368.

17 Jones D, Hassan HM (1987) Embedding of an inverted hard contact lens. *Am J Optom Physiol Opt* **64**: 879.

18 Smalling OH (1971) Embedment of inverted corneal contact lens. *J Am Optom Assoc* **42**: 755.

19 Nicolitz E, Flanagan JC (1978) Orbital mass as a complication of contact lens wear. *Arch Ophthalmol* **96**: 2238.

20 Yassin JG, White RH, Shannon GM (1970) Blepharoptosis as a complication of contact lens migration. *Am J Ophthalmol* **70**: 536.

21 Kelly JM (1994) Contact lens build-up (letter). *Optician* **207**: 13.

22 Kanski JJ (1999) *Clinical Ophthalmology*, 4th edition. Butterworth-Heinemann, Oxford.

23 Howitt DA, Goldstein JH (1969) Physiologic lagophthalmos. *Am J Ophthalmol* **68**: 355.

24 Müller FA, Müller AC (1910) *Das Künstliche Auge*. JF Bergmann, Wiesbaden.

25 Efron N, Pearson RM (1988) Centenary celebration of Fick's Eine Contactbrille. *Arch Ophthalmol* **106**: 1370.

# 3
# Meibomian gland dysfunction

Prevalence
Signs and symptoms
Pathology
Aetiology
Patient management
Differential diagnosis
Other contact lens-associated meibomian gland disorders

The meibomian glands in the upper and lower eyelids play a critical role in forming and maintaining a viable tear film. Specifically, these glands produce a clear, oily secretion that serves two main functions:

- Forming a hydrophobic lining along the lid margins which prevents epiphora.
- Forming a thin lipid layer over the surface of the aqueous tear phase which retards evaporative fluid loss.

There are approximately 25 meibomian glands in the upper eyelid and 20 meibomian glands in the lower eyelid, and the distribution of meibomian glands from inner to outer canthus is approximately uniform.

Meibomian gland dysfunction (MGD) (Figure 3.1) may be defined as a bilateral non-inflammatory clinical condition where there is a change in the lipid appearance from a normally clear state to a viscous and cloudy appearance, without any clinically observable meibomian gland abnormalities. However, some authors have adopted classification systems and definitions which suggest an inflammatory aetiology. For example, Bron et al[1] offer the following ambiguous definition of MGD: '...

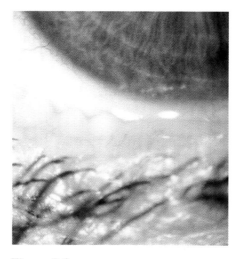

**Figure 3.1**
*Inspissated secretion from meibomian glands in the lower lid of a female rigid lens wearer*

an infection of the meibomian gland without necessarily implying that inflammation is present'. Wilhelmus[2] contends that MGD can also be termed 'posterior blepharitis'.

Although Wilhelmus[2] is correct in observing that meibomian gland secretions may be abnormal in posterior forms of sebor-

rhoeic blepharitis, it is best to consider posterior blepharitis (an inflammatory condition) to be a separate condition from MGD, which has a non-inflammatory aetiology. This view is shared by Ong,[3] who notes that many patients with MGD seen in primary eye care clinics are free of signs or symptoms of lid margin inflammation.

The question as to whether the relationship between meibomian gland dysfunction and contact lens wear is causal or casual has been investigated by Ong.[3] The eyes of 81 contact lens wearers and 150 age- and sex-matched non-lens wearers were examined for evidence of MGD. The prevalence of MGD was 49 per cent among the contact lens wearers and 39 per cent among the controls; this difference was not statistically significant, suggesting that contact lens wear is not a cause of MGD.

Although contact lens wear cannot be considered to be a cause of MGD, many problems relating to contact lens wear can be traced to problems in tear film function; it is in this regard that MGD can be of aetiological significance. Such problems are considered under the heading 'contact lens-associated meibomian gland dysfunction' (CL-MGD). This chapter will review the clinical ramifications of CL–MGD, and will conclude by briefly examining the implications for contact lens wear in association with other abnormalities of the meibomian gland.

## Prevalence

According to Ong and Larke,[4] 20 per cent of non-contact lens wearers show some loss of clarity of expressed meibomian oils, and opaque oils can be expressed from 6 per cent of non-wearers. These figures rise to 30 per cent and 11 per cent, respectively, in contact lens wearers. Among contact lens wearers, about 10 per cent of patients who complain of blurred vision and dryness can be demonstrated to have abnormal meibomian gland expressions.[4] The prevalence of MGD[5] and CL-MGD[4] is unrelated to gender.

Hom *et al*[5] conducted a survey of 398 normal patients presenting for a routine eye examination. Based on the principal clinical criterion of an absent or cloudy meibomian gland secretion upon expression, 39 per cent were found to have MGD. The prevalence of MGD was significantly increased with increasing age. Hom *et al*[5] reported that the prevalence of MGD was 41 per cent among contact lens wearers and 38 per cent among non-lens wearers; these figures broadly agree with those of Ong[3] of 49 per cent and 39 per cent, respectively.

## Signs and symptoms

The oily secretion from the normal meibomian gland is generally clear (Figure 3.2). The key diagnostic feature of CL-MGD is a change in the appearance of the clear oil expressed from healthy meibomian glands to a cloudy creamy yellow appearance.

This appearance is accompanied by symptoms of smeary vision, greasy lenses, dry eyes and reduced tolerance to lens wear. In severe cases, where the meibomian orifices are blocked, there may be an absence of gland secretion.

Figure 3.1 depicts the case of a 32-year-old female who was wearing gas permeable lenses and suffering from symptoms of dryness and reduced wearing time. Her lenses were wetting poorly and meibomian gland expression revealed a creamy, inspissated discharge, thus confirming a diagnosis of CL-MGD.

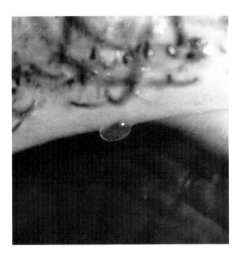

**Figure 3.2**
*Clear secretion expressed from a normal meibomian gland in the upper lid*

Long-standing cases of MGD may be associated with additional signs such as irregularity, distortion and thickening of eyelid margins, slight distension of glands, mild to moderate papillary hypertrophy, vascular changes (Figure 3.3) and chronic chalazia. The vascular changes have been described as neovascularisation, but it is more likely in the majority of cases where this change is observed that existing vessels have become distended and thus more visible.

Of the 155 patients found to have MGD in the survey of Hom *et al*,[5] 24 had blepharitis, four had chalazia and one meibomitis. None

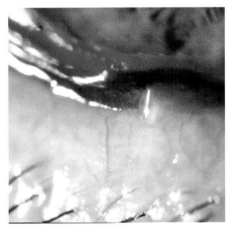

**Figure 3.3**
*Vessel enlargement and distortion of lid margin of a contact lens wearer. A blocked meibomian gland has just been expressed resulting in massive secretion of cloudy material, flooding the lacrimal river*

of the MGD-negative patients exhibited any of these conditions. Given that there is no difference in prevalence of MGD between contact lens wearers versus non-wearers, these associated conditions will often be observed in patients wearing contact lenses.

Examination of the lid margins using diffuse illumination at approximately × 20 magnification often reveals the presence of small oil globules at the orifices of the meibomian glands in patients suffering from CL-MGD. The clarity of the secretion will vary from slight murkiness to an almost opaque waxy milky-yellow colour. Viewing the lid margins against the dark background of the pupil or against a dark-coloured iris (see Figure 3.2) will enhance the view of the expressed material.[6]

Frothing or foaming of the lower tear meniscus is sometimes observed in CL-MGD (Figure 3.4), especially towards the outer canthus.[4] This may be due to a lowering of the surface tension of the tear film due to an absent or abnormal lipid layer.

The absence of oil globules at the meibomian gland orifices could indicate one of two extremes – normality or complete blockage. If oil globules are not observed on the lid margins of a symptomatic contact lens wearer, it may be necessary to conduct a provocative test in order to establish the state of health of the meibomian glands. This can be achieved by manual expression of the glands so that the nature of the expressed oils can be assessed.

Meibomian gland expression is a simple and rapid provocative test that is only mildly uncomfortable for the patient. Anatomical considerations dictate that expression of the meibomian glands in the lower lid is the preferred procedure. The patient is instructed to gaze superiorly. In cases of

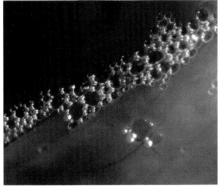

**Figure 3.4**
*Frothing of the tear film*

mild meibomian orifice blockage, gentle pressure with the finger or thumb immediately below the lower lid margin, together with a slight rolling action of the finger or thumb towards the lid margin, will generally result in the appearance of a small expression.

If nothing is expressed using the procedure described above, a more complete or even total meibomian blockage is indicated. In such cases, a support needs to be placed behind the lower lid margin so that increased pressure can be applied so as to force an expression of meibomian oils. This can be achieved by gently retracting the lower lid, placing a cotton-tipped bud behind the lid margin, and firmly squeezing the lid margin between the cotton-tipped bud and thumb.

Sudden release of the blockage at high pressure can result in a copious expression in the form of a thick stream of apparently dehydrated material, akin to the result of forcefully squeezing a toothpaste tube; this is referred to as an 'inspissated' secretion.

By careful observation and adopting the provocative tests described here, it is possible to grade the severity of CL-MGD on a clinical severity scale from 0 (normal) to 4 (severe). This grading system, which has been adapted from that described by Ong and Larke,[4] is presented in Table 3.1.

Associated signs of CL-MGD include all those which arise from clinical diagnostic procedures that are designed to indicate the integrity or otherwise of the lipid layer. Specifically, patients suffering from CL-MGD may display a reduced tear break-up time (measured either with fluorescein or non-invasively).[6] Examination of the tear layer in specular reflection using a Tearscope may reveal a contaminated lipid pattern, which is exacerbated by the use of cosmetic eye make-up (see Appendix B).[7]

Tear ferning analysis is likely to reveal a disrupted pattern in the form of minimal ferning, again indicating a contaminated and poorly formed tear layer.[8] Transillumination of meibomian glands during biomicroscopy can also assist in diagnosing CL-MGD by revealing the presence of distended or distorted glands.[9]

Hope-Ross *et al*[10] reported that in a series of 30 patients with recalcitrant recurrent corneal erosions, the prevalence of MGD was 100 per cent. Marren[11] reported a statistically significant link between MGD, contact lens wear and corneal staining. These findings suggest that increased corneal staining (that is, more than is typically observed in asymptomatic contact lens wearers) is associated with CL-MGD; however, neither Hope-Ross *et al* nor Marren could explain the basis for this link.

## Pathology

Changes to both the ductal lining of meibomian glands and the meibomian secretion in MGD have been reported in the literature. An increase in the turnover of epidermal epithelium around the orifices of the glands and an increase in the turnover of the epithelium lining of the ducts have been described; these changes can lead to mechanical clogging of the meibomian glands.[12,13]

Ong and Larke[4] failed to find any difference in the biochemical composition of meibomian secretions of contact lens wearers and non-wearers. They did, however, observe that abnormal meibomian oils began melting at 35°C (versus 32°C for normal meibomian oils) and that the melting profile of abnormal meibomian oils comprised five or six components (versus five to 12 components for normal meibomian oils). The results of this physical melting point analysis of meibomian secretions is consistent with the observation of a more free-flowing meibomian secretion in normals.

In a contact lens-wearing patient not suffering from MGD, the lipid layer is always separated from the lens surface by the aqueous phase of the tear layer. Some lipid can deposit on the lens surface – the magnitude and extent of which is determined in part by the polymeric nature of the lens material. Such lipid deposits are easily removed in practice using routine surfactant cleaning.

In CL-MGD, symptoms of blurred or greasy vision can probably be attributed to adhesion of waxy dysfunctional meibomian oils to the surface of the contact lens, which can more readily migrate down to the lens surface as a result of the disrupted nature of the tear layer.

As more lipid rapidly deposits on the lens, the surface becomes increasingly hydrophobic and is less able to sustain a continuous tear film. Also, the abnormal and irregular lipid layer is less capable of preventing evaporation of the aqueous tear fluid covering the lens and from exposed anterior ocular structures. These factors combine to dehydrate the lens and lead to a sensation of dryness.[14]

## Aetiology

Some interesting but largely unproved theories have been advanced as to the cause of CL-MGD. Rengstorff[15] suggested that CL-MGD may be attributed to the fact that contact lens wearers rub their eyelids less frequently than non-lens wearers for

| Grade | Clinical features |
|---|---|
| **Table 3.1** | **Grading system for contact lens-associated meibomian gland dysfunction (based on Ong and Larke[4])** |
| 0 | Normal<br>Clear fluid is expelled upon mild digital pressure from all gland orifices |
| 1 | Trace<br>One or two glands are partially obstructed |
| 2 | Mild<br>Three or more glands are partially obstructed<br>Glands tend to produce opaque fluid on digital pressure |
| 3 | Moderate<br>One or two glands are blocked<br>Many glands are partially obstructed<br>There is a tendency for foam to form in the tear film |
| 4 | Severe<br>More than three glands in each eye are blocked<br>Most of the remaining glands are partially obstructed<br>There is extensive foaming of the tear fluid |

fear of damaging or mechanically dislodging (and possibly losing) their lenses. This deprives the eyelid of the contact lens wearer of periodic rubbing which, Rengstorff claims, is essential to mechanically stimulate meibomian glands so that they will remain unblocked and free flowing.

This theory of Rengstorff[15] has been recently tested by Marren[11] who postulated that non-contact lens wearers using eye make-up would be similarly reluctant to rub their eyes for fear of disrupting the make-up. However, no difference was found in the prevalence of MGD between those who wear eye make-up versus those who do not.

An alternative 'eye rubbing' theory has been proposed to explain CL-MGD, but to opposite effect. Martin *et al*[16] suggested an association between CL-MGD and contact lens-associated papillary conjunctivitis (CL-PC). They proposed that the itching created by CL-PC stimulates eye rubbing which, rather than having a positive and stimulatory effect as proposed by Rengstorff,[15] causes mechanical damage to the meibomian glands and consequent dysfunction.

Since there is no difference in the prevalence of MGD between contact lens wearers versus non-wearers,[3,5] neither the meibomian stimulation theory of Rengstorff,[15] nor the meibomian trauma theory of Martin *et al*,[16] can be supported.

From a tissue pathology standpoint, the cause of MGD is an increased keratinisation of the epithelial walls of meibomian gland ducts.[12,13] This leads to the formation of keratinised epithelial plugs that form a physical blockage in meibomian ducts, which in turn restricts or prevents the outflow of meibomian oils. Increased levels of keratin proteins have been found in the meibomian oils of patients suffering from MGD.[17] It is thought that the creamy-yellow colour of meibomian oils is a result of the presence of keratin proteins.

It is not known why some patients suffer from increased keratinisation of meibomian ducts except to observe that it may be related to generalised systemic disorders; MGD is often observed in combination with seborrhoeic dermatitis and acne rosacea.

The increase in prevalence of MGD with age as reported by Hom *et al*[5] may be due to the fact that overall gland width decreases with age,[18] presumably due to a loss of gland acini. Other age-related factors that could

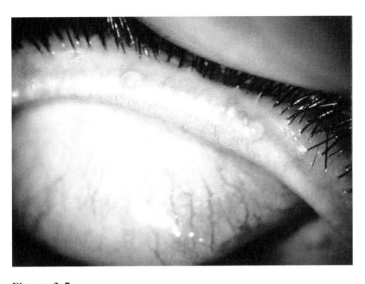

**Figure 3.5**
*Meibomian blockage of the upper lid in a 50-year-old female who reported contact lens intolerance. Increased visibility of vessels is apparent along the lid margin*

lead to MGD include general morphological changes[9] and orifice displacement (Figure 3.5).[19]

## Patient management

Although it is not possible to treat the underlying cause of meibomian gland dysfunction (epithelial keratinisation of meibomian gland ducts and consequent contamination of meibomian oils with keratin proteins), it is possible to provide symptomatic relief by adopting one or more of the following procedures. All of the procedures described below should be undertaken with contact lenses removed.

### Warm compresses
Henriquez and Korb[20] have advocated the use of warm compresses and lid scrubs to alleviate symptoms associated with CL-MGD. Cotton-wool pads soaked in hot water (boiled water that has been allowed to cool for a few minutes) are firmly massaged against the closed eyelids.

This procedure is intended to melt solidified lipids and thus unblock the meibomian orifices, allowing lipids to escape and reconstitute a trilaminate tear layer.

### Lid scrubs
The maintenance of clean and healthy lid margins is likely to be of benefit by:

- Preventing additional debris from blocking the meibomian orifices.
- Lessening the probability of contamination of meibomian glands, which could result in infection.

The patient is advised to clean the lid margins each morning and evening by gently rubbing or 'scrubbing' with a clean face cloth pre-soaked in mildly soapy water.

Alternatively, a cotton-tipped bud pre-soaked in weak baby shampoo may allow a more controlled lid clean. Commercially available lid hygiene kits are available. Proper attention to lid hygiene will lessen the likelihood of MGD developing into a meibomian cyst (chalazion).

Paugh *et al*[16] conducted a controlled, single-masked clinical trial examining the symptomatic and therapeutic benefits of a combined treatment of warm compresses and lid scrubbing in patients suffering from CL-MGD. These procedures were applied to one eye only, chosen at random, for 2 weeks, with the contralateral eye acting as a control.

After 2 weeks, the treated eye displayed a greater increase in tear break-up time (4.0 seconds greater than baseline) versus the non-treated eye (0.2 seconds greater than baseline).

Improved comfort was also reported in the treated eye, but it should be noted that the experiment was single-masked (i.e. the patient knew which eye was being treated) and the possibility of subject bias in recording comfort levels cannot be discounted.

### Mechanical expression

The patient can be instructed to express meibomian glands using the techniques described previously. If this procedure is adopted following the application of warm compresses, and lid hygiene procedures have been adopted, gentle pressure is usually all that will be required to facilitate expression of meibomian gland oils.

### Antibiotics

Although CL-MGD is not an inflammatory condition, it is thought that systemic antibiotics such as tetracycline may act by killing bacteria that normally split neutral lipids into irritating fatty acids.

### Artificial tears

Supplementing the tear film with artificial viscosity agents may help by increasing tear volume and prolonging the formation of a tear layer over the lens and ocular surface. This should at least provide symptomatic relief and lessen the 'dryness' sensation.

### Surfactant lens cleaning

Symptoms of blurred vision can be alleviated by ensuring that the contact lenses are being cleaned with an effective surfactant cleaning solution. Multi-purpose lens cleaning solutions that are designed to be compatible with the eye by necessity, contain relatively weak surfactant agents.

Although these solutions are perfectly adequate for the majority of contact lens wearers, patients suffering from conditions that can result in excessive deposition of abnormal lipids (such as CL-MGD) are best advised to use a separate surfactant cleaning agent.

In severe cases of CL-MGD, it may be necessary to advise the patient to use a surfactant cleaning agent every 4 hours. This should result in improved vision and comfort during lens wear.

### Prognosis

The underlying cause of MGD suggests that it is a chronic disorder with a poor prognosis for recovery. However, by adopting the procedures described above, CL-MGD can be kept under good control and adverse symptoms minimised.

Intensive therapy over several weeks might be required to bring the condition under control, but once this has been achieved, good comfort and vision can be attained by paying continued attention to lid hygiene and adopting occasional strategies to alleviate acute problems (e.g. physical expression, warm compresses etc.).

### Differential diagnosis

There are two aspects to differentiating CL-MGD from other disorders. Firstly, it is important to be able to differentiate CL-MGD from other possible disorders of the meibomian gland and indeed from other glands at the lid margin.

An external hordeolum (stye) is a small swelling at the lid margin associated with a staphylococcal infection and inflammation of a lash follicle, and involves the glands of Zeis or Moll. An internal hordeolum is a small abscess associated with a staphylococcal infection and inflammation of a meibomian gland, and is observed as a tender swelling of the tarsal plate (Figure 3.6). Patients suffering from these conditions complain of pain and tenderness; no such pain or tenderness is associated with MGD.

A meibomian cyst (chalazion) is a chronic lipogranulomatous inflammation of a meibomian gland secondary to an obstruction to the gland orifice. Thus, MGD and meibomian cyst formation may be considered as acute and chronic manifestations, respectively, of the same disease process.

Secondly, it is necessary to be able to differentiate the lipid irregularities and associated symptoms of dryness in patients with CL-MGD from other causes of tear film dysfunction in contact lens wearers. In general, this can be achieved by establishing the adequacy of the aqueous phase of the tear film; specifically, by applying tests of tear volume (e.g. Schirmer's test or cotton thread test) and lacrimal gland function (e.g. the Lactoplate test).

Symptoms of dryness and intermittent blurred vision in contact lens wearers in the presence of an adequate tear aqueous component should heighten suspicion of CL-MGD as being the cause of the problem.

### Other contact lens-associated meibomian gland disorders

As discussed above under the heading of 'Differential diagnosis', other disorders of the meibomian gland may be encountered, such as chalazion and internal hordeolum.

Figure 3.7 is a facial thermogram of a soft lens wearer suffering from an internal hordeolum of the right eye. The temperature distribution (red and yellow colours indicating higher temperatures) confirms the increased temperature associated with the

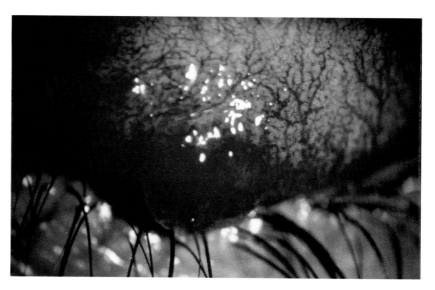

**Figure 3.6**
*Internal hordeolum in a soft lens wearer, which was surgically treated*

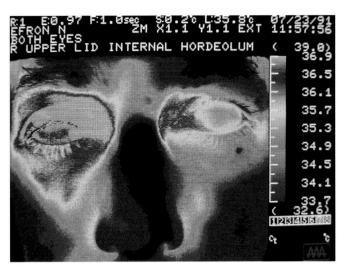

**Figure 3.7**
*Facial thermogram of a soft lens wearer suffering from an internal hordeolum of the right eye*

acute inflammation. In this case, lens wear was ceased until the condition resolved and the appearance of the tarsal plate returned to normal.

Contact lens wear should be suspended if a patient experiences either of these conditions, and should not be resumed until the condition has resolved. As a prophylactic measure, greater attention to lid hygiene should be reinforced in patients who have suffered from meibomian gland disease; this advice could include the prescription of lid scrub kits.

Sebaceous gland carcinomas involving the meibomian gland have also been described. These are the second most common form of malignancy of the eyelid, accounting for 2–7 per cent of all eyelid tumours and 1–5 per cent of eyelid malignancies. Sebaceous gland carcinomas are observed most commonly in elderly women and in Asians. There is no reason why patients suffering from such carcinomas should cease wearing contact lenses as long as the lenses are comfortable and the carcinoma remains under medical scrutiny.

## REFERENCES

1 Bron AL, Benjamin L, Sibson GR (1991) Meibomian gland dysfunction: classification and grading of lid changes. *Eye* **5**: 395.

2 Wilhelmus KR (1992) Inflammatory disorders of the eyelid margins and eyelashes. *Ophthalmol Clin North Am* **10**: 187.

3 Ong BL (1996) Relation between contact lens wear and meibomian gland dysfunction. *Optom Vis Sci* **73**: 208.

4 Ong BL, Larke JR (1990) Meibomian gland dysfunction: some clinical, biochemical and physical observations. *Ophthal Physiol Opt* **10**: 144.

5 Hom MH, Martinson JR, Knapp LL (1990) Prevalence of meibomian gland dysfunction. *Optom Vis Sci* **67**: 710.

6 Paugh JR, Knapp LL, Martinson JR (1990) Meibomian therapy in problematic contact lens wear. *Optom Vis Sci* **67**: 803.

7 Guillon JP (1997) Dry eye in contact lens wear. *Optician* **214**: 18

8 Golding TE, Brennan NA (1989) The basis of tear ferning. *Clin Exp Optom* **72**: 102.

9 Robin JB, Jester JV, Noble JR (1985) *In vivo* transillumination biomicroscopy and photography of meibomian gland dysfunction (a clinical study). *Ophthalmology* **92**: 1423.

10 Hope-Ross MW, Chell PB, Kervick GN (1994) Recurrent corneal erosion: clinical features. *Eye* **8**: 373.

11 Marren SE (1994) Contact lens wear, use of eye cosmetics, and meibomian gland dysfunction. *Optom Vis Sci* **71**: 60.

12 Korb DR, Henriquez AS (1980) Meibomian gland dysfunction and contact lens intolerance. *J Am Optom Assoc* **51**: 243.

13 Gutgesell VJ, Stern GA, Hood CI (1982) Histopathology of meibomian gland dysfunction. *Am J Ophthalmol* **94**: 383.

14 Efron N, Brennan NA (1988) A survey of wearers of low water content hydrogel contact lenses. *Clin Exp Optom* **71**: 86.

15 Rengstorff RH (1980) Meibomian gland dysfunction in contact lens wearers. *Rev Optom* **117**: 75.

16 Martin NF, Rubinfeld RS, Malley JD (1992) Giant papillary conjunctivitis and meibomian gland dysfunction blepharitis. *Contact Lens Assoc Ophthalmol J* **18**: 165.

17 Ong BL, Hodson SA, Wigham T (1991) Evidence of keratin proteins in normal and abnormal human meibomian fluids. *Curr Eye Res* **10**: 1113.

18 Pascucci SE, Lemp MA, Cavanagh HD (1988) An analysis of age-related morphologic changes in human meibomian glands. *Invest Ophthalmol Vis Sci* (Suppl) **29**: 213.

19 Norn M (1985) Meibomian orifices and Marx's line – studies by triple vital staining. *Acta Ophthalmol (Kbh)* **63**: 698.

20 Henriquez AS, Korb DR (1981) Meibomian glands and contact lens wear. *Br J Ophthalmol* **65**: 108.

# 4
# Eyelash disorders

External hordeolum (stye)
Marginal blepharitis
Parasitic infestation of eyelashes
Other contact lens-associated eyelash disorders

Disorders of the eyelashes (cilia), and of associated structures at the base of the eyelashes such as the eyelash follicles, glands of Zeis and skin of the lid margin, have implications for contact lens wear. Practitioners need to be aware of the possible existence of such conditions in contact lens wearers because they may explain ocular discomfort during lens wear, and in many instances will contraindicate lens wear until the condition is resolved. This chapter reviews eyelash-related problems as common as a dislodged eyelash entering the eye, and as uncommon as parasitic eyelash infestation by crab lice (Figure 4.1).

Eyelashes typically project from the anterior rounded border of the lid margin in two or three rows. They lie just anterior to the 'grey line' – an anatomical feature that indicates the position of the mucocutaneous junction. The superior eyelashes are longer and more numerous than those of the lower lid. Because upper lashes normally curl up and lower lashes normally curl down, lashes do not become tangled on eyelid closure. Eyelashes are typically darker than other hairs of the body except in conditions such as alopecia areata.[1]

## External hordeolum (stye)

An external hordeolum – commonly known as a 'stye' – presents as a discrete inflamed swelling of the anterior lid margin. It is extremely tender to touch, and may occur singly or as multiple small abscesses. A stye is an inflammation of the tissue lining the lash follicle and/or an associated gland of Zeis or Moll. It is typically an acute staphylococcal infection, and as such commonly presents in patients with staphylococcal blepharitis.

Styes have a typical time course of about seven days. Sometimes a stye will discharge spontaneously in an anterior direction. If a patient is in particular discomfort, resolu-

tion can be facilitated by removing the eyelash from the infected follicle and applying hot compresses to the affected area.[2]

Contact lens wear may add to the discomfort of a stye due to the mechanical effect of the lens. In soft lens wearers, mechanical pressure against the lens between the stye and the globe may effectively grip the lens and result in excessive lens movement during blinking. With a rigid lens fitted interpalpebrally, the lens may buffet against the lid margin with each blink. For these reasons, patients may prefer to cease lens wear during the acute phase of stye formation.

## Marginal blepharitis

Marginal blepharitis is typically classified as being either anterior or posterior. Anterior blepharitis is directly related to infections of the base of the eyelashes and manifests in two forms: staphylococcal blepharitis and seborrhoeic blepharitis.

Posterior blepharitis is a disorder of the meibomian glands and has been considered in Chapter 3.

### *Staphylococcal* anterior blepharitis
This condition is caused by a chronic staphylococcal infection of the eyelash folli-

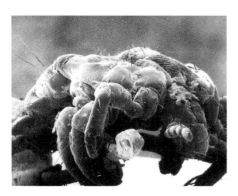

**Figure 4.1**
*Electron micrograph of a crab louse,* Phthirus pubis

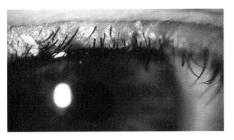

**Figure 4.2**
*Staphylococcal anterior blepharitis with the lid margin covered in brittle scales*

cles, and leads to secondary dermal and epidermal ulceration and tissue destruction. It is frequently observed in patients with atopic eczema and occurs more frequently in females and in younger patients.

Slit-lamp examination of patients suffering from this condition reveals the presence of hyperaemia, telangiectasis and scaling of the anterior lid margins. The scales are brittle (Figure 4.2) and when removed will leave a small bleeding ulcer. The lashes may appear stuck together and in severe cases a yellow crust can build around the base of cilia forming a collarette.

In long-standing cases, there may be a loss of some eyelashes (madarosis), some eyelashes may turn white (poliosis), and the anterior lid margin may become scarred, notched, irregular or hypertrophic (tylosis).

Hypersensitivity to staphylococcal exotoxins may lead to secondary complications such as low-grade papillary and bulbar conjunctivitis, toxic punctate epitheliopathy involving the inferior third of the cornea, and marginal corneal infiltrates. Patients suffering from staphylococcal anterior blepharitis may complain of burning, itching, foreign-body sensations and mild photophobia. Associated tear-film instability may also lead to symptoms of dryness, which are often worse in the morning.

The following management strategies may be employed:

- *Antibiotic ointment* – after removing crusts, antibiotic ointment is applied to the lid margins with a clean finger.
- *Promote lid hygiene* – crusts and toxic products can be removed by scrubbing the lids twice daily with a commercially available lid scrub. Alternatively, regular washing with a warm, moist face cloth and occasional rubbing with diluted baby shampoo should alleviate the condition.

- *Steroids* – weak topical steroids may be tried in more severe and protracted cases, especially if the strategies described above fail.
- *Artificial tears* – will provide symptomatic relief if the blepharitis is compromising the integrity of the tear film.

The treatment can be tailed off as the condition improves. However, staphylococcal anterior blepharitis is difficult to treat and the pattern of recovery is characterised by periods of remission and exacerbation.[2]

### Seborrhoeic anterior blepharitis
This condition is due to a disorder of the glands of Zeis and Moll, which connect with eyelash follicles. It is frequently associated with seborrhoeic dermatitis of the scalp, eyebrows, nasolabial folds, retroauricular areas and sternum. The symptoms are similar but less severe than for staphylococcal anterior blepharitis.

The anterior lid margin displays a shiny, waxy appearance with mild erythema and telangiectasis. Soft, yellow greasy scales are observed along the lid margin; these scales do not leave a bleeding ulcer when removed. The eyelashes may also become greasy and stuck together (Figure 4.3).

As with the staphylococcal form, secondary complications of seborrhoeic anterior blepharitis include mild papillary conjunctivitis and punctate epitheliopathy. The main form of treatment is lid hygiene and artificial tears.[2]

### Implications for contact lens wear
Contact lens wear is generally contraindicated during an acute phase of anterior marginal blepharitis, especially if the cornea is compromised. If contact lenses are worn during mild cases of staphylococcal

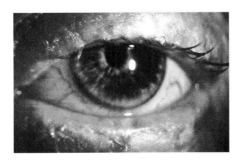

**Figure 4.3**
*Seborrhoeic anterior blepharitis in which the eyelashes have become greasy and stuck together*

anterior blepharitis, attention to lens cleaning is critical to prevent continued recontamination of the eye. Daily disposable contact lenses will eliminate the problem of recontamination by contact lenses.

Keys[3] conducted a 4-month study on 20 contact lens wearers and six non-lens wearing patients suffering from marginal blepharitis, to test the efficacy of various treatment regimens. These regimens were eyelid cleaning with hypoallergenic soap, lid scrubbing with dilute baby shampoo, and use of a commercial lid scrub. It was concluded that all three regimens resulted in improvement, and that about 85 per cent of patients preferred to use the commercial lid scrub.

## Parasitic infestation of eyelashes

Infestation of the eyelashes by mites or lice can lead to signs and symptoms that closely resemble marginal blepharitis. Clinicians must therefore be aware of this possibility, and be able to distinguish between the three species of parasite that most commonly infest human eyelashes and associated structures.[4] This is especially important in contact lens practice, as failure to identify parasitic eyelash infestation will almost certainly lead to patient dropout.

### Mites
Mite infestation is very common in humans, with a greater prevalence in older persons. In the US, the prevalence of lice has been reported to be 29 per cent in 0–25-year-olds, 53 per cent in 26–50-year-olds and 67 per cent in 51–90-year-olds.[5] Mite infestation in the eyelashes is ubiquitous and generally subclinical, but if present in excessive numbers, adverse signs and symptoms may develop. The mode of transmission of mites between humans is not clear but may arise from intimate contact. Mites are also more abundant in diabetic and AIDS patients, and in patients on long-term corticosteroid therapy, suggesting that compromised immunity can influence mite infestation.[4]

Two species of mite (*Demodex*) are found in the human pilosebaceous gland complex; these are from the family Demodicidae, order Acarina (mites and ticks), class Arachnida (spiders, scorpions, ticks and mites) and

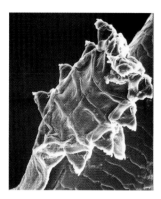

**Figure 4.4**
*Electron micrograph of a follicle mite,*
Demodex folliculorum, *lying on an epilated lash*

phylum Anthropoda. Infestation with *Demodex* species is termed 'demodicosis'.[4]

*Demodex folliculorum* is cigar-shaped with four evenly spaced stubby legs on the upper third of its body (Figure 4.4). It prefers to live in the space between the eyelash and the follicle wall, and in a single follicle will typically exist in small colonies of three to five mites. This species of mite is always located above the level of the gland of Zeis, primarily because of its size.[6]

*D. folliculorum* is much smaller in diameter than the base of the eyelash; it buries itself headfirst into the follicle and feeds off the cytoplasm of follicular epithelium by clawing away at, and puncturing, the epithelial cell walls with sharp mouth-parts. The shredded, hyperkeratinised cell material, combined with lipids and sebum, form a clear sleeve which covers the base of the eyelash; these sleeves are called 'cuffs' or 'collarettes' (Figure 4.5). Extensive mite activity can lead to an aggregation of cuffing material such that the mites are trapped within the hair follicle. This can lead to follicle distension, granulomas, telangiectasis, hyperplasia, erythema, madarosis, hyperaemia, burning and itching, which of course need to be dealt with clinically.[4]

*Demodex brevis* is found in human skin rich in sebaceous glands and sebum production. It prefers to infest the gland of Zeis, and can reach this gland because of its small size (0.18 mm long, versus *D. folliculorum* which is 0.38 mm long).[6] *D. brevis* has an almost identical structure to *D. folliculorum*, the former being shorter but stubbier. *D. brevis* is often found alone in a single sebaceous gland. In a similar manner to the actions of *D. folliculorum*, *D. brevis* can block the gland of Zeis and the

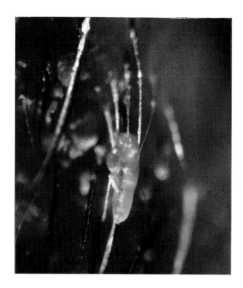

**Figure 4.5**
*Collarette surrounding an eyelash, providing evidence of mite infestation*

meibomian glands, leading to meibomian gland dysfunction and interference with lipid production, which in turn can result in dry-eye symptoms.

Because *D. brevis* prefers to live in an oily, sebaceous environment, it tends to thrive in the presence of oily cosmetics and facial preparations. This in turn can cause *D. brevis* to proliferate, and can lead to: meibomian glands, glands of Zeis and other facial sebaceous glands becoming blocked; the skin becoming dry; the patient applying more oily facial creams; *D brevis* profilerating; and the cycle continuing.[7]

*Demodex* species are typically nocturnal, but even during the day a busy migration of organisms can be observed passing between eyelash follicles. Patient symptoms typically parallel the life cycle of the organisms. Nests of *D. folliculorum* are laid around the base of lashes; they hatch after about 2–3 days and the adult lives from 5 to 14 days.[8]

Although they may be detected at high magnification ($\times$ 40) on a slit-lamp biomicroscope, mites are difficult to observe because they are very small (much narrower than the width of an eyelash). They withdraw into the follicle in bright light (being nocturnal in nature), and they are translucent. Diagnosis is confirmed by examination of epilated lashes under a light microscope; one or more mites observed on every two lashes is considered to be indicative of demodicosis.[9]

Additional signs of demodicosis include:

erythema of the lid margins, lid hyperplasia and madarosis (all of which give the impression of marginal blepharitis), conjunctival injection, cuffing around lashes, follicular distension and meibomian gland blockage. Eyelashes are more easily removed during active infestation due to damage to the eyelash follicles. Typical symptoms of demodicosis are pruritis, burning, crusting, itching, swelling of the lid margins and loss of lashes. The itching often parallels the 10-day reproductive cycle of *Denodex* species.[4]

**Lice**

Three species of lice infest the human body: the head louse (*Pediculus humanus capitis*), the body louse (*Pediculus humanus corpus*) and the pubic louse, or 'crab' (*Phthirus pubis*). These species are from the family Pediculidae, order Anoplura (the sucking lice), class Insecta and, like mites, they are classified as belonging to the phylum Arthropoda.[4]

*P. capitis* typically infests the scalp hair (especially the occipital region). During dense scalp infestation, *P. capitis* can be found in the eyelashes, but this is extremely rare. *P. corpus* inhabits seams and creases in clothing and feeds on the skin of patients. Infestation with these two species is termed pediculosis. The *Pediculus* species are typically 2.5–3.5 mm long, and are carriers for serious diseases such as typhus, relapsing fever and trench fever.[10]

The crab louse, *P. pubis*, is most commonly found in pubic hair, but also in other coarsely spaced hair such as on the chest and thighs (Figure 4.6). Infestation with this species is termed phthiriasis. The crab louse is about l.0–1.5 mm long, which is an ideal size for inhabitation among pubic hairs because these are spaced 2 mm apart and this corresponds to the anatomical grasping span of its legs. *P. pubis* can successfully infest eyelashes, which are also approximately 2 mm apart; indeed, of the three species of louse discussed above, it is the crab louse that is almost exclusively found among human eyelashes.[10] *P. pubis* has two pairs of strong grasping claws on the central and hind legs, allowing it to hold on to eyelashes with considerable tenacity.

Phthiriasis is considered to be a venereal disease because it is passed on by sexual contact. In adults, genital-to-eye transmission is the most probable cause of eyelash infestation, although infestation from contaminated bedding, towels etc. is another

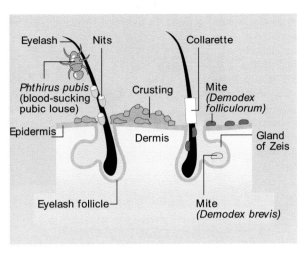

**Figure 4.6**
*Schematic diagram illustrating the preferred habitat of mites and lice that commonly infest the human pilosebaceous system*

possible mode of transfer. The eyelashes of children may be infested by eye-to-eye contact, and eyelashes of infants may be infested from contact with chest hair of parents or siblings who themselves are harbouring the lice.[4]

The three species discussed above are known as 'sucking lice' because of their mode of feeding, which is to anchor mouth hooklets to the host skin and to extend a long hollow tube (stylus) into the dermis. Anticoagulants are secreted to facilitate unimpeded sucking of blood and serum.[4]

All of these lice have internal fertilisation and lay eggs within 2 days of fertilisation. The eggs, or 'nits', are encapsulated in a cigar-shaped shell (Figure 4.7). Nit shells are cemented to eyelashes about 1–2 mm

from the base of the lash, and the nits hatch in 7–10 days. It takes lice about one month to reach adult stage, and the adult lives for a further month. Lice can survive for only 2 days if separated from the host.[4]

Signs of phthiriasis include pruritis of the lid margins, blepharitis, marked conjunctival injection and madarosis. Additional signs include pre-auricular lymphadenopathy and secondary infection along the lid margins at the site of lice bites. The most predominant symptom is intense itching, which is so severe that patients will also report insomnia, irritability and mental depression.[10]

The most obvious sign of phthiriasis is the presence of oval, greyish-white nit shells attached to the base of lashes, which are easily identifiable using high magnification (×40) slit-lamp biomicroscopy (Figure 4.8). Adult lice can be difficult to detect because they are almost completely transpar-

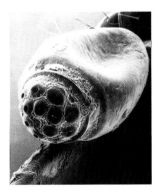

**Figure 4.7**
*Electron micrograph of lice eggs, or 'nits', encapsulated in a characteristic cigar-shaped shell*

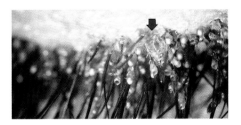

**Figure 4.8**
*Slit-lamp photomicrograph of a nearly transparent louse at the lid margin (arrow) surrounded by a mass of nits encapsulated in shells, and some empty shells which have already hatched*

ent. Reddish-brown deposits at the base of lashes also indicate the presence of lice; these deposits are a combination of blood from the host and faeces from the parasite. Blue spots may also be observed on the lid margins; these are due to enzymatic reactions from the digestive juices of the lice.[10]

**Treatment of mite infestation**
The main aim of treatment is to reduce the level of infestation to sub-clinical levels. In treating this condition, it should be assumed that there will be a concurrent bacterial infection. The initial course of action is to attempt to remove as many mites and mite eggs as possible. This can be achieved by applying a topical anaesthetic and swabbing the eyelid margins and eyelashes with a cotton-tipped applicator saturated in a contact lens cleaning solution, taking care to avoid contact with the cornea.[4]

Patients should be advised to engage in vigorous lid scrubbing twice daily using commercially available preparations, diluted baby shampoo, non-allergenic soap or hot flannels. Following the evening lid scrub, a viscous ointment should be applied to the upper and lower lid margins. This procedure will trap mites in their follicles, smother and kill the trapped mites, and prevent mites from migrating and cross-contaminating adjacent follicles. A lid scrub performed the following morning will remove dead lice and associated debris trapped in the ointment. Heavy metal ointments such as yellow mercuric oxide are usually prescribed because of their supplementary antimicrobial efficacy. Pilocarpine gel has been suggested as a more potent alternative. Treatment should be continued for at least 3 weeks, even if early symptomatic relief has been achieved.[4]

If the above measures are unsuccessful, more aggressive in-practice therapy may be needed. Vigorous scrubs with a cotton-tipped applicator soaked in alcohol or ether, performed weekly for 3 weeks, may control the condition.[4]

Patients experiencing symptoms of dryness due to demodectic infestation of the skin should be cautioned against the use of facial oils, and should be advised to wash the affected areas daily with soap.[4] Practitioners should be alert to the possibility of alarming patients about the existence of spider-like parasites on their body. It should be explained that this is a chronic condition that can be kept under control if the patient complies with the treatment protocol.

## Treatment of lice infestation

The initial course of action is to remove the crab lice mechanically from the lashes with forceps, while visualising the process using medium to high power on a slit-lamp biomicroscope. Removal may be difficult because the lice maintain a tight grasp on the lashes. Heavy infestations are best removed using cryotherapy (freezing) or argon laser photoablation. The latter technique effectively slices through the lashes; the result is initially unsightly, but the patient should be reassured that the lashes will quickly grow to full length. Lice and nits will also be killed by application of 20 per cent sodium fluorescein.[10]

Patients should apply yellow mercuric oxide ophthalmic ointment twice daily to the lid margins to smother and kill adult lice.[11] This therapy should be continued for 2 weeks to cover at least one complete lice life cycle. Anticholinesterase agents may also be tried. More potent insecticides are seldom used today because of the potential for serious corneal injury. Patients should be warned that symptoms may persist beyond effective eradication of lice due to residual lice-induced hypersensitivity reactions.[10]

Patients should be referred for treatment of pubic infestation and other possible sexually transmitted diseases. Sexual partners and family members should also be examined for eyelash infestation and counselled about the possibility of concurrent infestation of pubic hair. More potent pediculicidal ointment can be applied to regions of the body away from the eyes, offering the possibility of rapid and effective treatment.[10]

The home environment should also be sanitised to eradicate lice, with heat application being the most effective course of action. Lice will be killed if bed clothing, towels, sheets and clothes are washed at a temperature of 120°C for 30 minutes. Combs, brushes and hair accessories should be soaked in lice-killing products or in boiling water for 10 minutes. Isolation of blankets and other large items from the host for two weeks will ensure the death of all lice and nits.[10]

## Management in contact lens wearers

In general, contact lens wearers presenting with parasitic infestation of the eyelids should be treated in the same way as similarly infested non-lens wearers. Paradoxically, contact lenses (soft lenses in particular) serve a protective function during parasitic eyelash infestation because they prevent the cornea from mechanical effects of altered lid margins and lashes, and prevent toxins and debris from coming into contact with the cornea.[11] It is advisable to cease lens wear during the treatment period, which in severe cases may last up to one month. Contact lenses can theoretically serve as a vector for transmission of mites, lice, nits or other potentially toxic or allergenic by-products of the infestation process. The probability of such vectoral transmission increases if the patient is partially non-compliant by, for example, failing to surfactant clean and/or manually rub their lenses following removal. An intense cleaning regimen is indicated for patients with eyelash infestations. The best modality of lens wear for such patients is daily disposable lenses.

Caroline *et al*[12] have highlighted the sensitive nature of crab lice infestation in that it is primarily a sexually transmitted disease. They caution that loss to follow-up is to be expected in a significant number of patients who may well be embarrassed to return to their eye care practitioner for further care of the eyelash infestation or indeed for further contact lens management.

## Other contact lens-associated eyelash disorders

### Insects trapped in eyelashes

Dead flying insects are occasionally observed on the lid margins, just posterior to the base of the eyelashes. These insects perhaps land on the lid margin quite accidentally, realise that they have found a soft, moist and succulent environment (the conjunctiva and meibomian secretions), and take measures to anchor themselves in position. Another possibility is that they quickly become stuck in the oily lipid secretions of the lid margin. A strong reflex blink or eye rub by the host may then kill or incapacitate the insect, which remains in place until physically dislodged.

Figure 4.9 shows an insect trapped on the upper lid margin of a soft contact lens wearer who noticed discomfort in her left eye during a holiday in Spain. The patient attributed the consequent irritation to a split in her contact lens; she returned to her practitioner who detected the insect on slit-lamp examination. Figure 4.10 shows a larger flying insect trapped on the lower

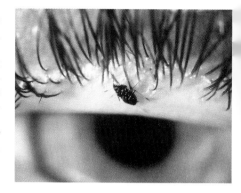

**Figure 4.9**
*Insect stuck on the upper lid margin just posterior to lashes*

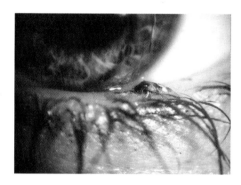

**Figure 4.10**
*Insect stuck on the lower lid margin just posterior to lashes*

lid margin of a rigid contact lens patient. The above cases highlight the importance of thoroughly examining the lid margins when trying to find the cause of discomfort that is apparently related to contact lens wear.

### Shedded eyelash entering the eye

The life cycle of an eyelash is about 5 months, and it takes about 2 months for a new eyelash to become fully grown.[1] Thus, there are frequent opportunities for a shedded eyelash to enter the eye. In non-lens wearers, an eyelash that enters the eye typically elicits an intense foreign body discomfort reaction, which causes increased lacrimation and results in the lash being flushed out. In contact lens wearers, the lash may become lodged beneath the lens; this is generally uncomfortable and the patient will remove the lens and attempt to remove the eyelash as well. Examination may reveal evidence of corneal epithelial trauma; if severe, lens wear should cease until the epithelium has recovered.

## Trichiasis

Trichiasis is a condition in which the eyelashes curl inwards towards the globe. This can manifest as a primary condition or be secondary to entropion. Whatever the cause, the result can be discomfort and persistent abrasion of the cornea by the eyelashes. In non-lens wearers this can lead to significant corneal decompensation in the form of a vascular pannus if left untreated for a significant length of time.[2]

Contact lenses can act as a protective buffer against corneal damage – with soft lenses offering more protection than rigid lenses due to their greater corneal coverage. However, the cornea can be damaged when lenses are not being worn, and subsequent lens wear in the presence of epithelial trauma is problematic because the epithelial breach may render the eye to be more susceptible to microbial infection. Inward growing eyelashes should therefore be treated by one of the following techniques:

- *Epilation* – eyelashes are mechanically removed with the aid of forceps.
- *Electrolysis* – the eyelash follicle is destroyed by passing an electrical current

through a fine needle inserted into the lash root.
- *Cryotherapy* – the lash follicle is frozen with a nitrous oxide cryoprobe at −20°C.[2]

## Distichiasis

Distichiasis is a condition whereby eyelashes emerge from regions of the lid margin other than their typical location. For example, eyelashes may emerge from between or even from within meibomian gland orifices. Distichiasis can be congenital or acquired, and typically causes the same problems of irritation and corneal trauma as occurs in trichiasis.[2] The implications for contact lens wear are also similar; the condition is usually treated using cryotherapy.

## REFERENCES

1 Bron AJ, Tripathi RC, Tripathi BJ (1997) *Wolff's Anatomy of the Eye and Orbit*, 8th edn. Chapman & Hall Medical, London.
2 Kanski JJ (1999) *Clinical Ophthalmology*, 4th edn. Butterworth-Heinemann, Oxford.
3 Keys JE (1996) A comparative study of eyelid cleaning regimens in chronic blepharitis. *Contact Lens Assoc Ophthalmol J* **22**: 209.
4 Edmondson W, Christenson MT (1992) Lid parasites. In: *Clinical Optometric Pharmacology and Therapeutics* (Ed. B Onefrey). Lippincott-Raven, Philadelphia, ch. 42.
5 Sengbusch HG, Hauswirth JW (1996) Prevalence of hair follicle mites, *Demodex folliculorum* and *D. brevis* (Acari: Demodicidae), in a selected human population in western New York, USA. *J Med Entomol* **23**: 384.
6 English FP, Nutting WB (1981) Demodicosis of ophthalmic concern. *Am J Ophthalmol* **91**: 362.
7 Heacock CE (1986) Clinical manifestations of demodicosis. *J Am Optom Assoc* **57**: 914.
8 Anderson PH, Jones WL (1988) A recalcitrant case of *Demodex blepharitis*. *Clin Eye Vis Care* **1**: 39.
9 Fulk GW, Clifford C (1990) A case report of demodicosis. *J Am Optom Assoc* **61**: 637.
10 Couch JM, Green WR, Hirst LW (1982) Diagnosing and treating *Phthirus pubis palpebrarum*. *Surv Ophthalmol* **26**: 219.
11 Holland BJ, Siderov J (1998) Phthiriasis and pediculosis palpebrarum. *Clin Exp Optom* **80**: 8.
12 Caroline PJ, Kame RT, Hatashida JK (1991) Pediculosis parasitic infestation in a contact lens wearer. *Clin Eye Vis Care* **3**: 82.

# Part II
# **Conjunctiva**

# 5
# Bulbar hyperaemia

Definitions
Prevalence
Signs and symptoms
Pathology
Aetiology
Observation and grading
Treatment
Prognosis
Differential diagnosis

Increased conjunctival redness in response to contact lens wear is so easily recognised that it serves as a fundamental indicator to clinicians of the physiological status of the contact lens wearing eye. It is not surprising that the first two clinical reports of contact lens wearing trials on humans – conducted independently in the late 1880s by Adolf Fick[1] and August Müller[2] – used conjunctival redness as a measure of the severity of reaction to, and time course of recovery from, the impact of lens wear.

Conjunctival redness is perhaps the only tissue reaction to contact lens wear that is also reported as a symptom by patients (Figure 5.1). Indeed, excessive eye redness is cosmetically unsightly and is generally perceived as a potential disadvantage of wearing contact lenses.

It is generally appreciated in eye care that the clinical presentation of a 'red eye' can be one of the most difficult cases to solve due to the numerous possible causes that are known. This problem may be even more complex in a contact lens wearer be-

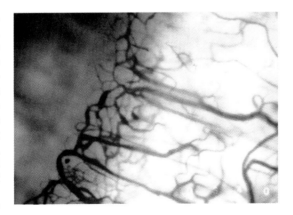

**Figure 5.1**
*Engorged conjunctival vessels resulting in the appearance of eye redness*

cause there are also many other contact lens-related causes of red eye.

## Definitions

Throughout the literature, the terms hyperaemia, injection, vascularity and red-

ness are used as synonyms. These terms are defined as follows:

- *Hyperaemia* – increased blood in a part, resulting in distension of the blood vessels.[3]
- *Injection* – a state of hyperaemia.[3]
- *Vascularity* – the quality of vessels.[3]
- *Redness* – of or approaching the colour

seen at the least-refracted end of the spectrum, of shades varying from crimson to brown and orange.[4]

Strictly speaking, hyperaemia or injection is the cause and redness is the effect. That is, an increased volume of blood in the conjunctival vessels (hyperaemia or injection) causes an increased appearance of redness. The term vascularity is somewhat ambiguous and could represent both the cause and effect.

## Prevalence

Most contact lens wearers will have experienced an episode of eye redness, no matter how mild, that may or may not have been related to lens wear. Conjunctival injection is such a common sign that few studies have documented its prevalence. According to Stapleton *et al*,[5] 37 out of 1104 contact lens wearers (3.4 per cent) attending the accident and emergency department at Moorfields Eye Hospital were primarily diagnosed as having 'contact lens-related red eye'.

However, this figure underestimates the true prevalence of red eye as a presenting symptom because many of the other patients in that study were diagnosed as having conditions that would certainly have been associated with eye redness, such as toxic disorders, keratitis, conjunctival abrasion etc. Virtually all patients who present to their eye care practitioner complaining of ocular discomfort will have associated eye redness.

## Signs and symptoms

The term 'conjunctival hyperaemia' is potentially confusing because it may not be clear whether this refers to redness of the bulbar, limbal or tarsal conjunctiva. Indeed, in his 1889 thesis on contact lenses, Müller[2] clearly differentiated between the extent of bulbar conjunctival redness, bulbar episcleral redness and limbal redness and he used the degree of redness in these three tissue types as the basis of his analysis of the likely pathophysiological effects of lens wear.

As with all adverse responses that can involve a wide expanse of tissue, there may be significant regional variations in the extent of hyperaemia with respect to a given conjunctival structure. Figure 5.2 illus-

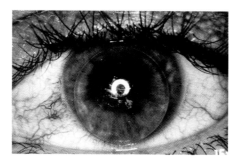

**Figure 5.2**
*Localised 3 and 9 o'clock bulbar conjunctival hyperaemia and circumlimbal hyperaemia in a rigid lens wearer*

trates severe bulbar conjunctival hyperaemia limited to the 3 and 9 o'clock position, associated with circumlimbal hyperaemia, in a patient wearing rigid lenses. The limbal engorgement suggests corneal involvement, which is consistent with the fact that this patient also displayed 3 and 9 o'clock staining.

There is also considerable variation in the magnitude of a hyperaemic response between individuals, as noted by Fick[1] in his 1888 paper. He observed: 'The degree of injection which manifests itself varies greatly...'. Fick[1] also used the conjunctival hyperaemic response to discover that the eye adapts to lens wear; he reported: 'The degree of injection ... is apt to be absent entirely in those ... eyes ... which have already been utilised in a long series of experiments. Apparently, therefore, a sort of toleration is established very soon.'

Conjunctival hyperaemia is generally asymptomatic, but patients may complain of itchiness, congestion, non-specific mild irritation or a warm or cold feeling. The existence of pain usually indicates corneal involvement or other tissue pathology (e.g. uveitis or scleritis).

Inferior bulbar conjunctival redness was assessed in asymptomatic contact lens wearers by McMonnies and Chapman-Davies.[6,7] The degree of redness was determined with reference to a photographic grading scale which contained six images of an eye displaying levels of redness ranging from grade 0 (no redness; 'white eye') to grade 5 (extreme redness). It can be determined from their data that the mean level of redness was as follows: no lenses – 0.78; RGP lenses – 0.96; soft lenses used in the absence of preservative-based care systems – 1.54; and soft lenses used in con-

junction with preservative-based care systems – 2.10.

As well as being statistically significant, these differences are undoubtedly clinically significant. Greater redness with soft lenses, compared with no lens wear or rigid lenses, is plausible because soft lenses impinge upon the conjunctiva, whereas rigid lenses generally do not. It should be noted that the study of McMonnies and Chapman-Davies[6,7] was conducted over a decade ago – at a time when relatively unsophisticated and potentially toxic preservatives (thimerosal and chlorhexidine) were included in contact lens solutions. The use of current generation preservatives is less likely to be associated with conjunctival hyperaemia.

The increasing availability of videocapture technology which can be interfaced with sophisticated computer-based image-analysis systems has led a number of researchers to develop objective techniques for measuring the level of conjunctival hyperaemia in response to contact lens wear.[8–12] Owen *et al*[10] used such a system and demonstrated that, over a four-month period, rigid lens wear was associated with an increase in conjunctival redness, whereas soft lens wear was not associated with increased hyperaemia.

These results do not necessarily conflict with those of McMonnies and Chapman-Davies,[6,7] who examined the conjunctivae of adapted lens wearers. The data of Owen *et al*[10] probably reflect the general ocular irritation experienced in the initial adaptive phase of rigid lens wear.

Holden *et al*[13] measured the extent of general conjunctival hyperaemia and limbal hyperaemia in a group of patients who had worn a high water content soft lens on an extended wear basis for an average of 5 years. Conjunctival hyperaemia was graded on a four-step scale from 0 (redness absent) to 3 (severe redness). General conjunctival hyperaemia was graded as 0.89 (vs 0.66 in non-lens wearing control eyes) and limbal hyperaemia was graded as 1.13 (vs 0.33 in non-lens wearing control eyes). From this data it can be inferred that extended wear of soft lenses has a much greater impact on limbal hyperaemia than on general conjunctival hyperaemia.

Guillon and Shah[11] used a computerbased video-capture system to objectively monitor diurnal changes in conjunctival redness in patients wearing soft lenses on a daily and extended wear basis. Non-lens wearers displayed similar levels of hyperaemia in the morning and evening, but less hyperaemia during the day. With daily wear lenses, conjunctival redness was greatest in the evening, whereas extended wear of soft lenses was associated with greatest levels of hyperaemia upon waking.

## Pathology

The bulbar conjunctiva contains a rich plexus of arterioles. Unlike arteries, arteriolar walls contain little elastic connective tissue. They do, however, contain a thick layer of smooth muscle that is richly enervated with sympathetic nerve fibres. The smooth muscle, as well as being under central autonomic control, can be influenced by numerous local changes.

Vasodilatation refers to enlargement in the circumference of a vessel due to relaxation of its smooth muscle layer, which leads to decreased resistance and increased blood flow through the vessel.[14] This is known as active hyperaemia. Since blood vessels can be observed directly through the transparent conjunctiva, reactive hyperaemia leads to an appearance of increased redness (less white sclera is visible).

Vasodilatation can also occur as a result of passive mechanisms, such as vessel blockages. Figure 5.3 shows a distended arteriole possibly due to a blockage near the limbus.

Arteriolar muscle normally displays a state of constriction known as vascular tone. This ongoing tonic activity is attributed to two factors: intrinsic myogenic activity due to fluctuating membrane potentials, and norepinephrine release from sympathetic fibres enervating the arterioles. Vessel circumference can thus be either increased or decreased by altering one or both of the above mechanisms.[14] This can be achieved by local control mechanisms or intrinsic controls; the latter mechanism relates more to blood pressure regulation and has relatively little influence on conjunctival redness.

## Aetiology

Eye redness, to a varying degree, is a sign and symptom of virtually every adverse response to contact lens wear. As a physical entity that comes into direct contact with the conjunctiva, a contact lens can have a local mechanical effect on the conjunctiva, resulting in hyperaemia. As a device that (a) can interfere with normal metabolic processes of the cornea and conjunctiva, and (b) is used in association with various solutions, a contact lens can also affect the level of conjunctival redness via a local chemical or toxic effect. Local infection and inflammation can also cause eye redness. Each of these influences will be considered in turn.

### Metabolic influences
Conjunctival arterioles are exposed to the chemical composition of the interstitial fluid in the tissue. During metabolic activity, the concentration of these chemicals can change, leading to vessel dilatation and an increase in blood flow. The following metabolic influences relax arteriolar smooth muscle:

- *Hypoxia* – caused by the lens; lenses of lower oxygen transmissibility (*Dk/L*) induce greater levels of hypoxia.
- *Hypercapnia* – caused by the lens; lenses of lower carbon dioxide transmissibility (*Dk/L*) induce greater levels of hypercapnia.
- *Acidic shift* – due to accumulation of lactic and carbonic acid as a consequence of hypoxia and hypercapnia, respectively.
- *Increased osmolarity* – due to an increased metabolic production of osmotically active particles.
- *Increased potassium* – due to repeated action potentials which cause a flood of potassium that cannot be removed by the sodium–potassium pump.

### Chemical influences
Non-toxic chemicals introduced into the eye either directly or indirectly (with contact lens insertion) can lead to conjunctival hyperaemia for the following reasons:

- *Acidic shift* – due to the introduction into the eye of a solution of different pH from that of conjunctival tissue.
- *Increased osmolarity* – due to the introduction into the eye of a hypertonic contact lens solution.

### Toxic reaction
A toxic reaction can occur due to exposure to noxious preservatives, buffers, enzymes, chelating agents or other chemical agents that are incorporated into contact lens solutions. Paugh *et al*[15] demonstrated an association between the concentration of hydrogen peroxide solution introduced into the eye and the degree of conjunctival redness, with a concentration of 800 ppm (the highest concentration tested) causing a mean degree of redness of 2.7 on the McMonnies–Chapman-Davies scale.[6] Figure 5.4 displays an acute circumlimbal toxic response to an experimental contact lens disinfecting solution; note the associated conjunctival haemorrhaging.

### Allergic reaction
The fact that the conjunctiva supports and reflects immunological activity is evidenced clinically by atopic patients who display variations in conjunctival hyperaemia that coincide with seasonal fluctuations in the concentration or airborne antigens such as pollen. Allergic reactions may also be triggered by chemicals in contact lens solutions or deposits on contact lenses.

### Neural control
The rich sympathetic enervation of conjunctival arterioles can exert an overall influence on conjunctival redness. Thus,

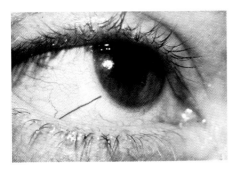

**Figure 5.3**
*Single distended conjunctival vessel presumed to be due to blockage at the limbus*

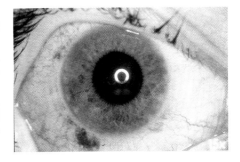

**Figure 5.4**
*Circumlimbal toxic response to an experimental contact lens disinfecting solution*

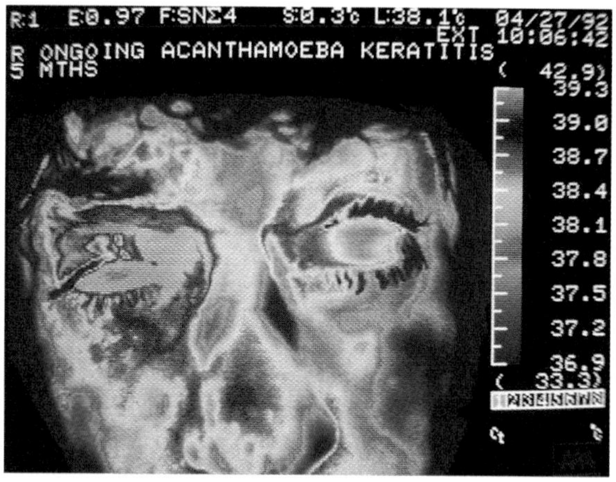

Figure 5.5
*Ocular thermogram of a patient suffering from Acanthamoeba keratitis, indicating increased temperature of the inflamed right eye*

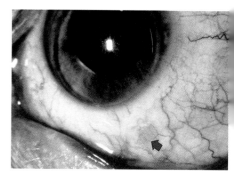

Figure 5.6
*Moderate chronic conjunctival hyperaemia due to RGP lens fragment imbedded in conjunctiva (arrow)*

pharmacological agents that modulate sympathetic enervation will affect eye redness. Such agents are generally not used in conjunction with contact lens care systems. In addition, the arteriolar system of the body in general is under sympathetic control for the regulation of blood pressure; however, variations in conjunctival redness as a result of this central control mechanism are likely to be minimal.

### Inflammation

Inflammation is the reaction of tissue to injury, and is characterised by heat, swelling, redness, pain and loss of function. In the conjunctiva, the association between heat and redness has been demonstrated by Efron *et al*,[16] who showed that a change of one grade on the McMonnies–Chapman-Davies conjunctival redness scale[6] corresponds to a change in conjunctival temperature of 0.15°C. Figure 5.5 is a graphic example of the association between ocular inflammation (primarily involving the cornea and conjunctiva – but also the surrounding facial tissues) and ocular temperature in a patient suffering from *Acanthamoeba* keratitis. This image, obtained using ocular thermography,[17,18] highlights the potential for this technique to monitor contact lens-related ocular inflammation in terms of the heat generated from a hyperaemic eye.

### The 'acute red eye' syndrome

A syndrome known as the 'acute red eye' (ARE) is observed from time to time in patients wearing extended wear contact lenses.[19] This is an inflammatory response in which the patient wakes in the morning with unilateral bulbar conjunctival and limbal injection, discomfort, lacrimation and photophobia. The severity of these signs and symptoms can vary from being mild to severe. On slit-lamp examination, anterior stromal infiltrates are usually observed near the limbus, but by definition there is no overlying epithelial staining or underlying stromal melt (ulceration).

This syndrome is generally attributed to the fact that an immobile lens covers the cornea, which can exacerbate one or more of the following possible aetiological factors: direct effects of hypoxia/hypercapnia (e.g. respiratory distress); indirect effects of hypoxia/hypercapnia (e.g. tissue acidosis); toxicity or inflammation due to trapped post-lens debris; infection due to trapped post-lens micro-organisms; mechanical effect of the lens; toxic, inflammatory, immunological or mechanical effect of lens deposits; tear film thinning; hypersensitivity or toxicity to preservatives re-released back into the eye from high water content lenses; or increased temperature.

### Mechanical influences

Contact lenses can come into direct contact with the conjunctiva and cause mechanical damage.[20] Trauma is known to cause mast cell degranulation, which results in histamine release. Histamine is the major cause of vasodilatation in an injured area, and can also lead to conjunctival chemosis (swelling).

Figure 5.6 shows the eye of a 35-year-old female who suffered a traumatic injury to this eye while wearing a rigid lens. The lens broke into many pieces and a small fragment became embedded in her conjunctiva (arrow), causing mild hyperaemia. The patient was asymptomatic and refused surgical treatment to remove the lens fragment. This case illustrates that chronic mechanical irritation, albeit asymptomatic, can induce conjunctival hyperaemia.

Many of the reactions described above are mediated by intrinsic substances in the body, such as prostaglandins, which are described as 'local hormones' in that they are synthesised locally, they have short half-lives, they exert a rapid and often profound effect, and they are finally metabolised to a biologically inactive form. Figure 5.7 is an illustration of a possible mechanism of prostaglandin-mediated vasodilatation caused by lens-induced hypoxia, as proposed by Efron *et al*.[21] Other intrinsic substances such as neutrophil chemotactic factor are released in traumatised tissue, which help establish an inflammatory reaction.

## Observation and grading

The extent of conjunctival redness can be graded with the assistance of grading scales such as those depicted in Appendix A. Although illustrative grading scales are not as accurate as computer-based image analysis systems, grading scales do offer sufficient sensitivity for general clinical use if practitioners are willing to estimate the grade of redness to the nearest 0.1 grade unit (see Chapter 19).

Because conjunctival redness typically displays regional variations, it is important

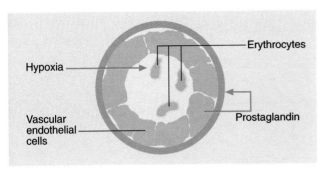

**Figure 5.7**
*Schematic illustration of a possible mechanism of prostaglandin-mediated vasodilatation caused by lens-induced hypoxia*

to indicate on the record card the area of conjunctiva being graded. It may also be worth noting the time of day that the observation is made in view of the normal diurnal variation in conjunctival hyperaemia.[11]

## Treatment

As described above, numerous factors may result in a red eye and the key factor in a given patient is rarely obvious. In some cases, a variety of actions may need to be taken, either sequentially or simultaneously.

Eye redness may be acute or chronic. Aside from the 'acute red eye syndrome',[19] most acute reactions are transient and self-limiting. Thus, eye redness as a key presenting complaint from a contact lens patient usually suggests a chronic problem requiring active intervention.

Treatment options fall into four broad categories:

- Alterations to the type, design and modality of lens wear.
- Alterations to care systems.
- Improving ocular hygiene.
- Prescription of pharmaceutical agents.

Each of these will be considered in turn.

### Alteration to the lens
All soft lenses develop deposits over time. Most of these deposits can be removed by daily surfactant cleaning, but some such as protein gradually build up regardless. Protein removal systems may slow the rate of protein build-up but they do not prevent it. Furthermore, it has recently been established that it is the quality of protein deposi-

tion, rather than the quantity, that will govern biocompatibility.[22] For example, with type IV (ionic high water) lenses the physiologic compatibility of the protein is preserved, whereas type I (non-ionic low water) lenses attract protein which readily denatures and is therefore more likely to be antigenic to the eye.

If it is true that bacteria adherent to protein deposits are the trigger for eye redness then the quantity of protein may be more important – less protein should mean less bacterial attachment.

Assuming protein accumulation to be one cause of red eye in soft lens patients, effective lens-related strategies would include:

- Changing to a lens material that deposits a protein film that is physiologically compatible with the eye.
- Changing to a lens material that deposits less protein.
- Changing to a rigid lens material.
- Replacing lenses more frequently, with daily disposability being the ultimate modality in this regard.

Alterations to soft lens design may alleviate eye redness if this has the effect of minimising the mechanical impact of the lens on the eye. Thus, the fitting of good quality thin lenses with restricted movement may be beneficial. Rigid lenses with thin interpalpebral designs, smooth edges and restricted movement are most likely to alleviate bulbar conjunctival redness because the lens will not usually come into physical contact with the bulbar conjunctiva.

Covey *et al*[23] have reported that new-generation silicone-hydrogel lenses, which are highly permeable to oxygen, cause vir-

tually no limbal redness, indicating that such lenses exert a minimal inflammatory or irritative effect upon the eye.

### Alteration to care systems
In the first instance, it is necessary to establish that the patient is being fully compliant with the prescribed care regimes, which for soft lenses could include surfactant cleaning, rinsing, disinfection and periodic protein removal treatment. Any deficiencies in this regard would need to be rectified.

A rigorous approach to protein removal may alleviate chronic eye redness. The introduction of protein removal systems into the regimen of those patients who do not use them, or an increase in frequency of usage (e.g. from weekly to bi-weekly or even daily) may be beneficial. This applies to both soft and rigid lens wearers.

If preservatives in contact lens solutions are thought to be of aetiological significance in a particular patient, then the employment of preservative-free systems (some hydrogen peroxide solutions fall into this category) may alleviate the condition.

### Improving ocular hygiene
Improvements to ocular hygiene begin with improvements to personal hygiene. Thus routine and thorough hand washing prior to lens handling and regular face washing have an impact in reducing eye redness. Some authors[24,25] have recommended the additional step of conjunctival irrigation with sterile unpreserved saline before and after lens insertion, and periodically during the day, as a means of diluting or removing antigens and generally enhancing patient comfort. Although this procedure was advocated for alleviating contact lens-induced papillary conjunctivitis, the principle can also be applied to the management of chronic red eye.

Attention to lid hygiene could also be of benefit. Encouraging patients to employ strategies such as lid scrubbing, warm compresses and expression could alleviate eye redness if lid involvement is suspected as being wholly or partially responsible for eye redness.

### Pharmaceutical agents
In certain cases, consideration can be given to prescribing ocular decongestants.[26] These drugs all contain vasoconstrictor agents that serve the dual purpose of reducing eye redness and alleviating symptoms. Of course, ocular disease and all other

possible lens-related causes of eye redness must be ruled out before prescribing decongestants, because they could end up exacerbating the problem by masking and prolonging the real cause of eye redness.

Ocular decongestants generally contain one of the following four vasoconstrictors: phenylephrine, naphazoline, tetrahydrozaline and ephedrine. Phenylephrine is used in concentrations of 0.12 to 0.2 per cent, which is insufficient to cause pupil dilatation. The side-effects of phenylephrine include reactive hyperaemia – an uncomfortable red eye that can occur following prolonged use, allergic reactions and soft lens discoloration.

The imidazole derivatives naphazoline and tetrahydrozaline, are more stable and longer-acting, and are less likely to cause an allergic reaction or rebound congestion, compared with phenylephrine. However, some patients – especially children – have apparently experienced a sedation effect following prolonged use.

Ephedrine is more stable than phenylephrine but may also cause reactive hyperaemia. It cannot be used in conjunction with solutions or lenses containing polyvinyl alcohol, as the two react to form a viscous precipitate.

In conclusion, ocular decongestants should generally be avoided and maximum effort be directed towards identifying and rectifying the primary cause of the problem. When all possible causes of eye redness have been ruled out, then decongestants can be prescribed for intermittent use with the primary cosmetic objective of alleviating an unsightly red eye appearance. Patients using decongestants should be monitored more frequently than normal (say, every 3 months).

## Prognosis

The prognosis for recovery from chronic contact lens-induced red eye after removal of lenses and cessation of wear is good. Holden *et al*[13] found that, following approximately five years of extended lens wear, general conjunctival hyperaemia resolved within 2 days (Figure 5.8); recovery from limbal hyperaemia had a slightly longer time course, taking about 7 days to resolve (Figure 5.9).

Recovery from acute lens-induced conjunctival hyperaemia is extremely rapid. In his early writings, Fick[1] recognised this

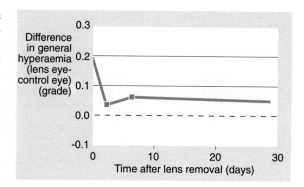

**Figure 5.8**
*Time course of resolution of general conjunctival hyperaemia following 5 years' extended wear of a high water content soft lens in one eye only, relative to non-lens wearing control eye (after Holden et al*[13]*)*

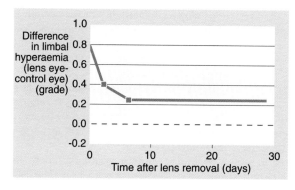

**Figure 5.9**
*Time course of resolution of limbal hyperaemia following 5 years' extended wear of a high water content soft lens in one eye only, relative to non-lens wearing control eye (after Holden et al*[13]*)*

and noted: 'The injection of the eyeball disappears with extraordinary rapidity after removal of the [haptic lens]' and '... any possible injection of the conjunctiva will disappear within half an hour ...'. Contemporary research has confirmed the observations of Fick that acute hyperaemia dissipates rapidly. For example, Paugh *et al*[15] demonstrated that, following instillation of 800 ppm hydrogen peroxide into the eye, it only took 5 minutes to recover from an eye redness grading of 2.7 down to a normal grading of 0.4.

In general, removal of any noxious stimulus, including a contact lens, will lead to a very rapid recovery of eye redness to normal levels.

## Differential diagnosis

When a contact lens wearing patient pre-

sents with a red eye as a primary complaint, the initial diagnostic step is to determine whether or not the problem is related to lens wear. This can often be simply solved by removing the lens, whereby eye redness should dissipate rapidly if the problem is purely lens-related. However, the possibility that the lens was somehow exacerbating a complication unrelated to lens wear itself should not be discounted.

Another differential diagnosis that may be necessary when presented with an extremely red eye is to determine to what extent the redness is due to conjunctival injection or ciliary flush. Two simple tests can be conducted. A sterile cotton bud can be applied to the bulbar conjunctiva in the region of redness and gently moved from side to side. The conjunctival vessels move but the ciliary vessels will remain in a fixed position. It can then be determined whether the redness relates primarily to the 'moving' vessels (indicating conjunctival involvement) or the 'static' vessels (indicating ciliary involvement).

An alternative test is to instil a decongestant into the eye.[26] The effect of a decongestant is limited to the superficial conjunctival vessels; these drugs have no effect on the deeper ciliary vessels. Thus if the instillation of a decongestant alleviates eye redness, the condition is primarily conjunctival. If the decongestant has no impact on eye redness, then the redness can be attributed to excessive ciliary flush.

A subconjunctival haemorrhage can be easily differentiated from conjunctival and/or ciliary hyperaemia because of the stark appearance of an intensely 'blood red' eye. Small haemorrhages of individual conjunctival vessels can also increase conjunctival redness (Figure 5.10), but the redness is diffuse and differential diagnosis from vascular engorgement is clear.

Assuming that a given case of eye redness is lens-related, it is necessary to determine whether the source of the problem is the cornea or conjunctiva. Conjunctival redness associated with a quiet limbus and absence of pain indicates a primary conjunctival problem. Conjunctival redness associated with an injected limbus and corneal pain indicates corneal involvement, or indeed a problem that is related exclusively to the cornea. Careful slit-lamp examination of the anterior ocular structures, and inspection of the lens at high magnification, should reveal the cause of the problem. It may also be necessary to prescribe different care systems and differentially diagnose the effects of various solutions over time.

If the red eye is deemed to be unrelated to lens wear, then all other possible causes of red eye must be investigated. This may involve a full ocular examination including the use of direct and indirect ophthalmoscopy, tonometry etc. A full account of the differential diagnosis of the red eye in a general ophthalmic context is beyond the scope of this chapter.

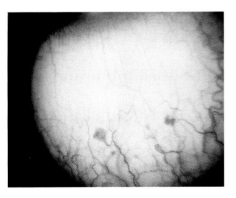

**Figure 5.10**
*Localised conjunctival haemorrhages in a soft lens wearer*

## REFERENCES

1 Efron N, Pearson RM (1988) Centenary celebration of Fick's Eine Contactbrille. *Arch Ophthalmol* **106**: 1370.
2 Pearson RM, Efron N (1989) Hundredth anniversary of August Müller's inaugural dissertation on contact lenses. *Surv Ophthalmol* **34**: 133.
3 Osol A, ed. (1973) *Blakiston's Pocket Medical Dictionary*, 3rd edn. McGraw-Hill, New York.
4 Sykes JB ed. (1976) *The Concise Oxford Dictionary of Current English*, 6th edn. Clarendon Press, Oxford.
5 Stapleton F, Dart J, Minassian D (1992) Nonulcerative complications of contact lens wear. *Arch Ophthalmol* **110**: 1601.
6 McMonnies CW, Chapman-Davies A (1987) Assessment of conjunctival hyperaemia in contact lens wearers Part I. *Am J Optom Physiol Opt* **64**: 246.
7 McMonnies CW, Chapman-Davies A (1987) Assessment of conjunctival hyperaemia in contact lens wearers Part II. *Am J Optom Physiol Opt* **64**: 251.
8 Villumsen J, Rinquist J, Alm A (1991) Image analysis of conjunctival hyperaemia. *Acta Ophthalmol* **69**: 536.
9 Willingham FF, Cohen KL, Coggins JM (1995) Automated quantitative measurement of ocular hyperaemia. *Curr Eye Res* **14**: 1101.
10 Owen CG, Fitzke FW, Woodward G (1996) A new computer-assisted objective method for quantifying vascular changes of the bulbar conjunctiva. *Ophthal Physiol Opt* **16**: 430.
11 Guillon M, Shah D (1996) Objective measurement of contact lens-induced conjunctival redness. *Optom Vis Sci* **73**: 595.
12 Cox I, Potvin R (1996) Quantification of ocular bulbar conjunctival redness using computer-based image analysis. *Optom Vis Sci* **73**(12S): 231.
13 Holden BA, Sweeney DF, Swarbrick HA (1986) The vascular response to long-term extended contact lens wear. *Clin Exp Optom* **69**: 112.
14 Sherwood L (1989) *Human Physiology – from Cells to Systems*. West Publishing Company, New York.
15 Paugh JP, Brennan NA, Efron N (1988) Ocular response to hydrogen peroxide. *Am J Optom Physiol Opt* **65**: 91.
16 Efron N, Brennan NA, Hore J (1988) Temperature of the hyperemic bulbar conjunctiva. *Curr Eye Res* **7**: 615.
17 Efron N, Young G, Brennan NA (1989) Ocular surface temperature. *Curr Eye Res* **8**: 901.
18 Morgan PB, Soh MP, Efron N (1993) Potential applications of ocular thermography. *Optom Vis Sci* **70**: 568.
19 Holden BA, Zantos SG (1979) The ocular response to continuous wear of contact lenses. *Optician* **177**: 50.
20 Efron N, Veys J (1992) Defects in disposable contact lenses can compromise ocular integrity. *Int Contact Lens Clin* **19**: 8.
21 Efron N, Holden BA, Vannas A (1984) The prostaglandin-inhibitor naproxen does not affect contact lens induced changes in the human corneal endothelium. *Am J Optom Physiol Opt* **61**: 741.
22 Sack RA, Jones B, Antiguani A (1987) Specificity and biological activity of the protein deposited on the hydrogel surface. *Invest Ophthalmol Vis Sci* **28**: 842.
23 Covey MA, Papas E, Austen R (1995) Limbal vascular response during daily wear of conventional and high Dk soft lenses. *Optom Vis Sci* **72**: 12S, 171.
24 Allansmith MR, Ross RN, Greiner JV (1985) Giant papillary conjunctivitis: diagnosis and treatment. In: *Contact Lenses* (ed. OH Dabezies). Little, Brown and Company, Boston, MA, p. 43.1.
25 Farkas P, Kasalow TW, Farkas B (1986) Clinical management and control of giant papillary conjunctivitis secondary to contact lens wear. *J Am Optom Assoc* **57**: 197.
26 Jose JG, Polse KA, Holden EK (1984) *Optometric Pharmacology*. Grune & Stratton, Orlando, FLA.

# 6
# Papillary conjunctivitis

Prevalence
Normal tarsal conjunctiva
Signs and symptoms
Pathology
Aetiology
Observation and grading
Treatment
Prognosis
Differential diagnosis

Australian ophthalmologist Tom Spring is widely credited as being the first to observe an allergic-like reaction of the upper tarsal conjunctiva to contact lens wear, which was later to become known as 'giant papillary conjunctivitis'. In his 1974 letter to the editor of the *Medical Journal of Australia*, Spring noted the presence of large tarsal papillae, accompanied by discomfort and excessive mucus production, in 43 per cent of patients wearing soft lenses.[1]

The term 'giant papillary conjunctivitis' was coined by Allansmith *et al*[2] to describe papillary changes on the tarsal conjunctiva that were likened to a cobblestone formation (Figure 6.1). However, this condition can take on a variety of different appearances, depending on the level of severity and whether it relates to soft or rigid lens wear. In its mild form, this condition has been termed 'lid roughness' and 'papillary hypertrophy'. Even in advanced stages the papillary formations may be extensive but not necessarily 'giant'. Thus, a more appropriate term that encompasses all of the possible manifestations of the same condition is 'con-

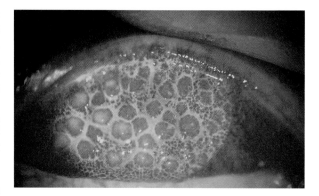

**Figure 6.1**
*'Giant' papillae in a patient wearing soft lenses on a daily wear basis*

tact lens-induced papillary conjunctivitis' (CLPC).

## Prevalence

In soft lens wearers, CLPC may develop as soon as 3 weeks, or take as long as 4 years, to manifest. In rigid lens wearers, CLPC typically appears after 14 months.

It is difficuilt to characterise the prevalence of a condition that:

- Has a variable time of onset.
- Varies in severity throughout the seasons of the year (because of its allergic nature).
- Varies over the years as different lens care regimens and lens wear modalities change.

It is also apparent that the definition of CLPC has changed over time, with the earlier literature (say, pre-1985) focusing on the appearance of very large papillae (consistent with the notion of 'giant' papillae) and the later literature paying more attention to CLPC in its more subtle variants.

The prevalence of overt CLPC in wearers of conventional soft lenses (non-planned replacement) on a daily wear basis (CSDW lenses) has been reported by various authors to be 1.8 per cent,[3] 12 per cent[4] and 15 per cent.[5] The reason for these figures being much lower than that reported by Spring[1] (43 per cent) is probably a reflection of changing times – most of Spring's patients were likely to have been using thermally disinfected HEMA lenses, whereas the patients surveyed in more recent studies[3–5] were using modern lens care regimens (such as hydrogel peroxide and designer-preservative multi-purpose disinfection systems).

Grant[6] reported a prevalence of CLPC of 19 per cent in patients using conventional soft (non-planned replacement) extended wear (CSEW) lenses, versus 3 per cent with disposable soft extended wear (DSEW) lenses. On the other hand, Poggio and Abelson[3] found no difference in CLPC between patients wearing CSEW lenses (1.9 per cent) versus DSEW lenses (2.0 per cent). Other authors have reported somewhat higher incidence figures of 4.2 per cent,[7] 6.7 per cent[8] and 6–12 per cent[9] for disposable extended wear lenses.

Alemany and Redal[5] found a lower incidence of overt CLPC in patients wearing daily wear rigid lenses compared with conventional daily wear soft lenses. Grant *et al*[9] reported that the incidence of CLPC in patients wearing rigid lenses on an extended wear basis was 2 per cent versus 6–12 per cent for soft disposable extended wear.

## Normal tarsal conjunctiva

In normals, the tarsal conjunctiva can take on a variety of forms, which may be categorised in different ways. Allansmith[10] maintains that there are three forms of normal tarsal conjunctival appearance: satin or smooth (14 per cent); small, uniformly sized 'micropapillae', which are less than 0–3 mm in diameter (85 per cent); and non-uniform papillae (<1 per cent), where

some papillae can be as large as 0.5 mm in diameter.

An alternative model for classifying the normal tarsal conjunctiva has been proposed by Potvin *et al*,[11] who conducted a computer assisted morphometric examination of photographic images of the fluorescein-stained tarsal conjunctiva of eight asymptomatic non-lens wearers. The eight subjects were classified into two distinct groups – those displaying 'small feature' tarsal plates (with a modal feature area of 25 000 to 35 000 μm² and a restricted range of areas) and those displaying 'large feature' tarsal plates (with a modal feature area of 50 000 to 70 000 μm² and a wide range of areas). The cells generally appear to be pentagonal and hexagonal in shape.

The three-category model of Allansmith[10] is of more relevance to clinicians because it is based upon the appearance of the tarsal conjunctiva under low magnification using the slit-lamp biomicroscope.

## Signs and symptoms

It is important that an assessment is made only of the central region of the tarsal plate, for the following reasons:

- There is often increased 'roughness' of the conjunctiva at the lateral extremities of the everted lid that is unrelated to lens-induced pathology.
- The process of lid eversion causes the conjunctiva artificially to appear distorted and irregular along the margin of the lid eversion fold (ie anatomically superior to the tarsal plate, but paradoxically 'inferior' as the everted lid is viewed).
- The conjunctiva just inside the lid margin (i.e. anatomically inferior to the tarsal plate) is rarely affected by lens wear.

Allansmith[10] noted that the appearance of CLPC was different in soft vs rigid lens wearers. In soft lens wearers, papillae are more numerous; they are located more towards the upper tarsal plate (that is, closer to the fold of the everted lid); and the apex of the papillae take on a rounded, flatter form (Figure 6.1). In rigid lens wearers, papillae take on a crater-like form and are located more towards the lash margin with few papillae being present on the upper tarsal plate (Figure 6.2). Papillae often appear as round light reflexes, giving an irregular specular reflection.

In the early stages of development, the tarsal conjunctiva in patients suffering from CLPC may be indistinguishable from the normal tarsal conjunctiva. An important early distinguishing feature is increased hyperaemia of the tarsal conjunctiva (Figure 6.3). This change can be detected with reference to the lower palpebral conjunctiva which is usually unaffected and can therefore act as a 'baseline' against which any change is measured.

In advanced cases, papillae can exceed 1 mm in diameter and often take on a bright red/orange hue. The hexagonal/pentagonal shape is lost in favour of a more rounded appearance. The pattern of distribution of papillae may reflect the underlying anatomy of the tarsus; for example, Figure 6.4 is a non-uniform CLPC that has developed in a soft lens wearer. Three-dimensionally,

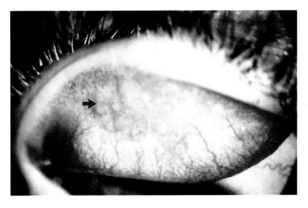

**Figure 6.2**
*CLPC in a rigid lens wearer, with more papillae observed (arrow) towards the lash margin*

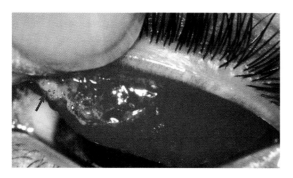

**Figure 6.3**
*Gross hyperaemia of tarsal conjunctiva with mucus formation (arrow) in CLPC*

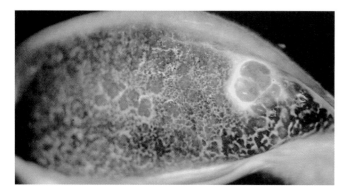

**Figure 6.4**
*Non-uniform CLPC in a soft lens wearer*

giant papillae can be said to take on a 'mushroom' form, with a flattened or even slightly depressed apex or tip.

Because the conjunctiva is thickened, oedematous and often hyperaemic, fine vessels which can normally be observed to traverse the conjunctival surface are obscured, although deep vessels remain visible over the tarsal plate. A tuft of convoluted capillary vessels is often observed at the apex of papillae; this vascular tuft will sometimes stain with fluorescein.

Other signs that can be observed in severe manifestations of CLPC include conjunctival oedema and excessive mucus (see Figure 6.3), which usually forms into strands that lie in the valleys between papillae. Excess mucus will also accumulate at the inner and outer canthus at night and can sometimes be observed floating across the cornea. Prolonged oedema may result in a mild ptosis, which is often asymmetric.

Giant papillae can display infiltrates, and if the condition persists for some time, the

conjunctival surface at the apex of the papillae can become scarred and appear a cream/white colour (Figure 6.5). The cornea may also be compromised and display superficial punctate staining and infiltrates superiorly. Injection of the superior limbus may also be apparent.

There is general concordance between the severity of signs and symptoms. In the early stages of CLPC, patients may complain of discomfort towards the end of the wearing period and slight itching. Patients may report an increase in mucus production upon awakening. Intermittent blurring is sometimes noted; this is due to mucus being periodically smeared across the lens surface. A slight but non-variable vision loss is attributable to more tenacious lens deposits such as protein, which is of aetiological significance in this condition (see later).

In more severe cases, the itching and discomfort can become so marked that the patient is forced to remove the lens. Excessive lens movement and decentration can result from a combination of:

- The large papillae creating greater contact and friction with the coated lens surface.
- Excess mucus acting as an 'adhesive' between the tarsal conjunctival and lens surfaces.

## Pathology

The conjunctiva becomes thicker in CLPC (0.2 mm in CLPC vs 0.05 mm in normals). Greiner *et al*[12] observed dramatic ultrastructural changes in the conjunctival surface in patients with CLPC. Conjunctival surface area is increased by two-fold and epithelial cells are enlarged and distorted, becoming elongated in

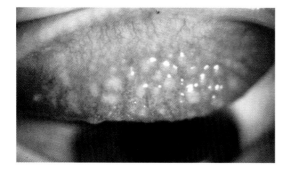
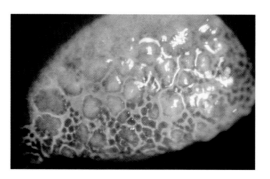

**Figure 6.5**
*Scarring at the apex of papillae, seen here in white light (left) and cobalt blue light (right)*

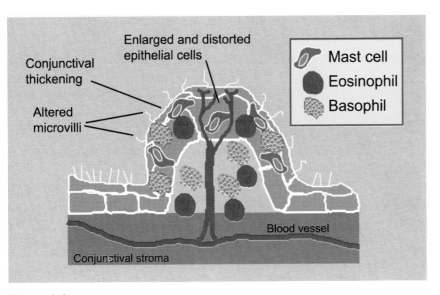

**Figure 6.6**
*Schematic diagram of pathological changes that characterise a papilla*

shape. The microvilli are reduced in number and become distorted, forming aggregated tufts on the surface of papillae. Normally present Crypts of Henle are not observed. The number of mucus-secreting non-goblet cells is increased. More dark cells are observed at the apices of the papillae.

CLPC is associated with a dramatic redistribution of inflammatory cells between the epithelium and stroma of the conjunctiva. Mast cells, eosinophils and basophils are found in the epithelium (they do not normally reside there) and there is an increase in the number of neutrophils and lymphocytes in the epithelium. Eosinophils and basophils are found in the stroma, with an increase in the number of mast cells, plasma cells and neutrophils (Figure 6.6).

## Aetiology

A number of factors have been suggested as playing a role in the aetiology of CLPC, and it is unlikely that any one causative factor can account for all cases. These factors are summarised below.

### Mechanical trauma
Papillary conjunctivitis of an apparently identical form to that induced by contact lenses has been observed in patients who do not wear contact lenses but whose tarsal conjunctivae have been exposed to various types of mechanical trauma, such as:

- Plastic ocular prostheses[13]
- Extruded scleral buckle[14]
- Excessive cyanoacrylate glue used to close a perforated cornea[15]
- Protruding nylon sutures[16]
- Rigid contact lens imbedded in upper fornix[17]
- Elevated corneal deposits[18]
- Epithelialised corneal foreign body[19]

In many of these cases, the papillary conjunctivitis resolved and patient symptoms were alleviated upon removal of the trauma. The reports of Dunn *et al*[18] and Greiner[19] are particularly noteworthy because, unlike the other cases which involve trauma induced by man-made materials, the papillary conjunctivitis was induced by trauma from inert epithelial irregularities.

Trauma is known to cause mast cell degranulation, so the presence of large numbers of degranulated mast cells in the conjunctival epithelium and stroma of patients with CLPC[20] is consistent with trauma being a factor of aetiological significance in this condition. Furthermore, the conjunctivae of patients with CLPC have significantly higher levels of neutrophil chemotactic factor[21] – a substance which is generally released in traumatised tissue.

### Immediate hypersensitivity
This anaphylactic reaction is mediated by immunoglobulin type E (IgE) antibodies which proliferate when the conjunctiva is exposed to certain antigens. The IgE anti-

bodies set off a chain reaction leading to mast cell degranulation, and the release of inflammatory mediators and other substances that can affect tissue damage repair. Patients with CLPC exhibit large numbers of degranulated mast cells in the conjunctival epithelium,[22] and elevated levels of IgE in tears.[23]

Protein deposition on the lens has been implicated as the antigenic stimulant to IgE production. More specifically, deposits that form on the anterior lens surface are likely to be more significant in that this surface lies in direct apposition with the tarsal conjunctiva. In support of this lens deposition theory, Ballow *et al*[24] demonstrated that when contact lenses from patients suffering from CLPC were placed in the eyes of monkeys, a frank papillary conjunctivitis ensued, with elevated IgE levels. These changes did not occur in monkeys that wore new lenses or lenses from patients who did not suffer from CLPC.

A critical issue in formulating strategies to treat or prevent CLPC is to determine the specific causative antigens. Protein deposition on the lens surface is the most popular candidate; however, protein on lenses of patients with CLPC is indistinguishable from protein on lenses of patients without CLPC. The antigenic stimulus could also be one of a number of other potential lens contaminants, such as lipids, calcium and mucus. Micro-organisms such as bacteria (and bacterial endotoxins) may also trigger CLPC.

The type of plastic used to fabricate the contact lens could theoretically have an antigenic role. However, this is difficult to prove. The success or otherwise of various polymers in alleviating or preventing CLPC probably relates more to the propensity of different materials to become deposited rather than any real differences in their intrinsic antigenic potency.

Early-generation preservatives such as thimerosal and benzalkonium chloride are known to have a causative role in the development of CLPC.[25] Certainly, treatment is more likely to succeed if care systems are free of such preservatives.[26]

### Delayed hypersensitivity
In their initial writings, Allansmith *et al*[12] likened CLPC to vernal conjunctivitis in view of the similar inflammatory cell profiles of the two conditions. The unusual presence of large numbers of basophils led Allansmith *et al*[2] to suggest that these diseases were of

the cutaneous basophilic type. This is classically a skin reaction which has a delayed time course and is mediated by sensitised T lymphocytes and antibodies. In support of this proposed aetiology, Hann et al[27] induced a CLPC-type reaction in guinea pigs following injection of various antigens into the tarsal plate.

Despite the evidence cited above, the proportion of basophils to the total pool of inflammatory cells in CLPC is significantly less than that observed in a typical cutaneous basophilic hypersensitivity reaction. In view of this, Begley[28] suggests that CLPC may better reflect the classic tuberculin type of delayed hypersensitivity reaction in which variable numbers of basophils can be present.

The antigens discussed in the previous section on the immediate hypersensitivity reaction are likely to be the same as those that mediate the delayed hypersensitivity reaction.

### Individual susceptibility

There is disagreement in the literature as to whether atopic individuals are more susceptible to developing CLPC. Some authors have found no connection between atopy and CLPC[2,22] whereas others have reported an increased prevalence of allergies in patients exhibiting CLPC.[29] Buckley[30] found elevated serum IgE levels in patients suffering from CLPC, suggesting the presence of an IgE-mediated atopy in these patients.

Indirect evidence of the association of atopy with CLPC comes from the work of Begley et al,[31] who reported that the onset of this condition was seasonal in a population of 68 patients. The condition peaked during the 'allergy seasons' in mid-western USA, where the study was conducted. These patients reported significantly more overall

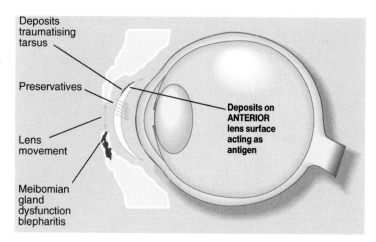

**Figure 6.7**
*Factors of aetiological significance in CLPC*

allergies, in addition to CLPC, than did a control group.

### Meibomian gland dysfunction

Recent research suggests an association between CLPC and meibomian gland dysfunction (MGD).[32,33] Martin et al[32] found that 42 consecutively presenting patients were also suffering from MGD blepharitis, and that the severity of the conditions was positively correlated. After treating the MGD blepharitis and refitting new lenses to 32 patients, 28 were judged to be successful 21 months later.

Figure 6.7 is a schematic illustration describing the various factors thought to be of aetiological significance in CLPC.

## Observation and grading

As CLPC manifests in the superior palpebral conjunctiva, it is necessary to evert the lid to detect this condition. This is best performed with the patient positioned in the head and brow rest of a slit-lamp biomicroscope, so that the everted lid can be readily observed at low magnification (×10–15) and high illumination. The extent of hyperaemia and oedema, and the general position and distribution of papillae, should be noted. High magnification can then be employed to examine the conjunctival surface, with particular attention to the distribution of vessels over the surface of the papillae.

After observing the tarsal conjunctiva in white light, the lid should be reverted back to its normal form and fluorescein instilled. Following a few blinks, the lid should be everted once again and observed under white light and then cobalt blue light (Figure 6.8). Fluorescein pools at the base of the papillae, allowing individual papillae to be resolved and the overall pattern of papillary formation to be more readily appreciated.

The lower lid should be everted by simply

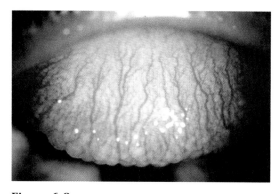
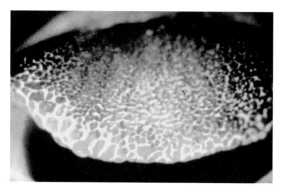

**Figure 6.8**
*CLPC observed under white light (left) and cobalt blue light (right). Observation with cobalt blue reveals a more extensive pattern of papillae*

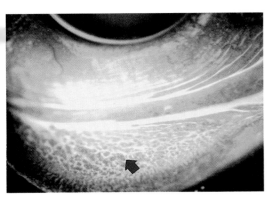

**Figure 6.9**
*An unusual case of CLPC of the lower palpebral conjunctiva (arrow) in response to rigid lens wear*

pulling downwards on the skin just beneath the lashes on the lower eyelid. The exposed lower palpebral conjunctiva will generally be clear and forms a useful baseline reference for assessing the level of hyperaemia and oedema of the superior palpebral conjunctiva. However, a mild CLPC will very occasionally be observed in the lower lid (Figure 6.9).

It is important to examine the superior cornea carefully as CLPC can be associated with superior limbal hyperaemia, corneal staining, corneal infiltrates and excess tear mucus.

As with all conditions described in this book, the severity of CLPC can be quantified by assigning gradings of 0 (normal), 1 (trace), 2 (mild), 3 (moderate) or 4 (severe). Pictorial grading scales can assist this task; see the grading scales in Appendix A. Table 6.1 gives a guide to these grading levels by defining the signs and symptoms that correspond to each grading step.

Because there are many possible factors involved in the aetiology of CLPC – and the key factor in a given patient is rarely obvious – a variety of treatment options may need to be employed, either sequentially or simultaneously. As a general rule, the earlier the condition is detected and treated, the better is the prognosis for an effective and speedy cure.

In many respects, CLPC is a condition that is best managed with reference to patient symptoms rather than signs. Many patients will be motivated to continue lens wear even in the presence of low-grade CLPC (grades 1 and 2), and they should be allowed to do so. Subtle non-intrusive strategies should be introduced in an attempt to alleviate the condition while at the same time maintaining

patient motivation. The tarsal plate of patients who are largely asymptomatic should be monitored carefully to detect the development of chronic tissue compromise.

## Treatment

Treatment options fall into four categories:

- Alterations to the lens type, lens design and modality of lens wear
- Alterations to care systems
- Improving ocular hygiene
- Prescribing pharmaceutical agents

Each of these will be considered in turn.

### Alteration to the lens

All soft lenses develop deposits over time. Most of these deposits can be removed by daily surfactant cleaning, but some deposits such as protein gradually build up regardless. Protein removal systems may slow the rate of protein build-up but they do not prevent it. Furthermore, it has recently been established that it is the quality of protein deposition, rather than the quan-

| Table 6.1 | Descriptive grading scale for papillary conjunctivitis | |
|---|---|---|
| Grade | Signs | Symptoms |
| 0 | • Normal tarsal conjunctiva:<br>　(a) smooth<br>　(b) uniform micropapillae<br>　(c) non-uniform micropapillae | • None |
| 1 | • Slight hyperaemia of upper tarsus | • Occasional itching |
| 2 | • Slight papillary roughness<br>• Slight hyperaemia of upper tarsus<br>• Slight increase in lens movement | • Mild itching<br>• Mild lens awareness |
| 3 | • Moderate papillary roughness<br>• Small papillae along lid fold<br>• Moderate hyperaemia of upper tarsus<br>• Infiltrates in vascular tuft<br>• Moderate lens movement<br>• Moderate lens decentration<br>• Fine mucus strands on tarsus<br>• Some mucus in tears<br>• Slight coating apparent<br>• Vision variable | • Moderate itching<br>• Moderate lens awareness<br>• Wearing time reduced<br>• Some mucus noted<br>• Aware of moderate lens movement<br>• Aware of moderate lens decentration<br>• Slight intermittent blur with lens |
| 4 | • Severe papillary roughness<br>• Large papillae extending over tarsus<br>• Severe hyperaemia of upper tarsus<br>• Infiltrates may mask vascular tuft<br>• Central scarring of papillae<br>• Excessive lens movement<br>• Excessive lens decentration<br>• Mucus pooling between papillae<br>• Mucus strands on cornea<br>• Mucus strands and clumps in tears<br>• Heavy lens coating<br>• Vision variable<br>• Vision slightly reduced<br>• Superficial limbal hyperaemia<br>• Superficial corneal staining<br>• Superficial corneal infiltrates | • Severe itching<br>• Severe lens awareness<br>• Wearing time minimal<br>• Excess mucus noted<br>• Aware of excessive lens movement<br>• Aware of excessive lens decentration<br>• Frequent intermittent blur with lens<br>• Slight vision loss with lens |

tity, that will govern biocompatibility. For example, Sack[34] has demonstrated that although type IV (ionic high water) lenses attract significant amounts of protein, the conformational integrity (i.e. physiological compatibility) of the protein is preserved. Type I lenses (non-ionic low water) attract much less protein but the protein is denatured and therefore is more likely to be antigenic to the eye.

If it is true that bacteria adherent to protein deposits are the trigger for CLPC then the quantity of protein may be more important – less protein should mean less bacterial attachment.

Assuming protein accumulation to be one cause of CLPC in soft lens patients, effective lens-related strategies would include:

- Changing to a lens material that deposits a protein film which is physiologically compatible with the eye.
- Changing to a lens material that deposits less protein.
- Changing to a rigid lens material.
- Replacing lenses more frequently.

Alterations to soft lens design may alleviate CLPC if the mechanical impact of the lens is minimised. Thus, the fitting of good quality thin lenses with restricted movement may be beneficial.

The ophthalmic literature is devoid of descriptions of properly controlled studies that prove the efficacy of the various treatments described above. Even the ultimate form of regular lens replacement – daily disposable lenses – will not necessarily solve the problem. For example, daily disposable lenses made from type IV materials deposit significant levels of protein within 15 minutes of insertion.[35] The success or otherwise of such lenses in the prevention or cure of CLPC will depend on the physiological compatibility of the protein that rapidly accumulates and/or the rate of attachment of bacteria to the protein.

Cessation of lens wear will certainly result in a complete cure, but such an option is generally met with little enthusiasm by patients. In more severe cases (grade 3 or 4), ceasing lens wear for a brief period of one week, say, will enhance the prospect of success of subsequent treatment. Similarly, a reduction in wearing time in the early phase of treatment will optimise the prospect for recovery.

Certain rigid lenses may attract deposits in such a way that is less antigenic to the

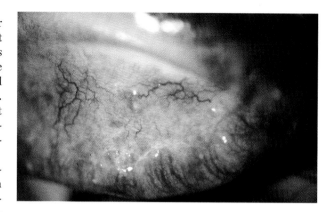

**Figure 6.10**
*Deformities in the tarsal plate of an atopic individual who had never worn contact lenses and had used cromolyn sodium for over 10 years*

patient (e.g. less protein and/or protein that is physiologically compatible). However, rigid lenses potentially have a greater physical impact on the eye, which could exacerbate CLPC. Lenses with thin interpalpebral designs, smooth edges and restricted movement are most likely to yield a successful outcome. Douglas *et al*[36] reported that the onset of CLPC could be delayed or prevented by fitting lenses of higher oxygen transmissibility.

**Alteration to care systems**
In the first instance, it is necessary to establish that the patient is being fully compliant with the prescribed care regimes, which for soft lenses could include surfactant clearing, rinsing, disinfection and periodic protein removal treatment. Any deficiencies in this regard will need to be rectified.

A rigorous approach to protein removal may alleviate CLPC. The introduction of protein removal systems into the regimen of those patients who do not use them, or an increase in frequency of usage (e.g. from weekly to bi-weekly or even daily) may be beneficial. This applies to both soft and rigid lens wearers.

If preservatives in contact lens solutions are thought to be of aetiological significance in a particular patient, then the employment of preservative-free systems (some hydrogen peroxide solutions fall into this category) may alleviate the condition.

**Improving ocular hygiene**
Improvements to ocular hygiene begin with improvements to personal hygiene. Thus, routine and thorough hand washing

prior to lens handling and regular face washing should mitigate against developing CLPC. Some authors[26,37] have recommended the additional step of conjunctival irrigation with sterile unpreserved saline before and after lens insertion, and periodically during the day, as a means of diluting or removing antigens to CLPC and generally enhancing patient comfort.

If one accepts the association between CLPC and MGD described earlier,[32,33] then attention to lid hygiene should be of benefit. Encouraging the patient to employ strategies such as lid scrubbing, warm compresses and expression will alleviate MGD and presumably have some positive outcome with respect to the CLPC.

**Pharmaceutical agents**
A variety of medications have been advocated for the treatment of CLPC and the provision of symptomatic relief. The agent that has received most attention is ocular cromolyn sodium, which acts by stabilising mast-cell membranes, thus preventing the release of inflammatory mediators such as histamine. Prescription of this drug is generally used to supplement alternative strategies such as those described above. An initial dosage of 2 per cent or 4 per cent cromolyn sodium four times a day, tapering off to once a day as the condition improves, has been advocated by various authors.[38,39] The preservative-free form of this drug should be used if there is a poor initial response.

Figure 6.10 is the tarsal conjunctiva of an atopic individual who presented requesting contact lenses but who had never worn lenses previously. She had been using cromolyn sodium daily for over 10 years. The scarring and abnormal vascular changes present may reflect a combination of long-term ocular compromise and drug induced alterations to the normal inflammatory and tissue repair processes.

Suprofen is another non-steroid anti-inflammatory agent that has been used to treat CLPC. This drug, which inhibits prostaglandin synthesis, was found by Wood *et al*[40] to have a significant effect on signs and symptoms of CLPC after 2–3 weeks. Patients instilled two drops of 1 per cent suprofen solution four times daily.

Steroidal agents are sometimes used for short duration in severe cases of CLPC (grade 4); however, in view of the risks of cataract formation, increased intraocular pressure and corneal infection, their use is generally avoided.

A 'soft steroid' known as loteprednol etabonate (a chemical analogue of prednisolone) has been found to be as effective in treating CLPC as conventional steroids but without the untoward side-effects. Specifically, Howes and Asbell[41] found that this drug resulted in a significant reduction both in the size of papillae and the extent of itching and lens intolerance in patients with CLPC.

Butts and Rengstorff[42] claimed that an aqueous preparation containing the antioxidant 'polysorbate 80' and vitamin A alleviated CLPC in a population of 19 patients; however, the experiment was not masked and lacked controls, and the results were not subjected to statistical analysis. Thus, the efficacy of this therapy is not proven.

## Prognosis

The prognosis for recovery from CLPC after removal of lenses and cessation of wear is good. Even in the most severe conditions (grade 4), symptoms will disappear within 5 days to 2 weeks of lens removal,[2,40] and hyperaemia and excess mucus will resolve over a similar time course. Resolution of papillae takes place over a much longer time course – typically many weeks and as long as 6 months. The more severe the condition, the longer the recovery period.

In the longer term, however, the prognosis is less good. The condition can recur, especially in atopic patients who appear to have a propensity for developing the condition. Fortunately, such patients will have a lower threshold for noticing the early 'warning signs', and will typically seek

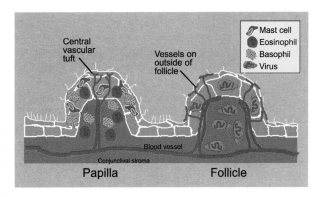

**Figure 6.11**
*Schematic diagram of pathological changes that characterise a papilla (left) and follicle (right)*

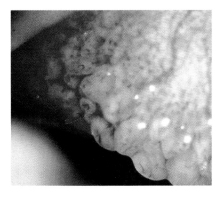 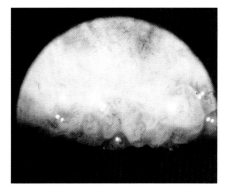

**Figure 6.12**
*Magnified view of papillae (left) and follicles (right). Note the presence of vascular tufts (arrow) at the apex of papillae*

prompt attention, which will in turn enhance the probability of successful treatment.

## Differential diagnosis

A key issue in the accurate diagnosis of CLPC is the capacity to differentiate between papillae and follicles (Figure 6.11). Papillae are observed in allergic diseases such as CLPC and vernal conjunctivitis, whereas follicles are indicative of viral or chlamydial conjunctival infections. There is generally little to distinguish between the two conditions and careful history-taking will provide the most important diagnostic clues.

The appearance of papillae has been described in detail previously in this chapter. According to Allansmith *et al*,[26] the side walls of papillae may be perpendicular to the plane of the tarsal plate and not pyramidal like follicles (Figure 6.12). Other key distinguishing features are as follows: some deep vessels can be observed traversing the surface of papillae, whereas vessels may be more obvious on the surface of follicles. Papillae often display a rich plexus of convoluted vessels (vascular tuft) at the apex; follicles generally do not display this feature. Follicles tend to be more pale.

In advanced stages, the apex of papillae may fill with infiltrates, thus masking the vascular tuft and taking on a whitish centre. Subsequent scarring also tends to be whitish, making it easy to distinguish papillae from follicles which usually do not display scar-like areas.

In vernal conjunctivitis that is unrelated to lens wear, the papillae can be truly gigantic (Figure 6.13) and thus differentiated from CLPC. Its other distinguishing features are the characteristic thick yellow discharge consisting of mucus, epithelial cells, neutrophils and eosinophils. The condition is usually bilateral and a bilateral

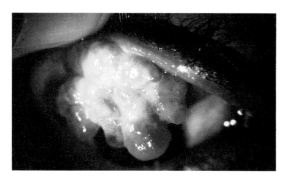

**Figure 6.13**
*Advanced vernal conjunctivitis with characteristic thick yellow discharge*

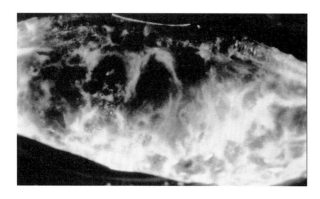

**Figure 6.14**
*Long-standing vernal conjunctivitis with distorted papillae and disorganised scarring*

ptosis may be present. Longstanding vernal conjunctivitis may result in distorted papillae and disorganised scarring (Figure 6.14).

Other pathologies of the tarsal conjunctiva will present from time to time, but these are easily distinguishable from the classic cobblestone appearance of multiple papillae formations.

## REFERENCES

1 Spring TF (1974) Reaction to hydrophilic lenses. *Med J Aust* **1**: 499.

2 Allansmith MR, Korb DR, Greiner JV (1977) Giant papillary conjunctivitis in contact lens wearers. *Am J Ophthalmol* **83**: 697.

3 Poggio EC, Abelson M (1993) Complications and symptoms in disposable extended wear lenses compared with conventional soft daily wear and soft extended wear lenses. *Contact Lens Assoc Ophthalmol J* **19**: 31.

4 Nason RJ, Boshnick EL, Cannon WM (1994) Multisite comparison of contact lens modalities. Daily disposable wear vs conventional daily wear in successful contact lens wearers. *J Am Optom Assoc* **65**: 774.

5 Alemany AL, Redal AP (1991) Giant papillary conjunctivitis in soft and rigid lens wear. *Contactologia* **13**: 14.

6 Grant T (1991) Clinical aspects of planned replacement and disposable lenses. In *The Contact Lens Year Book.* (ed. C Kerr). Medical and Scientific Publishing Ltd, p. 7.

7 Soni PS, Hathcoat G (1983) Complications reported with hydrogel extended wear contact lenses. *Int Contact Lens Clin* **10**: 144.

8 Rao GN, Naduvilath TJ, Sankaridurg PR (1996) Contact lens related papillary conjunctivitis in a prospective randomised clinical trial using disposable hydrogels. *Invest Ophthalmol Vis Sci* **37**: S1129.

9 Grant T, Holden BA Rechberger J (1989) Contact lens related papillary conjunctivitis (CLPC): influence of protein accumulation and replacement frequency. *Invest Ophthalmol Vis Sci* **30**: 166.

10 Allansmith MR (1987) Pathology and treatment of giant papillary conjunctivitis. The US perspective. *Clin Ther* **9**: 443.

11 Potvin RJ, Doughty MJ, Fonn D (1994) Tarsal conjunctival morphometry of asymptomatic soft contact lens wearers and non-lens wearers. *Int Contact Lens Clin* **21**: 225.

12 Greiner JV, Covington HI, Allansmith MR (1978) Surface morphology of giant papillary conjunctivitis in contact lens wearers. *Am J Ophthalmol* **85**: 242.

13 Srinivasan BK, Jakobiec FA, Iwamato T (1979) Giant papillary conjunctivitis with ocular prostheses. *Arch Ophthalmol* **97**: 892.

14 Robin JB, Regis-Pacheco LF, May WN (1987) Giant papillary conjunctivitis associated with an extruded scleral buckle. *Arch Ophthalmol* **105**: 619.

15 Carlson AN, Wilhelmus KA (1987) Giant papillary conjunctivitis associated with cyanoacrylate glue. *Am J Ophthalmol* **104**: 437.

16 Reynolds RMP (1978) Giant papillary conjunctivitis: a mechanical aetiology. *Aust J Optom* **61**: 320.

17 Stenson S (1982) Focal giant papillary conjunctivitis from retained contact lens. *Ann Ophthalmol* **14**: 881.

18 Dunn JP, Weissman BA, Mondino BJ (1990) Giant papillary conjunctivitis associated with elevated corneal deposits. *Cornea* **9**: 357.

19 Greiner JV (1988) Papillary conjunctivitis induced by an epithelialized corneal foreign body. *Ophthalmologica* **196**: 82.

20 Greiner JV Peace DG, Baird RS (1985) Effect of eye rubbing on the conjunctiva as a model of ocular inflammation. *Am J Ophthalmol* **100**: 45.

21 Ehlers WH, Fishman JB, Donshik PC (1991) Neutrophil chemotactic factors derived from conjunctival epithelial cells: preliminary biochemical characterisation. *Contact Lens Assoc Ophthalmol J* **17**: 65.

22 Henriquez AS, Kenyon KR, Allansmith MR (1981) Mast cell ultrastructure. *Arch Ophthalmol* **99**: 1266.

23 Donshik PC, Ballow M (1993) Tear immunoglobulins in giant papillary conjunctivitis induced by contact lenses. *Am J Ophthalmol* **96**: 460.

24 Ballow M, Donshik PC, Rapacz P (1989) Immune response in monkeys to lenses from patients with contact lens induced papillary conjunctivitis. *Contact Lens Assoc Ophthalmol J* **15**: 64.

25 Roth HW (1991) Studies on the etiology and treatment of giant papillary conjunctivitis in contact lens wearers. *Contactologia* **13E**: 55.

26 Allansmith MR, Ross RN, Greiner JV (1985) Giant papillary conjunctivitis: diagnosis and treatment. In: *Contact Lenses* (ed. OH Dabezies). Little, Brown and Company, Boston, MA, p. 43.1.

27 Hann LE, Cornell-Bell AH, Marten-Ellis C (1986) Conjunctival basophil hypersensitivity lesions in guinea pigs. *Invest Ophthalmol Vis Sci* **27**: 1255.

28 Begley CG (1992) Giant papillary conjunctivitis, In: *Complications of Contact lens Wear* (ed. A Tomlinson). Mosby, St Louis, p. 237.

29 Barishak Y, Aavaro A, Samra Z (1984) An immunological study of papillary conjunctivitis due to contact lenses. *Curr Eye Res* **3**: 1161.

30 Buckley RJ (1987) Pathology and treatment of giant papillary conjunctivitis: II The British perspective. *Clin Ther* **9**: 451.

31 Begley CG, Riggle A, Tuel JA (1990) Association of giant papillary conjunctivitis with seasonal allergies. *Optom Vis Sci* **67**: 192.

32 Martin NF, Rubinfeld RS, Malley JD (1992) Giant papillary conjunctivitis and meibomian gland dysfunction blepharitis. *Contact Lens Assoc Ophthalmol J* **18**: 165.

33 Mathers WD, Billborough M (1992) Meibomian gland dysfunction and giant papillary conjunctivitis. *Am J Ophthalmol* **114**: 188.

34 Sack RA, Jones B, Antiguani A (1987) Specificity and biological activity of the protein deposited on the hydrogel surface. *Invest Ophthalmol Vis Sci* **28**: 842.

35 Leahy CD, Mandell R, Lin ST (1990) Initial in vivo tear protein deposition on individual hydrogel contact lenses. *Optom Vis Sci* **67**: 504.

36 Douglas JP, Lowder CY, Lazorik R (1988) Giant papillary conjunctivitis associated with rigid gas permeable contact lenses. *Contact Lens Assoc Ophthalmol J* **14**: 143.

37 Farkas P, Kasalow TW, Farkas B (1986) Clinical management and control of giant papillary conjunctivitis secondary to contact lens wear. *J Am Optom Assoc* **57**: 197.

38 Donshik PC, Ballow M, Luistro A (1984) Treatment of contact lens induced giant papillary conjunctivitis secondary to contact lens wear. *Contact Lens Assoc Ophthalmol J* **10**: 346.

39 Meisler DM, Berzins UJ, Krachmer JH (1982) Cromolyn treatment of giant papillary conjunctivitis. *Arch Ophthalmol* **100**: 1608.

40 Wood TS, Stewart RH, Bowman RW (1988) Suprofen treatment of contact lens associated giant papillary conjunctivitis. *Arch Ophthalmol* **95**: 822.

41 Howes JF, Asbell PA (1995) A double-masked placebo-controlled evaluation of the efficacy and safety of loteprednol etabonate in the treatment of contact-lens associated giant papillary conjunctivitis. *Invest Ophthalmol Vis Sci* **36**: S630.

42 Butts BL, Rengstorff RH (1990) Antioxidant and vitamin A drops for giant papillary conjunctivitis. *Contact Lens J* **18**: 40.

# 7
# Superior limbic keratoconjunctivitis

Prevalence
Signs and symptoms
Pathology
Aetiology
Treatment
Prognosis
Differential diagnosis

Unlike the other contact lens complications that are described in this book, contact lens-induced superior limbic keratoconjunctivitis (CLSLK) is a syndrome comprising a combination of tissue pathologies. Tissues affected include the corneal epithelium and stroma, the limbus and the bulbar and tarsal conjunctiva. Although this condition was first fully described in the literature in the early 1980s,[1–10] a similar syndrome unrelated to contact lens wear (Theodore's superior limbic keratoconjunctivitis; 'Theodore's SLK') had been known to exist for about 20 years prior to this.[11]

Because of the strong association between the development of CLSLK and the use of contact lens care solutions containing thimerosal, this condition has also been called 'thimerosal keratoconjunctivitis'[1] or 'thimerosal keratopathy'.[12]

In its mild form, CLSLK is easy to overlook (Figure 7.1). The condition is confined to the superior limbal area and as such is hidden by the upper lid in primary gaze. The proper procedure for observing this condition is to lift the upper lid while the patient gazes down. Such an examination technique should be part of the routine proce-

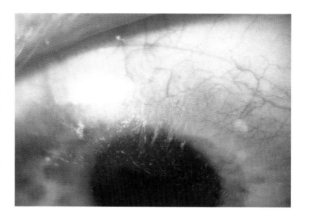

**Figure 7.1**
*Mild case of CLSLK displaying superior conjunctival hyperaemia*

dure during every contact lens aftercare examination.

## Prevalence

Although the prevalence of CLSLK in the general population is not known, the prevalence of this condition among symptomatic contact lens wearers has been investigated. In 1989, Wilson-Holt and Dart[1] reported the results of a retrospective

evaluation of the record cards of 312 patients with contact lens-related complications presenting consecutively to an eye clinic. They found that 42 patients (13.5 per cent) presented with a typical CLSLK and 13 (4.1 per cent) presented with an atypical CLSLK. Thus, a total of 55 patients (17.6 per cent) were affected with this condition.

Dart reported the results of a similar study (conducted with different colleagues)[13] in 1992. Of 1104 patients with contact lens-related disorders presenting to an eye clinic, only five (0.5 per cent) displayed a classic CLSLK; however, 67 patients (6 per cent) displayed what was described as 'thimerosal keratopathy/conjunctivitis'. The description given by these authors[13] of the pathological changes at the superior limbus that characterised this latter condition indicated that they were observing an atypical form of CLSLK. Thus, combining these figures gives a prevalence of CLSLK-associated disease among symptomatic contact lens wearers of about 6.5 per cent.

Thimerosal was commonly used as a preservative in contact lens solutions up until the mid-1980s; its use declined thereafter as a result of practitioners and industry taking note of the increasing number of reports linking thimerosal to CLSLK. This probably explains why the prevalence of this condition declined from 17.6 per cent[1] to 6.5 per cent[13] between 1989 and 1992. It is likely that the prevalence of CLSLK has reduced even further since the introduction onto the UK market in 1994 of chlorhexidine-based designer preservatives such as Dymed and Polyquad that do not contain thimerosal, or indeed any other preservatives that could be toxic or allergenic to the cornea. Such products, together with hydrogen peroxide-based disinfecting systems, now dominate the market. Noxious preservatives such as thimerosal are now used infrequently. Data is not yet available to confirm the expectation of a very low prevalence of CLSLK in patients using modern disinfection systems devoid of thimerosal.

## Signs and symptoms

Symptoms of CLSLK include increased lens awareness, lens intolerance, foreign-body sensation, burning, itching, photophobia, redness and increased lacrimation. Although an occasional slight mucus secretion might be observed, there is no heavy discharge such as that seen in bacterial conjunctivitis. Some loss of vision (by three or more lines of Snellen acuity[1,3]) has been reported in advanced cases such as with extensive pannus formation.

A myriad of signs are observed in patients with CLSLK; these include:

- Punctate epithelial fluorescein staining (Figure 7.2) – typically in the upper third to half of the cornea, which can be

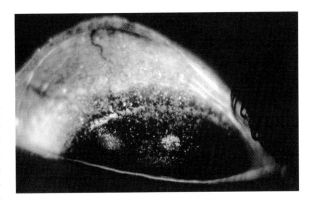

**Figure 7.2**
*Corneal, limbal and conjunctival fluorescein staining in CLSLK in a patient wearing bifocal hydrogel contact lenses*

coarse in some patients, and sometimes in a swirled pattern.[2]
- Epithelial rose bengal staining of the superior cornea.
- Intra-epithelial opacities.
- Sub-epithelial haze in the superior cornea – extending in a V-shaped pattern towards the pupil.
- Epithelial dulling, microcysts, infiltrates (Figure 7.3) and irregularity of the superior cornea.
- Stromal opacification.
- Fibrovascular micro-pannus – a plexus of vessels advancing from the superior cornea in the form of a V-shape, with the apex towards the pupil and an even linear leading edge parallel with the upper lid margin (see Figures 7.1 and 7.4).
- Fine sub-epithelial linear opacities at the

periphery of the superior cornea – aligned with the general direction of blood vessels in the pannus.
- Superior limbal oedema, hypertrophy, fluorescein staining and vascular injection.
- Poor wetting of the superior bulbar conjunctiva.
- Superior bulbar conjunctival punctate staining.
- Superior bulbar conjunctival hyperaemia.
- Superior bulbar conjunctival chemosis – described as a 'boggy apron' of bulbar conjunctiva that forms redundant folds over the superior limbus.[3]
- Papillary hypertrophy of the upper tarsal conjunctiva – in 25 per cent of cases.[3]
- Follicular hypertrophy, hyperaemia and scattered petechiae on the upper tarsal conjunctiva.
- Corneal filaments – said to be present in

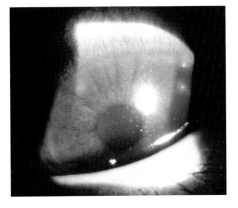

**Figure 7.3**
*A mild case of CLSLK displaying superior limbal hyperaemia, focal infiltrates and increased lacrimation. The hazy corneal reflex indicates an uneven epithelium*

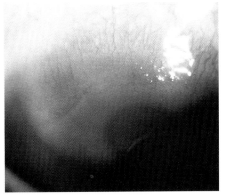

**Figure 7.4**
*Fibrovascular pannus in CLSLK stained with rose bengal*

13 per cent of patients suffering from CLSLK.[3]

- Corneal warpage and astigmatism.
- Pseudo-dendrites – bilateral dendritic corneal lesions that lack the terminal bulbs characteristic of herpetic disease.

CLSLK is almost always bilateral and the specific signs often display symmetry between the eyes. There is considerable variability in the time course of onset of the condition; signs usually becomes manifest between 2 months and 2 years of commencement of lens wear.[3,4]

It is interesting to compare the clinical presentation of CLSLK with that of Theodore's SLK which also occurs in non-contact lens wearers. Table 7.1 is a summary of the similarities and differences between the two conditions.

There have been a few reports of CLSLK in patients wearing rigid contact lenses. Wilson-Holt and Dart[1] report two cases in which the patients were using a wetting solution containing thimerosal. One patient had previously worn soft lenses. Both patients suffered from lens intolerance and red eyes, although the overall signs and symptoms were less severe compared with those observed in patients wearing soft lenses.

## Pathology

Sendele *et al*[3] used light microscopy to examine biopsy material from the superior bulbar conjunctiva of five patients suffering from CLSLK and of five normal control subjects. The following observations were made of the affected specimens:

- Epithelial keratinisation (2 patients).
- Intracellular epithelial oedema (3 patients).
- Acanthosis (3 patients).

- Pseudoepitheliomatous hyperplasia (3 patients).
- Acute inflammatory ceils in the epithelium (3 patients).
- Acute inflammatory cells in the stroma (3 patients).
- Plasma cells in the stroma (indicating chronic inflammation) (5 patients).
- Mononuclear cells in the stroma (indicating chronic inflammation) (5 patients).
- Absence of goblet cells (4 patients).

Transmission electron microscopy of the same tissue samples revealed the following additional pathological changes:

- Flattening of surface microvilli.
- Accumulation of intracytoplasmic keratin filaments.
- Condensed cytoplasm.
- Fibrillogranular inclusions (probably lipoproteinaceous).
- Epithelial infiltration of polymorphonuclear leukocytes.

Sendele *et al*[13] pointed out that although their findings provided evidence of acute and chronic inflammation typical of Theodore's SLK, they did not observe marked epithelial keratinisation, nuclear degeneration or glycogen accumulation – which have been reported by other researchers to be representative of Theodore's SLK. However, Stenson[4] observed prekeratinised epithelial cells as well as a neutrophilic response in conjunctival and corneal scrapings of CLSLK patients.

Figure 7.5 is a schematic diagram highlighting the differences between the normal bulbar conjunctiva and the bulbar conjunctiva of a patient suffering from CLSLK.

## Aetiology

Despite claims to the contrary throughout the literature, the primary aetiological factor in the development of CLSLK is thimerosal hypersensitivity. However, other factors must be involved. Provocative tests in thimerosal-sensitised patients result in general conjunctival hyperaemia[1,3] (not just confined to the superior limbus), meaning that contact lens wear has impacted on the clinical presentation.

Although other factors perhaps play a minor role by initiating, modulating or exacerbating the condition, it is unlikely that

---

### Table 7.1 Comparison of Theodore's SLK and CLSLK

| Feature | Theodore's SLK | Contact lens-induced SLK |
|---|---|---|
| Age | Usually middle-aged (over 40) | Younger (under 40) |
| Sex | More common in females | Equal male/female distribution |
| Associated factors | Linked to thyroid disease | Usually soft contact lens wear<br>Increased lens movement<br>Soiled lenses<br>Thimerosal in lens solutions |
| Symptoms | Mild to severe irritation without lenses<br>Vision rarely affected | Mild to severe irritation with lenses<br><br>Vision can be reduced |
| Signs | Mild superior corneal staining<br>Superior bulbar conjunctival injection<br>Superior bulbar conjunctival chemosis<br>Limbal injection<br>Grade 3 papillary hypertrophy<br>Corneal filaments frequently observed | Severe superior corneal staining<br>Superior bulbar conjunctival injection<br>Superior bulbar conjunctival chemosis<br>Limbal injection<br>Grade 1 papillary hypertrophy<br>Corneal filaments rarely observed |
| Staining | Superior corneal fluorescein staining | Superior corneal rose bengal staining |
| Pathology | Epithelial keratinisation<br>Nuclear degeneration | Epithelial keratinisation<br>Neutrophilic response<br>Reduced number of goblet cells |
| Management | Lubricants<br>Silver nitrate application<br>Bandage lens therapy<br>Pressure patching<br>Conjunctival resection<br>Conjunctival cauterisation | Temporary cessation of lens wear<br>Interim steroids<br>Interim lubricants<br>Interim prostaglandin inhibitors<br>Change lens design<br>Use non-thimerosal regimen |

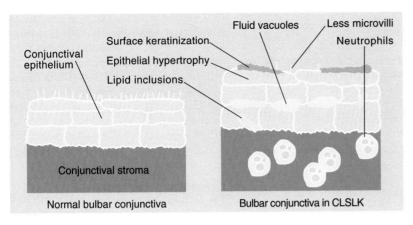

Fluid vacuoles    Less microvilli
Neutrophils
Surface keratinization
Conjunctival epithelium
Epithelial hypertrophy
Lipid inclusions

Conjunctival stroma

Normal bulbar conjunctiva          Bulbar conjunctiva in CLSLK

**Figure 7.5**
*Schematic diagram of the normal bulbar conjunctiva and the bulbar conjunctiva in CLSLK*

CLSLK will develop in the absence of ocular contact with thimerosal. Evidence relating to the significance of these and other aetiological factors will be considered in turn.

**Thimerosal hypersensitivity**
Thimerosal is an organic mercury compound that interacts with living tissue (such as bacteria or corneal epithelial cells) by binding to sulphydryl groups of enzymes and other proteins. Compared with other traditional preservatives such as chlorhexidine, thimerosal has relatively inferior antibacterial potency but superior anti-fungal potency.[14]

There is some confusion in the literature concerning the use of the word 'thimerosal', which sometimes appears as 'thiomersal'. These are in fact different solutions – thimerosal being the US formulation, and thiomersal (or thiomersolate) being the UK formulation.[15] Because the US formulation is used almost universally in solutions, 'thimerosal' is the preferred spelling (and is thus used in this book).

The key evidence linking thimerosal to CLSLK comes from clinical studies that have sought to identify a common causative factor in patients presenting with this condition. Wright and Mackie[5] observed that all 61 patients suffering from CLSLK in their sample were using solutions containing thimerosal. All of 10 patients subjected to a provocative test (a challenge dose of 0.005 per cent thimerosal 'in normal saline' applied topically) showed a rapid adverse response. Sendele et al[3] reported 40 cases of CLSLK; in every case, patients were using thimerosal-preserved care solutions. In all 40 CLSLK patients of Sendele et al,[3] all six

CLSLK patients of Miller et al,[6] all 15 CLSLK patients of Fuerst et al[7] and all 31 CLSLK patients of Wilson et al,[8] thimerosal was a component of care solutions being used.

Other evidence implicating thimerosal in the aetiology of CLSLK includes:

• The condition is always bilateral.
• Signs and symptoms resolve when the patient ceases using thimerosal-preserved solutions.[1,3]
• The syndrome recurs if thimerosal is reintroduced into the care regimen.
• The syndrome does not recur if thimerosal-free solutions are used.

The results of 'patch testing' have confounded the thimerosal argument. For example, Sendele et al[3] applied three challenge tests to patients suffering from CLSLK:

• Two drops of 0.001 per cent and 0.01 per cent thimerosal (the latter being 10 times the concentration usually used in contact lens solution formulations), balanced in saline, instilled into the eyes of 15 patients every hour during waking hours.
• An occlusive skin patch test soaked in 0.001 per cent thimerosal applied to the forearm.
• 0.1 ml of 0.001 per cent thimerosal injected into the forearm.

Only five of the 15 patients tested (and none of the control subjects) developed a reaction to the thimerosal within 72 hours. Similarly, Miller et al[6] noted a positive skin

test reaction to thimerosal in only one of six patients examined.

Wilson-Holt and Dart[1] adopted a different approach to provocative testing. They instilled one drop of a saline solution containing 0.005 per cent thimerosal into the eye, four times each day. Conjunctival hyperaemia was observed in all patients – usually within 12 hours but sometimes taking up to 72 hours to develop. The inconclusive nature of patch testing results may be due to the thimerosal molecule being too small for skin testing of an antibody mediated response.[2]

There have been reports of patients who have recovered from CLSLK but have suffered a recurrence when lens wear has been resumed in the absence of thimerosal.[7] Such reports are inconclusive because in many cases the same lens' has been reused. Despite thorough cleaning, not all of the offending antigen may have been completely purged from the lens.

Of the four patients in the study of Stenson,[4] three experienced a resolution of signs of CLSLK after lens removal and were able to resume a limited wearing schedule with thinner lenses, presumably while still using thimerosal-preserved solutions. However, the fact that it was necessary to restrict wearing time suggests that the condition was not fully resolved. A shorter wearing schedule would have minimised the time of contact of thimerosal with the ocular surface, thus reducing the severity of the condition. Any additional strategy to minimise the overall physiological challenge of lens wear such as the use of thinner lenses (of necessarily superior oxygen performance) would be expected to have a general beneficial effect on ocular signs and symptoms (such as eye redness) independently of any direct effect in curing CLSLK.

Thimerosal has long been known to cause an intense delayed hypersensitivity reaction. The mechanism of a delayed hypersensitivity reaction requires that affected patients have been previously sensitised to an offending antigen and are then re-exposed to that antigen for a prolonged period before the condition flares up. Likely mechanisms for pre-sensitisation which involve thimerosal include previous vaccine injections (such as those for diphtheria and tetanus), topical antiseptics and ophthalmic preparations.

Once a patient has been sensitised to thimerosal, a re-exposure of minute concentrations later in life results in the onset of symptoms and signs over a period of weeks or months. This is typical of a hypersensitivity reaction, as distinct from a toxicity reaction which is dose-dependant and immediate. Furthermore, Langerhans cells are present in the limbus and adjacent tissues; such cells are known to mediate cutaneous hypersensitivity reactions to a variety of chemicals.[12] Patch testing studies have revealed that the incidence of skin hypersensitivity to thimerosal is about 7 per cent in the US[16] and 25 per cent in Sweden.[17]

Mackie[12] argues that CLSLK can present as a Type I (immediate) or Type IV (delayed) hypersensitivity reaction, primarily based upon clinical evidence that some patients display an immediate reaction and some display a delayed response.

The precise mechanism by which thimerosal induces a hypersensitivity reaction in CLSLK is not known, but Wilson-Holt and Dart[1] have advanced the following theory: hydrogel lenses absorb thimerosal (which is highly water-soluble) during the disinfection procedure, and the thimerosal is slowly re-released back into the eye during lens wear. This prolonged ocular contact with thimerosal induces a local delayed hypersensitivity reaction initiated by sensitised T lymphocytes.

### Thimerosal toxicity

Thimerosal is only mildly cytotoxic – to a degree that is much less than other preservative systems.[18] A true toxicity reaction would affect all of the ocular surface and would not be restricted to the superior cornea and conjunctiva as occurs in CLSLK. It is for these reasons that CLSLK is not considered to be a toxic reaction.

### Mechanical effects

Evidence that there is a significant mechanical component to the aetiology of CLSLK is weak and largely anecdotal. Stenson[4] noted that some of her CLSLK patients displayed excessive lens movement. Abel *et al*[9] noted lens movement of greater than 1.5 mm in the majority of their patients. Excessive movement indicates a poor fit and may be associated with increased mechanical influences.

Stenson[4] also reported that refitting with thinner lenses resulted in some alleviation of CLSLK; however, as explained earlier, the reason for this improvement may be

more physiological (increased oxygen) than physical (mechanical).

Abel *et al*[9] reported one case where a patient had apparently been successfully wearing spin-cast lenses cared for with thimerosal-based preservatives. CLSLK developed after switching to a lathe-cut design. These authors surmised that the new lens may have created a mechanical heaping of the superior bulbar conjunctiva, resulting in poor wetting of the superior cornea and eventual epithelial pathology.

The fact that CLSLK occurs at the site of the superior limbus lends some support to the theory of mechanical aetiology because of the physical bearing of the upper lid against the lens which would exacerbate any ocular irritation due, for example, to lens surface deposits. Ocular lubricants provide some symptomatic relief,[9] suggesting that mechanical irritation is a component of the CLSLK syndrome.

### Lens deposits

Lens deposits such as protein are of potential significance in the aetiology of adverse ocular reactions to lens wear because these deposits can (a) act as a mechanical abrasive, (b) support bacterial colonisation and (c) absorb or attract extraneous contaminants such as metal ions, preservatives and other components of care systems. It is thought that the latter mechanism in particular may be relevant to CLSLK because of possible absorption of the mercuric component of thimerosal into deposits on the posterior lens surface and subsequent release on to the ocular surface during wear.

To examine the role of lens deposition in

CLSLK, Barr *et al*[19] conducted a thorough protein and elemental analysis of contact lenses worn by 12 patients suffering from this condition. Apart from one case in which high levels of mercury were found in a lens, no clear association between deposit type and the genesis of CLSLK could be demonstrated. Thus, the role of lens spoliation in the aetiology of CLSLK remains unclear.

### Hypoxia beneath upper lid

The fact that the ocular response in CLSLK is confined to the region of the superior limbus suggests that upper lid-induced hypoxia may be a contributing factor to the aetiology of this condition. The upper lid normally covers the superior third of the cornea. The oxygen supply to the superior limbus during normal open eye lens wear comes from the capillary plexus of the superior palpebral conjunctiva. The partial pressure of oxygen at the lens surface beneath the upper eyelid is 55 mmHg,[20] versus 155 mmHg in the absence of the eyelid.

Of course, lid-induced hypoxia cannot be the sole or primary cause of CLSLK, otherwise all contact lens wearers would be affected. Nevertheless, partial oxygen deprivation may be an exacerbating factor that compromises the physiological status of the superior cornea and limbus so that this region is more prone to immunological challenge. Holden *et al*[21] have provided evidence for this by demonstrating that lens-induced hypoxia inhibits respiration and growth of the corneal epithelium and stroma.

Figure 7.6 is a schematic diagram illustrating the various aetiological factors that

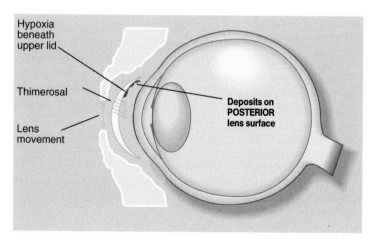

**Figure 7.6**
*Factors of aetiological significance in CLSLK*

are thought to lead to the development of CLSLK.

## Treatment

The accumulated clinical evidence implicating thimerosol as the prime cause of CLSLK provides an excellent focus for treating this condition.

### Suspension of lens wear

Following suspension of lens wear, the signs and symptoms of CLSLK will immediately begin to resolve because the ocular surface will no longer be in contact with thimerosal. The recommended period of cessation of lens wear is related to the severity of the condition. Patients suffering from CLSLK may be advised to cease lens wear for 2–4 weeks in mild cases and for up to 3 months in severe cases. The time course of resolution is discussed under 'Prognosis'.

Boruchoff and Bajart[22] have suggested the following criteria for resumption of lens wear: there must no longer be any epithelial haze, surface irregularity or peripheral neovascularisation. These criteria may be a little too stringent. Certainly it would be prudent to wait until corneal haze has largely resolved and the corneal surface is smooth; however, a vascular pannus may be permanent. Lens wear can be resumed in the presence of a vascular pannus as long as the patient is monitored closely to the check that vascularisation does not progress.

### Elimination of thimerosal

Total elimination of thimerosal will almost certainly cure CLSLK, and when the patient recommences lens wear it is essential that none of the lens care solutions contains thimerosal (see Table 7.2 for a list of solutions containing thimerosal, bearing in mind that this list is not necessarily complete). The patient should also be carefully interrogated as to whether they use any other topical ocular medications – even those not related to contact lens wear. If thimerosal is an ingredient of any product being used, the patient should be advised to cease using them. In cases where the patient is using a prescription product containing thimerosal, the prescribing practitioner should be notified.

Patients should be warned of their allergy to thimerosal and should be told always to check that thimerosal is not an ingredient of any product to be applied to the eye in the future.

### Alteration to the lens

Any lens that has been worn by a patient suffering from CLSLK should be discarded and a new lens prescribed, because no matter how thoroughly such a lens is cleaned, it only takes a trace amount of residual thimerosal to induce a reaction.

Assuming that subsequent lens wear is prescribed in the absence of thimerosal-preserved solutions, there are no constraints on the design of the replacement lenses or the modality of lens wear. However, for patients who are commencing lens wear after having not completely recovered from CLSLK, it would be advisable to prescribe a lens of superior oxygen performance (i.e. high water content and/or thin design) and minimum thickness profile (so as to reduce the potential for mechanical irritation). Changing over to rigid lenses is unlikely to be of any additional benefit, as CLSLK is known to occur also in patients wearing rigid lenses.[1]

Frequent replacement or disposable lenses are not essential in the management of CLSLK, notwithstanding the numerous distinct advantages of such lenses in a general sense. This is because deposit accumulation is of secondary importance in the aetiology of CLSLK; that is, deposit formation in respect of this condition is only problematic if thimerosal-preserved solutions are being used.

### Pharmaceutical agents

Because there is no infectious component to CLSLK, there is no point in prescribing

**Table 7.2  Contact lens solutions containing thimerosal**

| Product | Manufacturer | Thimerosal concentration |
|---|---|---|
| *Cleaning solutions for soft lenses* | | |
| Alcon | Preflex | 0.004% |
| Allergan | Hyrocare | 0.001% |
| CIBA Vision | Hydroclean | 0.0025% |
| Wesley Jessen–PBH | Cleaner No. 4 | 0.004% |
| Wesley Jessen–PBH | Hexidin | 0.001% |
| Sauflon | Daily Cleaner | 0.004% |
| *Saline solutions for soft lenses* | | |
| Ciba Vision | Lensrins | 0.001% |
| *Preserved chemical disinfection systems for soft lenses* | | |
| Alcon | Flex-Care | 0.001% |
| Allergan | Hydrocare | 0.002% |
| *Combined solutions for soft lenses* | | |
| AKI Lens | AKI Soft All-in-One Solution | 0.004% |
| Pilkington Barnes–Hind | Combi Comfort | 0.04 mg |
| *In-eye preparations for soft lenses* | | |
| Alcon | Adapettes | 0.004% |
| CIBA Vision | Hydrosol | 0.0025% |
| Pilkington Barnes–Hind | Soft Comfort | 0.004% |
| *Cleaning solutions for rigid lenses* | | |
| Pilkington Barnes–Hind | Combi Clean | not stated |
| Pilkington Barnes–Hind | Combi Sol | not stated |
| Sauflon | Steri-Clens | 0.004% |
| *Wetting solutions for rigid lenses* | | |
| Sauflon | Sterifresh | 0.0021% |
| *Combined solutions for rigid lenses* | | |
| Alcon | Soaclens | 0.004% |

Extracted from the 1995 *International Contact Lens Yearbook*[25]

antibiotics or anti-viral agents etc. Opinion is divided as to the value of prescribing corticosteroids to dampen the immunological response. Abel *et al*[9] were of the opinion that corticosteroids helped in severe cases, whereas others[1,3,12] found that such drugs had no beneficial effect. Wilson-Holt and Dart[1] did not use any other therapeutic agents in the management of their CLSLK cases.

For patients whose eyes are particularly hyperaemic and uncomfortable, Mackie[12] has recommended the prescription of oxy-tetracycline 250 mg twice daily or oral doxycycline 100 mg on alternate days for their anti-inflammatory effect on the conjunctiva.

In severe cases, the cornea can be treated with silver nitrate to remove affected cells and to promote regrowth of a new, healthy epithelium.

Ocular lubricants in the form of drops or ointments may provide symptomatic relief during the recovery phase,[9] further to a positive placebo effect in a naturally anxious patient.

### Bandage lenses and pressure patching

Paradoxically, bandage lenses have been advocated for patients suffering from Theodore's SLK.[23] Adapting this approach to CLSLK would mean rapid resumption of lens wear in the absence of thimerosal-preserved care systems. The main beneficiary of such an approach would be a patient suffering from a concurrent tarsal hypertrophy whose limbus would be protected from mechanical insult from the roughened tarsus. Similarly, pressure patches provide symptomatic relief by limiting eye movement and consequent mechanical irritation.[23]

### Surgery

Sendele *et al*[3] removed the involved superior corneal epithelium in two CLSLK patients with incapacitating reduction of vision attributed to corneal epithelial irregularity. This was achieved by mechanical scraping with a scalpel blade. They reported that although this procedure may have hastened visual recovery, it did not seem to otherwise affect the clinical course.

Kenyon and Tseng[24] described three severe cases of CLSLK in which two free grafts of limbal tissue were transplanted from the most affected to the least affected eye, the latter having been prepared by limited conjunctival resection and superficial dis-section of the fibrovascular pannus. Subsequent impression cytology confirmed restoration of the corneal epithelium. It is curious that this procedure is possible in view of the perfect symmetry that is encountered in virtually all cases of CLSLK.[12]

With increased knowledge and understanding of CLSLK coupled with the rapidly declining use of thimerosal in contact lens care solutions, such radical surgical procedures are unlikely to be necessary in the future.

## Prognosis

In the 42 patients suffering from CLSLK examined by Wilson-Holt and Dart,[1] the time of resolution of clinical signs following cessation of lens wear took from 3 weeks to 9 months, with a mean of 4.2 months. Sendele *et al*[3] reported a similar time course of resolution, as did Abel *et al*,[9] who noted that recovery took from 5 days to 10 months in the eight patients they followed. In these patients, oedema and injection subsided first, followed by clearing of the epitheliopathy. Papillary changes took the longest to resolve and persisted for months in several cases. Sendele *et al*[3] reported that one patient took 2 years to recover in the absence of lens wear; fortunately, such a prolonged period of recovery is rare.

Recovery of visual acuity following severe cases of CLSLK was reported by Sendele *et al*[3] to be 'gradual'. These authors inferred that visual acuity had only recovered to 6/9 in some subjects, even after several months.

## Differential diagnosis

Wilson-Holt and Dart[1] reported that they had misdiagnosed two CLSLK patients as having bacterial conjunctivitis; these patients were unfortunately treated with thimerosal-preserved topical antibiotics, which of course exacerbated the condition.

In the early stages, CLSLK may be mistaken for regional limbal injection that could be caused by a variety of insults. For example, Figure 7.7 depicts superior limbal irritation in a 24-year-old asymptomatic male wearing rigid lenses. The edge of the lens was chipped, leading to irritation of the superior limbus between the 8 and 12 o'clock positions. This appearance is very similar to that in CLSLK.

CLSLK can also be mistaken for infiltrative keratitis. A culture-positive scraping would provide verification of an infectious keratitis. True CLSLK should be suspected if thimerosal-preserved care solutions are being used.

The key difference between CLSLK and Theodore's SLK is that the latter generally occurs in the absence of lens wear. Theoretically, a contact lens wearer can coincidentally develop Theodore's SLK in the presence or absence of thimerosal-preserved care systems. The distinguishing features between these two conditions are outlined in Table 7.1.

In general, the clinical presentation of a severe case of CLSLK is unambiguous, with a host of corneal, limbal and conjunctival pathologies confined to the region of the superior limbus.

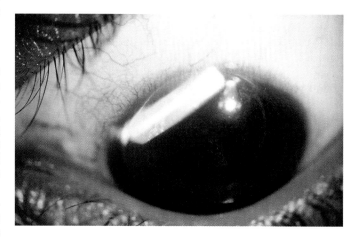

**Figure 7.7**
*Injection of the superior limbus caused by irritation from the edge of a chipped rigid lens, which takes on a similar appearance to CLSLK*

## REFERENCES

1 Wilson-Holt N, Dart JKG (1983) Thiomersal keratoconjunctivitis, frequency, clinical spectrum and diagnosis. *Eye* **3**: 581.

2 Wallace W (1985) Soft contact lens associated superior limbic keratoconjunctivitis. *Int Eyecare* **1**: 302.

3 Sendele DD, Kenyon KR, Mobilia EF (1983) Superior limbic keratoconjunctivitis in contact lens wearers. *Ophthalmol* **90**: 616.

4 Stenson S (1983) Superior limbic keratoconjunctivitis associated with soft contact lens wear. *Arch Ophthalmol* **101**: 402.

5 Wright P, Mackie I (1982) Preservative-related problems in soft contact lens wearers. *Trans Ophthalmol Soc UK* **102**: 3.

6 Miller RA, Brightbill FS, Slama SL (1982) Superior limbic keratoconjunctivitis in soft contact lens wearers. *Cornea* **1**: 293.

7 Fuerst DJ, Sugar J, Worobec S (1983) Superior limbic keratoconjunctivitis associated with cosmetic soft contact lens wear. *Arch Ophthalmol* **101**: 1214.

8 Wilson LA, McNatt J, Reitschel R (1981) Delayed hypersensitivity to thiomersal in soft contact lens wearers. *Ophthalmol* **8l**: 804.

9 Abel R, Shovlin JP, DePaolis MD (1985) A treatise on hydrophilic lens induced superior limbic keratoconjunctivitis. *Int Contact Lens Clin* **12**: 116.

10 Binder PS, Rasmussen DM, Gordon M (1981) Keratoconjunctivitis and soft lens solutions. *Arch Ophthalmol* **99**: 87.

11 Theodore FH (1963) Superior limbic keratoconjunctivitis. *Ear Nose Throat J* **42**: 25.

12 Mackie IA (1993) Thiomersal keratopathy. In: *Medical Contact Lens Practice, A Systematic Approach* Butterworth-Heinemann, Oxford.

13 Stapleton F, Dart J, Minassian D (1992) Nonulcerative complications of contact lens wear. *Arch Ophthalmol* **110**: 1601.

14 Tragakis MP, Brown SI, Pearce DB (1973) Bacteriological studies of contamination associated with soft contact lenses. *Am J Ophthalmol* **75**: 496.

15 Stewart-Jones JH, Hopkins GA, Phillips AJ (1989) Drugs and solutions in contact lens practice and related microbiology. In: *Contact Lenses* (eds AJ Phlllips and J Stone), 3rd edn. Butterworth-Heinemann, London, p. 130.

16 Rudner EJ, Clendenning WE, Epstein E (1973) Epidemiology of contact dermatitis in North America. *Arch Dermatol* **108**: 537.

17 Hansson H, Moller H (1970) Patch test reactions to merthiolate in healthy young subjects. *Br J Dermatol* **83**: 349.

18 Gasset AR, Ishir Y, Kaufman HE (1974) Cytotoxicity of ophthalmic preservatives. *Am J Ophthalmol* **78**: 98.

19 Barr JT, Dugan PR, Reindel WR (1989) Protein and elemental analysis of contact lenses of patients with superior limbic keratoconjunctivitis or giant papillary conjunctivitis. *Optom Vis Sci* **66**: 133.

20 Efron N, Carney LG (1979) Oxygen levels beneath the closed eyelid. *Invest Ophthalmol Vis Sci* **18**: 93.

21 Holden BA, Sweeney DF, Vannas A (1985) Effects of long-term extended contact lens wear on the humun cornea. *Invest Ophthalmol Vis Sci* **26**: 1489.

22 Boruchoff SA, Bajart AM (1989) The superior limbic manifestations of contact lens intolerance, Vol 2. In: *Contact Lenses. The CLAO Guide to Basic Science and Clinical Practice* (ed. OH Dabezier Jr), 2nd edn. Little, Brown and Co, Boston, MA.

23 Mondino BJ, Zaidman GW, Salamon SW (1982) Use of pressure patching and soft contact lenses in superior limbic keratoconjunctivitis *Arch Ophthalmol* **100**: 1932.

24 Kenyon KR, Tseng SCG (1989) Limbal autograft transplantation for ocular surface disorders *Ophthalmology* **96**: 709.

25 Efron N (1995) *The International Contact Lens Yearbook 1995.* Saunders, London.

# Part III
# Tear Film

# 8
# Tear film dysfunction

Normal tear film
Tear film function during contact lens wear
Signs of tear film dysfunction during contact lens wear
Symptoms
Pathology and aetiology
Treatment
Prognosis
Differential diagnosis

The integrity of the tear film is critical for safe and comfortable contact lens wear. The consequences of a tear film of insufficient quantity or quality include dry eye, lens deposition, reduced vision, tissue damage, infection, poor lens fit and intolerance to lens wear.

The tear film in contact lens wear differs in many ways from the normal, undisturbed tear film. The most obvious difference, from a clinical perspective, is a necessary structural reorganisation, whereby the tears are compartmentalised into the pre-lens tear film and post-lens tear film.

This chapter will consider the key clinically relevant features of the tear film during contact lens wear, and will review important tests of tear film integrity.

## Normal tear film

Appreciation of the structure of the tear film in the contact lens-wearing eye is confounded by the ongoing uncertainty of the structure of the normal tear film. The description of the tear film originally proposed by Wolff,[1] although perhaps simplistic, is regarded as providing the most useful model of tear film structure (Figure 8.1). According to this model, tear film is about 7 μm thick and is composed of an outer lipid layer (approximately 0.1 μm thick), an intermediate aqueous phase (7 μm), and an inner mucus layer (0.05 μm).

Subsequent research has suggested refinements of the original Wolff model and has provided important insights into the

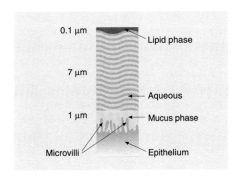

**Figure 8.1**
*Structure of the pre-corneal tear film*

fine structure of the component layers of the tear film. Tiffany[2] accepts the basic structure as outlined by Wolff but argues that the interfaces between the air, lipid, aqueous, mucus and epithelium have their own peculiar physicochemical properties; he thus concludes that tear film should technically be considered as being composed of six layers. Prydal and Campbell[3] suggest that the Wolff model does not take into account the true thickness of the mucus layer and argue that the tear film should be thought of as being 34–45 μm thick, but with the same tri-laminate structure as originally proposed.

More radical theories have been proposed by others. Baier and Thomas[4] argue from a theoretical standpoint (based on the appearance of oil slicks on the ocean as viewed from space) that the structure of the tear film is the reverse of that proposed by Wolff; that is, the outer layer of tear film is a mucinous glycoprotein gel and an inner lipid layer lines the epithelium. Hodson and Earlam[5] suggest that the tear film has no defined structure, but instead is composed of a loose fibronectin gel in which the lipid, mucus and aqueous

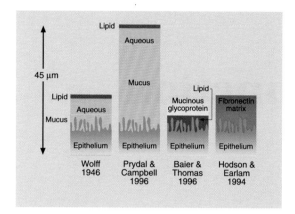

**Figure 8.2**
*Alternative theories of tear film structure*

components are intermixed. Alternative models of tear film structure are illustrated in Figure 8.2.

## Tear film function during contact lens wear

The functions of the tear film during contact lens wear can be described as follows:

- *Optical* – maintaining an optically uniform interface between the air and the anterior surface of the lens.
- *Mechanical* – acting as a vehicle for the continual blink-mediated removal of intrinsic and extrinsic debris and particulate matter from the front of the lens and from beneath the lens.
- *Lubricant* – ensuring a smooth movement of the eyelids over the front surface of the lens, and of the lens over the globe, during blinking.
- *Bacteriocidal* – containing defence mechanisms in the form of proteins, antibodies, phagocytotic cells and other immuno-defense mechanisms that prevent ocular infection.
- *Nutritional* – supplying the corneal epithelium with necessary supplies of oxygen, glucose amino acids and vitamins via the lid-activated tear pump.
- *Waste removal* – acting as an intermediate reservoir for the removal of by-products of metabolism from the cornea, such as carbon dioxide and lactate, that are flushed out from beneath the lens via the lid-activated tear pump.

## Signs of tear film dysfunction during contact lens wear

### General appearance

The most fundamental test that a clinician can apply when investigating tear film dysfunction in a lens wearer is to observe the tear film using a slit-lamp biomicroscope. Similar techniques used for examining the non-lens wearing eye can also be applied to the lens wearing eye. The overall integrity of tears during lens wear can be assessed by observing the general flow of tears over the lens surface following a blink, as indicated by the movement of tear debris. A 'sluggish' movement may indicate an aqueous-deficient, mucus-rich and/or lipid-rich tear film, and the amount of debris provides an indication of the level of contamination of the tears – perhaps, for example, from over-use of cosmetics, A sluggish and/or contaminated tear film is potentially problematic, and could result in increased deposit formation, intermittent blurred vision and discomfort.

### Tear volume

The volume of tears in prospective and current contact lens wearers can be assessed by observing the height of the lower lacrimal tear prism (Figure 8.3). Mainstone *et al*[6] found that measurements of tear meniscus radius of curvature and height correlated well with results of the cotton thread test, non-invasive tear break-up time (NITBUT), and ocular surface staining scores, demonstrating the value of such an assessment in diagnosing dry-eye conditions.

Tear film volume can be measured in the non-lens wearing eye using the Schirmer Test, or the preferred and less invasive

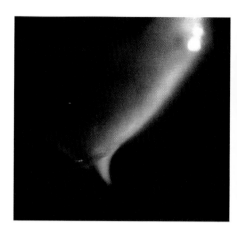

**Figure 8.3**
*Full inferior tear meniscus stained with fluorescein*

cotton-thread tear test. The Schirmer test involves the placement of one end of a strip of filter paper into the lower fornix and measuring the length of paper that becomes wetted over a given time period (Figure 8.4). The greater the length of wetting, the greater the tear volume (assuming that there has been no reflex stimulation).

The cotton-thread test, as adapted by Hamano *et al*,[7] involves impregnating fine cotton threads with the pH-reactive dye phenolsulphophthalein, which turns the thread yellow in air. One end of a cotton thread is looped over the lower lid margin, with one end resting in the lower lid cul-de-sac (Figure 8.5). As a result of a tear-induced shift in pH, the yellow thread turns red as it soaks up the tears. The greater the passage of redness down the thread, the greater the tear

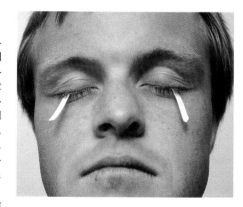

**Figure 8.4**
*Schirmer test*

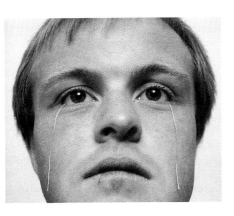

**Figure 8.5**
*Cotton-thread tear test*

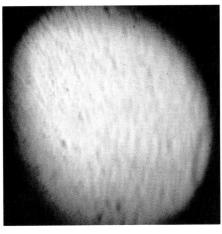

**Figure 8.6**
*Open marmorial lipid formation viewed in specular reflection*

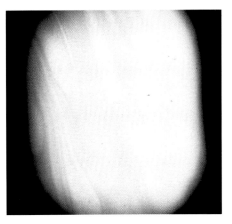

**Figure 8.7**
*Flow pattern lipid formation viewed in specular reflection*

volume (again assuming that there has been no reflex stimulation).

Hamano *et al*[7] applied this test to 1600 asymptomatic PMMA, RGP and HEMA lens wearers, and observed a mean wetting length of 16.9 mm over 15 seconds. This result was no different from that of normal non-lens wearing subjects, suggesting that, from a clinical perspective, contact lenses do not alter tear production in normal subjects.

## Tear film structure and quality

It was established in 1921 that certain structural aspects of the tear film can be assessed clinically by observing the corneal surface in specular reflection.[8] This can be achieved using the slit-lamp biomicroscope by setting the angle of the illumination arm equal to the angle of the microscope arm (say, 30° to the normal) and observing a thin vertical beam at ×30–40 magnification. The limitations of this approach – such as the necessity of using a narrow beam and the generation of heat from the light source – can be overcome by using a wide-field, cold cathode light source, which is available as a hand-held instrument known as a tearscope.[9]

As discussed above, component layers of the tear film are extremely thin. The refractive index differences between the air–lipid and lipid–aqueous boundaries cause destructive interference within the lipid layer resulting in the appearance of coloured fringes, from which can be inferred the thickness of the lipid layer. The aqueous layer of the pre-corneal tear film cannot be observed using this technique because of an insufficient refractive index difference between the aqueous–mucus and mucus–epithelium interfaces.

These coloured fringe patterns, coupled with the general morphological appearance and dynamic characteristics of the lipid layer when viewed in specular reflection, led Guillon and Guillon[9] to devise the following six-category lipid layer classification scheme. The various appearances described below are ranked in order of increasing lipid layer thickness:

- Open marmorial ('marble-like') (13–50 nm thickness; observed in 21 per cent of the population) – grey, marble-like appearance with a sparse open-meshwork pattern; may represent a contraindication for contact lens wear in some patients because the thin lipid layer may lead to rapid evaporative tear loss (Figure 8.6).
- Closed marmorial – (30–50 nm; 10 per cent) – grey, marble-like appearance

with a more compact meshwork pattern; thought to represent a stable lipid layer satisfactory for lens wear.
- Flow pattern – (50–80 nm; 23 per cent) – also termed 'wave pattern', with a pattern of vertical or horizontal grey waves, but constantly flowing and changing between blinks; thought to represent a full lipid layer that is generally satisfactory for contact lens wear (Figure 8.7).
- *Amorphous pattern* – (80–90 nm; 24 per cent) – a more or less even pattern with a whitish, highly reflective appearance; this pattern is thought to represent an ideal, well-mixed lipid layer.
- *First-order colour fringe pattern* – (90–140 nm; 10 per cent) – discrete fringes of brown and blue, superimposed on an amorphous whitish background – thought to represent a full lipid layer (Figure 8.8).
- *Second-order colour fringe pattern* – (140–180 nm; 5 per cent) – discrete fringes of

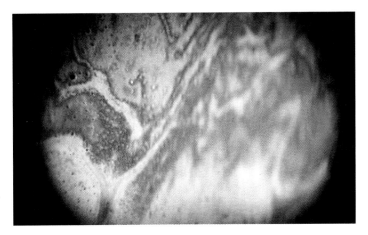

**Figure 8.8**
*First-order colour fringe lipid pattern viewed in specular reflection*

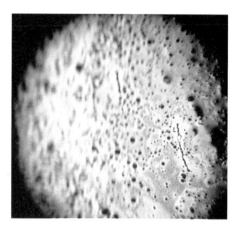

**Figure 8.9**
*Second-order colour fringe lipid pattern viewed in specular reflection*

green and red, superimposed on an amorphous whitish background; thought to represent a full lipid layer that will be problematic for contact lens wear, because an excess lipid coating on the lens can reduce wettability (Figure 8.9).

- *Globular* – (variable thickness; 7 per cent) – highly variable coloured patterns, sometimes forming as globules or pockets of intense fringe formation (Figure 8.10), probably represent heavy lipid contamination and thus may contraindicate contact lens wear.

Although the aqueous phase of the precorneal tear film cannot be observed using a tearscope, it is often visible on the front surface of a contact lens because the pre-lens lipid layer is generally poorly formed or absent. The thicker the pre-lens lipid

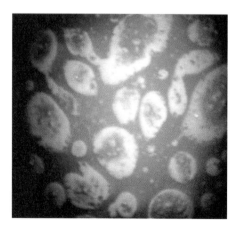

**Figure 8.10**
*Discrete islands of colour fringes, in the form of lipid globules, viewed in specular reflection*

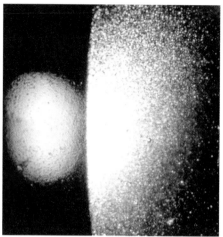

**Figure 8.11**
*Haze on the surface of a high-Dk RGP lens, observed four seconds after a blink*

layer the less visible are the aqueous fringes. When fringes can be observed, it is possible to estimate the thickness of this layer by counting the number across the tearscope field. Less than five fringes indicates an aqueous layer thickness of < 1 μm, and more than 10 fringes indicates an aqueous layer thickness of 2 μm. An aqueous without fringes is probably more than 3.5 μm thick.

Using a tearscope, Young and Efron[10] evaluated the structure of the tear film on the surface of a range of hydrogel lenses of various water contents. They observed that the lipid layer was either absent or thin on all lenses, although there was a tendency for higher water content lenses to support a thin lipid layer. The aqueous phase was generally found to be thicker on lenses of higher water content.

As with hydrogel lenses, the lipid layer is extremely thin or absent on the surface of RGP lenses.[11] The aqueous phase over such lenses is also thin, typically between 2 and 3 μm thick; this variation in thickness is thought to be patient-dependent. A poorly wetting hydrophobic surface of an RGP lens takes on a hazy appearance if the surface is allowed to dry (Figure 8.11). The haziness is thought to be due to a rapidly drying mucoprotein coating.

**Tear film stability**
The structural integrity of the pre-lens tear film can be assessed by measuring the time elapsed from the execution of a normal blink until the tear film breaks up; this is

known as the tear break-up time (TBUT). The classical method of measuring TBUT, by instilling fluorescein into the eye and observing the break-up of the fluorescein pattern, cannot be applied to the contact lens-wearing eye because fluorescein will be absorbed into the lens, thus discolouring (and perhaps destroying) the lens and confounding the estimated time of break-up. In addition, fluorescein is known to destabilise the tear film.

Non-invasive techniques are preferred for measuring break-up of the pre-ocular and pre-lens tear film.[12] A black and white grid in an illuminated hemispherical dome can be optically projected on to the eye and observed (Figure 8.12); the time taken for the reflected grid to begin breaking up is referred to as the non-invasive tear break-up time (NITBUT) (Figure 8.13). When contact lenses are being worn, the pre-lens tear film non-invasive break-up time (PLTF NITBUT) is recorded.

In the non-lens wearing eye, the tear film remains stable for at least 30 seconds. In many patients NITBUT may be considerably greater than this but such measurements are not possible because few patients can voluntarily refrain from blinking for periods longer than 30 seconds. Young and Efron[10] demonstrated that tear break-up occurs within 3–10 seconds on the front surface of hydrogel lenses, and that longer PLTF NITBUTs were generally associated with higher water content lenses. This latter finding is consistent with the thicker aqueous layer present on higher water content lenses observed by Young and Efron[10] in the same study. The PLTF NITBUT of rigid lenses typically ranges from 4 to 6 seconds.[13]

**Ocular surface staining**
Tissue disruption to the surface of the cornea and conjunctiva can occur during contact lens wear as a consequence of disruption of the tear layer. This can be readily detected by instilling fluorescein and observing the eye in cobalt blue light on a slit-lamp biomicroscope. Perhaps the most common manifestation of this problem in patients wearing rigid lenses is 3 and 9 o'clock staining. This is a form of desiccation staining, which may also be observed in association with soft lens wear, particularly in regions where the cornea has become intermittently exposed, or in regions of the cornea where the overlying lens has become dehydrated.

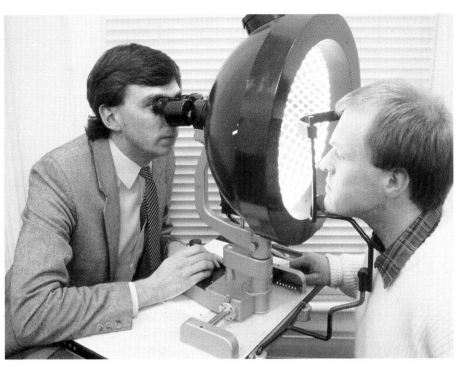

**Figure 8.12**
*System for projecting a grid on to the eye for measuring NITBUT*

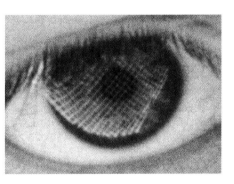

**Figure 8.13**
*Reflection of grid on the ocular surface*

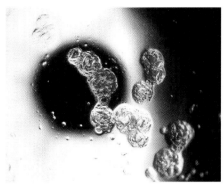

**Figure 8.14**
*'Jelly bumps' on a soft lens*

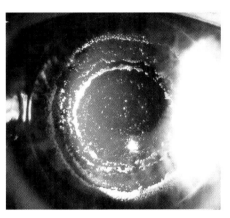

**Figure 8.15**
*Calcium ring deposits on a soft lens*

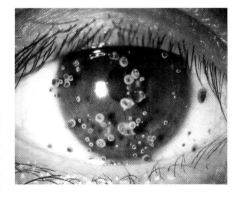

**Figure 8.16**
*Iron deposits on a soft lens*

## Lens deposits

Numerous factors, many of which are inter-active, are involved in the formation of deposits on the front or back surface of contact lenses. These factors include lens wear modality, replacement frequency, bulk chemical composition, water content, physicochemical nature of the lens surface (such as ionicity), chemical composition of lens maintenance solutions, adequacy of lens maintenance procedures (a measure of patient compliance), hand contamination, proximity to environmental pollutants, and intrinsic properties of the patient's tears. The most common tear-derived components of lens deposits are proteins, lipids and calcium.

Visible lens deposits take months or years to form, and are thus rarely encountered in modern contact lens practice as lenses (particularly soft lenses) are disposed of and replaced regularly. The most common form of visible deposition derived from the tear film is known as 'jelly bumps' or 'mulberry deposits'. These consist of various layered combinations of mucus, lipid, protein, and sometimes calcium (Figure 8.14). Barnacle-like calcium carbonate deposits, also derived from the tear film, can project anteriorly and be a source of discomfort (Figure 8.15). Iron deposits, derived from exogenous sources, appear as small red–orange spots or rings and form when iron particles become embedded in the lens and oxidise to form ferrous salts (Figure 8.16).

It is clear that proteins and lipids from tears can deposit on contact lenses within minutes of insertion. Although these rapidly forming deposits cannot be seen and do not generally compromise vision or comfort, they can reduce lens surface wettability.[14]

Both tear quality and composition have a bearing on deposit formation. An excess of a particular tear component, coupled with compromised structural integrity of the tears leading to rapid tear break-up and excessive surface drying, are factors thought to be conducive to deposit formation. Indeed, there is some clinical evidence to support the notion that lens deposition is a particular problem in dry-eye patients wearing contact lenses.[15]

### Post-lens tear film thinning

The tear film between a contact lens and the cornea can be viewed with a slit-lamp biomicroscope.[16] As for the pre-lens tear film, the thickness of the post-lens tear film can be inferred from the appearance of the specular reflection; an amorphous appearance indicates a relatively thick, aqueous film, and coloured patterns and striated formations (texture without colour) indicate thinner tear films (Figure 8.17). Patterned appearances occur in 25 per cent of soft lens wearers, irrespective of lens type, and are associated with reduced lens movement.[16]

## Symptoms

Of all the symptoms experienced by contact lens wearers, that of 'dryness' is reported most frequently.[17,18] Indeed, in one survey of over 100 contact lens wearers[18] only 25 per cent reported never having experienced this symptom. Brennan and Efron[18] reported that, in a group of contact lens

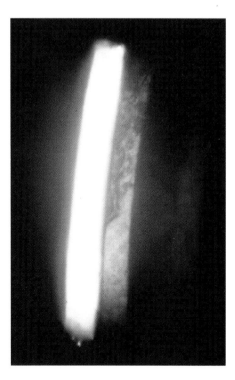

**Figure 8.17**
*Colour fringe patterns in the post-lens tear film observed in specular reflection*

wearers, all the females using oral contraceptives reported experiencing 'dryness' at times, versus 63 per cent of females not using oral contraceptives and 76 per cent of males. These differences were statistically significant.

A major difficulty in assessing the symptom of 'dryness' is that there may be many stimuli that elicit this sensation; that is, it cannot be assumed that 'dryness' is due to the eye being dry. Because there are no specific 'dryness receptors' in human tissue, ocular dryness must be a response to specific coding of afferent neural inputs. Aside from an actual dry eye, reports of 'dryness' may arise from the neural misinterpretation of stimuli that are unrelated to dry eye, such as vasodilatation induced by mechanical irritation of ocular tissues by the lens. Lowther[19] reported a more rapid tear break-up (lower TBUT) in a group of contact lens wearers with dry-eye symptoms versus a group of contact lens wearers without dry-eye symptoms, but Bruce *et al*[19] failed to demonstrate such an association in a similar experiment. Little and Bruce[15] found no relationship between post-lens tear film morphology and hydrogel lens comfort.

A prudent approach in dealing with a tentative diagnosis of contact lens-induced dry-eye is to apply a comprehensive questionnaire[17] that draws in other systemic correlates of dryness, such as dryness of other mucous membranes of the body, use of medications, effect of different challenging environments, and times when dryness is noted. Such questionnaires are time-consuming, although they can be conducted by ancillary staff. Dry-eye questionnaires can help identify a true dry-eye situation in prospective or current contact lens wearers and thus form a clinical rationale for more detailed assessment.

## Pathology and aetiology

Alterations to tear chemistry, composition and structure may be responsible for various adverse signs and symptoms during contact lens wear. Certain aspects of tear physiology during lens wear have been explored through the development and application of existing and experimental methodologies. The results of some of these tests, which have more immediate clinical relevance, will be reviewed here.

### Tonicity

Immediately after the insertion of either rigid[21] or soft[22] lenses, reflex tearing creates a hypo-osmotic tear film that returns to normal or to slightly hyperosmotic levels once adaptation is complete. Martin[22] observed symmetric binocular changes in tear osmolarity during monocular lens wear, suggesting that bilateral reflex lacrimation is responsible for post-lens insertion changes in tear tonicity.

In adapted patients, daily rigid lens wear and extended soft lens wear are associated with elevated levels of tear osmolarity, whereas tear osmolarity is normal in adapted daily soft lens wear.[23] Three mechanisms could explain these hyperosmotic shifts: (a) reduced tear stimulation due to reduced corneal sensitivity, (b) increased lens-induced tear evaporation, or (c) leaching of deposits from the lens into the tears.

### Acid–base balance (pH)

Theoretically an acidic shift in tear pH might be expected with contact lens wear due to a retardation by the lens of the normal carbon dioxide efflux into the atmosphere; the carbon dioxide would then dissolve in the tears and reduce to carbonic acid, inducing an acidic pH shift.

Although Norn[24] reported that all lens types induce an acidic pH shift during lens wear, other studies have failed to arrive at a consensus on the direction of the pH shift (if any). Tapasztó *et al*[25] observed an acidic shift during rigid lens wear, but Carney and Hill[26] found no such change. With soft lenses, various authors have reported acidic shifts,[27] alkaline shifts,[28] and no shifts in pH.[25] Carney *et al*[29] reported that the buffering capacity of tears (i.e. the intrinsic capacity of tears to dampen down pH change) is unaffected by lens wear.

### Composition

Contact lenses only appear to alter the composition of tears during the adaptation phase of lens wear. When lenses are worn for the first time, the increased reflex lacrimation tends to dilute the concentration of those components of the tears that are not secreted from the lacrimal gland (i.e. serum-derived components). This phenomenon is particularly evident during adaptation to rigid lenses, which induce a more intense lacrimation response. Tear components that display increased levels during adaptation, but not during subsequent adapted lens wear, include serum-derived proteins (such as albumin, IgG and trans-ferrin), sodium, chloride, potassium and cholesterol.

Certain components of tears alter during inflammation, metabolic stress and mechanical trauma, and in many cases these changes are linked to contact lens wear. For example, Vinding *et al*[30] reported decreased tear concentrations of secretory IgA in long-term wearers of daily wear and extended wear soft contact lenses, a finding thought to indicate a higher prevalence of subclinical corneal and conjunctival inflammation in such patients. Fullard and Carney[31] noted an increase in the ratio of lactate dehydrogen-ase (LDH) to malate dehydrogenase (MDH) during soft lens wear, and Imayasu *et al*[32] observed increased LDH levels in the tears of rabbits fitted with contact lenses of low oxygen transmissibility; these findings are consistent with the known anaerobic shift in the corneal epithelium due to hypoxia during lens wear.

When a small sample of tears is taken from the eye and allowed to dry on a micro-scope slide, fern-like crystallisation pat-terns may form which indicate certain characteristics of the tear film, including the salt-to-macromolecule ratio, lipid con-tamination of mucus and altered tear rheology.[33] A well-structured ferning pat-tern (Figure 8.18) represents a good or even excessive supply of mucus, whereas a disrupted pattern with few or absent ferns (Figure 8.19) may indicate mucus defi-ciency. Kogbe and Liotet[34] have recom-mended that the tear ferning test be used in contact lens practice to diagnose marginal dry-eye as the cause of contact lens intoler-ance. However, such an approach requires further clinical validation.

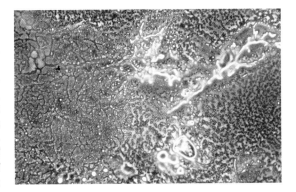

**Figure 8.19**
*Tear sample displaying an absence of ferning*

### Temperature

Morgan *et al*[35] have demonstrated how infra-red ocular thermography can provide a measure of the thickness of the tear film overlying the cornea. Soh[36] has adapted this technique to explore the apparent tempera-ture of the tear film on the surface of rigid contact lenses. Figure 8.20 is a thermogram of an eye wearing a rigid lens. Warmer colours appear red and cooler colours blue. Lower temperatures (blue) are thought to indicate a thinner tear film.[35] Thinning is evident towards the inferior of the lens, which is where tear break-up would be expected to occur first. Martin and Fatt[37] demonstrated that contact lens wear induces a small increase in the temperature of the post-lens tear film.

### Tear film turnover

The turnover rate of the tear film is about 16 per cent of the total tear volume per minute.[38] The main determinants of tear turnover are aqueous tear production – pri-marily from the main lacrimal gland – and tear loss via drainage and/or evaporation. Tear turnover rate can be determined by measuring the decay over time of the fluor-escence of tears that have been stained with fluorescein. Such studies have failed to detect any contact lens-induced change in tear production, except during the initial adaptation phase where increased lacrimation is observed. Tomlinson and Cedarstaff[39] found that tear evaporation is increased during wear of all contact lens types. This is presumably due to a compro-mise of the integrity of the lipid layer of the tear film during lens wear.

### Tear break-up

The precise mechanism leading to tear film break-up is not known. The most popular theory is that advanced by Holly.[40] Accord-ing to his theory, tear break-up occurs

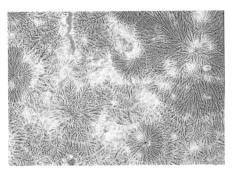

**Figure 8.18**
*Well structured tear ferning pattern*

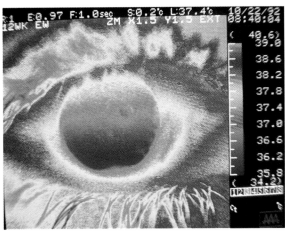

**Figure 8.20**
*Ocular thermogram presumably showing tear thinning on the inferior portion of a rigid lens*

68 ■ *Tear Film*

when lipid, which is hydrophobic in nature, migrates down to the mucus layer and compromises the hydrophilicity of the epithelial surface. Tears recede from this region of poor wettability and a dry spot forms. As the tears continue to recede, there is further intermixing of lipid and mucus at the receding edge, and the field of hydrophilicity increases, thus increasing the dry area – and the process continues. Alternative theories propose that tear break-up is due to rupture of the mucus layer[41] or disturbance of the superficial epithelial glycocalyx.[42]

Figure 8.21 is an illustration of the clinical appearance of the thinning and breaking up of the tear film using a projected grid, together with a schematic representation of the process of disruption of the tear film according to the model of Holly.[40]

The mechanism of tear break-up on the surface of contact lenses must be different from that on the surface of the eye because of the absence of properly formed lipid or mucus layers on the lens surface. Rapid pre-lens tear break-up times[10] suggest that tear thinning occurs as a result of evaporation and lateral surface tension forces that draw tear fluid from the lens surface into the surrounding tear meniscus at the lens edge. Tear break-up is likely to be expedited by the presence of surface deposition.

## Treatment

Most of the strategies applied to alleviating signs and symptoms of dry eye of the non-lens wearing eye can also be applied to the eye during contact lens wear. This section will review these strategies, with particular emphasis on their application in contact lens wear.

### Choice of lens and solution

The most fundamental choice to make when attempting to solve a contact lens-related dry eye problem is whether to fit soft or rigid lenses. This choice will depend on a number of factors, such as the precise nature of the problem. For example, rigid lens-induced 3 and 9 o'clock staining can be solved by changing the patient from rigid to soft lenses, to prevent epithelial drying at the 3 and 9 o'clock positions. Problems related to surface drying with a low water content soft lens can be solved by fitting a lens of higher water content, which will have a longer TBUT.[10]

Efron and Brennan[43] demonstrated that patients wearing soft lenses were more likely to complain of 'dryness' the more the lens has dehydrated. Not withstanding uncertainty as to the pathophysiological meaning of the subjective complaint of dry-

ness, as discussed above, this finding suggests that, for a given category of material, patients will be most comfortable wearing a lens that dehydrates the least. Research to date has failed to reveal the material characteristics that determine lens dehydration in-eye, so practitioners must rely on comparative date published in the literature.[44] Frequent lens replacement is also desirable because the pre-lens tear film will more readily break up in the presence of lens surface contamination.

As a general rule, the characteristics of a contact lens that is most suited for a patient experiencing dry-eye problems is as follows:

- a soft lens – for full corneal coverage;
- a high water content lens – to maximise the volume of water in front of the lens;
- a lens that displays minimal in-eye dehydration – to prevent ocular surface desiccation; and
- a lens that is replaced frequently – for optimal, deposit-free surface characteristics.

Discomfort and symptoms of dryness are usually associated with the use of solutions containing early generation preservatives such as thimerosal and chlorhexidine. Changing to a solution system that contains new-generation large molecular weight preservatives, or one that contains no preservatives, will typically solve solution-related problems. The use of solutions containing re-wetting or lubrication agents will also help alleviate dry-eye symptoms.

### Re-wetting drops

A commonly used strategy in the management of contact-lens related dry eye is to supplement the tear film with viscous substitutes and gels. The most popular form of delivery of these agents is via the periodic instillation of rewetting drops; alternative delivery systems include ointments and inserts (solid pellets that dissolve slowly over time). Golding et al[45] found that rewetting drops improve pre-lens tear film stability for a period of only 5 minutes following instillation, and that saline performs no differently from specially formulated products containing viscoelastic lubrication agents. The same authors[46] also found that saline drops provide short-term symptomatic relief that is indistinguishable from that of re-wetting drops. None of these solutions was found to

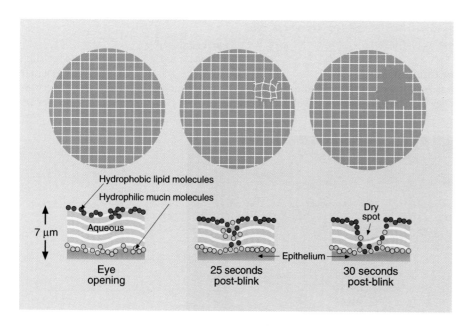

**Figure 8.21**
*Schematic representation of the intact tear film observed at eye opening (left), followed by tear thinning at 25 secs (middle) and tear break-up at 30 secs (right). The top row illustrates this sequence as observed using a projected grid (NITBUT measurement). The bottom row illustrates how a dry spot forms*

reduce lens dehydration. From these studies it can be surmised that there is a psychological rather than a physical or physiological basis for the perception of long-term symptomatic relief (i.e. enhanced comfort for greater than 5 minutes) provided by saline or re-wetting drops.

Caffrey and Josephson[47] evaluated the performance of 10 different commercially available re-wetting drops and found little difference between them, except that non-preserved solutions were preferred to those containing preservatives.

### Soft lens soaking

Based upon the observation of Efron and Brennan[43] that lens dehydration leads to complaints of dryness, it stands to reason that removal of the lens from the eye and re-hydration in saline solution can redress the problem. Although such a procedure has yet to be experimentally validated, Lowther[48] has advocated that patients be advised to adopt the following soaking procedure if lens-related symptoms of dryness occur: first, remove the lens; second, soak in unit-dose preservative-free saline in the palm of the hand for 10 to 20 seconds, and third, reinsert the lens.

### Nutritional supplements

Some researchers[49,50] have suggested that systemic malnutrition, and consequent malnutrition of the tear film and ocular surface, can be a source of dry-eye problems. While it is clear that gross Vitamin A deficiency can cause serious disease of the ocular surface, there is no evidence that Vitamin A drops, or indeed other such nutritional supplements, can alleviate contact lens-related dry-eye problems. Of interest, however, is the recent claim of Patel *et al*[50] that pre-corneal tear film stability can be enhanced by systemic ingestion of vitamin and trace element dietary supplements.

### Control of evaporation

Various approaches to reducing tear evaporation in patients suffering from contact lens-related dry-eye symptoms can be adopted. One strategy is to modify the local environment around the eye. This can be achieved by having the patient wear spectacles with a tightly fitting side-shield. The use of tightly fitting swimming goggles represents a more extreme treatment. Clearly, such approaches will be rejected by most contact lens wearers because the very reason they are wearing contact lenses is to avoid wearing spectacles. Alternatively, the use of a room humidifier may provide some relief.

Patients can be given the following advice about the environment in which they are spending most of their time:

- air conditioners tend to have a dehumidifying effect on the local atmosphere;
- the environment in aeroplanes is generally of low humidity; and
- certain regions of the world have a temperature–humidity relationship that results in a low atmospheric water vapour pressure, which in turn is conducive to rapid lens dehydration. To assist practitioners in offering appropriate advice in this regard, Fatt and Rocher[51] tabulated the time of year when patients could be expected to experience dryness problems related to lens dehydration in various cities throughout the world.

### Reduction of tear drainage

Tear volume can be preserved by blocking the puncta with punctal plugs. Lowther and Semes[52] inserted temporary dissolvable collagen plugs into one eye of 32 soft lens patients with dry-eye problems and conducted a 'sham' procedure in the other eye. They found improvement in both the plugged eye and the control eye, demonstrating a powerful placebo effect, and suggested that dissolvable implants were not effective as a provocative test of the efficacy of permanent punctal plugs.

Giovagnoli and Graham[53] reported that symptomatic soft lens patients enjoyed a 35 per cent increase in comfortable wearing time after insertion of permanent punctal plugs into the lower puncta. This finding suggests that punctal plugs are a viable alternative in contact lens patients suffering from discomfort due to tear insufficiency.

### Tear stimulants

Pharmacological stimulation of residual tear function is a relatively new approach for treating dry-eye related problems. A variety of agents that can enhance basal lacrimal secretion, such as pilocarpine, 3-isobutyl-1-methylxanthine, eledoisis, bromhexine and cyclosporin A, have been investigated for possible commercial development.[54] Some of these substances are administered topically, and some systemically. Further research is required to determine whether such an approach will be of benefit to symptomatic contact lens wearers.

### Management of associated disease

It is beyond the scope of this chapter to review all of the possible disease states that can adversely affect the tear film, except to say that practitioners need to be alert to the various possibilities. Perhaps the most common ocular disease state in contact lens wearers associated with lens dryness is meibomian gland dysfunction (see Chapter 3). Severe blockage of the meibomian gland orifices can result in a lipid deficiency in the tear film, leading to a more rapid tear loss. Abnormal lipid may also be secreted from diseased meibomian glands, leading to lipid deposition on lenses that can result in intermittent blurred vision and discomfort. Treatment strategies such as warm compresses, lid scrubs and mechanical expression can be applied to alleviate this condition.

### Bandage lenses

It may seem paradoxical to be considering the prescription of soft contact lenses for patients with intractable dry-eye problems in a review of problems associated with, or induced by, contact lenses. However, it is clear that patients with severe aqueous deficiency can benefit from bandage lenses. The best type of lens is one with characteristics described previously (see 'Choice of lens and solution'). It may also be necessary to supplement bandage lenses with re-wetting drops. Rigorous aftercare monitoring of patients wearing bandage lenses is essential in view of the known increase in susceptibility to corneal ulceration in such patients because of the underlying disease state.[55]

### Reduced wearing time or cessation of lens wear

Symptoms of dryness typically become worse throughout the daytime wearing period to the point where the lenses are so uncomfortable that they are removed; indeed, discomfort due to dryness is often the limiting factor in determining maximum lens wearing time. If all other strategies to alleviate extreme dryness fail, then the only advice, albeit unsatisfactory, that can be offered to patients is that the strategy that they have already been forced to adopt – that of reducing lens wearing time – is both the problem itself and the solution to the problem.

The ultimate sanction in the management of intractable contact lens-related tear film dysfunction is to advise the patient to cease lens wear. In such cases, refractive surgery may provide a suitable solution.

## Prognosis

The prognosis for recovery from tear film dysfunction related to contact lens wear will depend on the specific cause of the problem. If the symptoms relate to the wearing of inappropriate lenses or the use of unsuitable solutions, then the prognosis may be good if the right lens and/or solution can be found. Similarly, a good prognosis can be advised if the problem is due to an associated disease state that can be managed successfully – for example meibomian gland dysfunction. In cases where the underlying cause is difficult to treat – such as aqueous deficiency due to keratoconjunctivitis sicca – the prognosis is poor, although further research into new strategies such as the clinical application of tear stimulating agents[54] does hold future promise of a better prognosis for some patients.

An additional consideration of prognostic interest is whether the tear film is disrupted following lens removal, and if so, how long it takes before tear film returns to normal. This question was addressed by Kline and DeLuca,[56] who documented a 54 per cent decrease in TBUT measured within 10 minutes of removal of a hydrogel lens (compared with pre-fitting estimates of TBUT). Faber *et al*[57] made a similar observation, and noted that the TBUT had recovered within 25 minutes of lens removal. Thus, lens-induced disruption to the precorneal tear film is short-lived following lens removal.

## Differential diagnosis

As has already been discussed, practitioners need to be alert to the myriad of associated disease states that can occur concurrently with contact lens wear so that these can be differentiated from conditions due to the contact lens alone. Differential diagnosis between contact lens-associated tear film dysfunction versus tear film dysfunction due to associated disease can be effected by ceasing lens wear for one month; if problematic signs and symptoms persist for this period, then it is unlikely that contact lenses are the cause of the problem.

Albietz and Golding[58] have classified the various non-lens related dry-eye subtypes, which are listed below together with common causes and prevalence (shown in parentheses):

- *Aqueous tear deficiency* – due to lacrimal gland dysfunction (0.5–3.0 per cent).
- *Lipid anomaly* – due to meibomian gland dysfunction (40 per cent).
- *Lid surfacing anomalies* – due to eyelid or blinking dysfunction (1.5–3.0 per cent).
- *Mucus deficiency* – due to conjunctival goblet cell disorder (rare).
- *Primary epitheliopathy* – due to epithelial disorder (rare).
- *Allergic dry eye* – due to non-goblet epithelial cell disorder (unknown).

Attempts should, of course, be made to treat associated ocular pathology that is identified as a possible cause of dry-eye symptoms in a contact lens wearer. Whether or not the associated pathology is cured completely, the practitioner will be in a much better position to devise a viable management plan and to formulate an accurate prognosis for ongoing contact lens wear success.

## REFERENCES

1 Wolff E (1946) The muco-cutaneous junction of the lid margin and the distribution of the tear fluid. *Trans Ophthalmol Soc UK* **66**: 291.

2 Tiffany JM (1988) Tear film stability and contact lens wear. *J Br Contact Lens Assoc* **11**: 35.

3 Prydal JI, Campbell FW (1992) Study of precorneal tear film thickness and structure by interferometry and confocal microscopy. *Invest Ophthalmol Vis Sci* **33**: 1996.

4 Baier RE, Thomas EB (1996) The ocean: the eye of earth. *Contact Lens Spectrum* **11**: 37.

5 Hodson S, Earlam R (1994) Of an extracellular matrix in human pre-corneal tear film. *J Theor Biol* **168**: 395.

6 Mainstone JC, Bruce AS, Golding TR (1996) Tear meniscus measurements in the diagnosis of dry eye. *Curr Eye Res,* **15**: 653.

7 Hamano H, Hori M, Hamano T (1983) A new method for measuring tears. *Contact Lens Assoc Ophthalmol J*, **9**: 281.

8 Koby ES (1924) *Microscopie de l'Oeil vivant.* Paris, Masson et Cie p. 47.

9 Guillon JP (1998) Non-invasive Tearscope plus routine for contact lens fitting. *Contact Lens Ant Eye* **21**: S31.

10 Young G, Efron N (1991) Characteristics of the pre-lens tear film during hydrogel contact lens wear. *Ophthal Physiol Opt* **11**: 53.

11 Guillon M, Guillon JP, Mapstone V (1989) Rigid gas permeable lenses in vivo wettability. *Trans Br Contact Lens Assoc* Conference Proceedings: 24.

12 Mengher LS, Bron AJ, Tonge SR (1985) A non-invasive instrument for clinical assessment of the pre corneal tear film stability. *Curr Eye Res* **4**: 1.

13 Guillon M, Guillon JP (1988) Pre-lens tear film characteristics of high Dk rigid gas permeable lenses. *Am J Optom Physiol Opt* **65**: 73.

14 Jones L, Franklin V, Evans K (1996) Spoliation and clinical performance of monthly vs three monthly group II disposable contact lenses. *Optom Vis Sci* **73**: 16.

15 Dougman DJ (1975) The nature of 'spots' on soft lenses. *Ann Ophthalmol* **7**: 345.

16 Little SA, Bruce AS (1994) Postlens tear film morphology, lens movement and symptoms in hydrogel lens wearers. *Ophthal Physiol Opt* **14**: 65.

17 McMonnies CW, Ho A (1986) Marginal dry eye diagnosis: history versus biomicroscopy. In: *The Pre-ocular Tear Film in Health, Disease and Contact Lens Wear* (ed. FJ Holly). Dry Eye Institute. Lubbock, Texas.

18 Brennan NA, and Efron N (1989) Symptomatology of HEMA contact lens wear. *Optom Vis Sci* **66**: 834.

19 Lowther GE (1993) Comparison of hydrogel contact lens patients with and without the symptoms of dryness. *Int Contact Lens Clin* **20**: 191.

20 Bruce AS, Golding TR, Au SWM (1995) Mechanisms of dryness in soft lens wear. *Clin Exp Optom* **78**: 168.

21 Terry JE, Hill RM (1977) Osmotic adaptation to rigid contact lenses. *Arch Ophthalmol* **37**: 785.

22 Martin DK (1987) Osmolality of the tear fluid in the contralateral eye during monocular contact lens wear. *Acta Ophthalmol* **65**: 551.

23 Farris RL, Stuchell RN, Mandel ID (1981) Basal and reflex human tear analysis. 1. Physical measurements: osmolarity, basal volumes, and reflex flow rate. *Ophthalmology* **88**: 852.

24 Norn MS (1988) Tear fluid pH in normals, contact lens wearers and pathological cases. *Acta Ophthalmol* **66**: 485.

25 Tapasztó I, Koller A, Tapasztó Z (1988) Biochemical changes in the human tears of hard and soft contact lens wearers. II. The pH variations in the human tears of hard and soft contact lens wearers. *Contact Lens J* **16**: 265.

26 Carney LG, Hill RM (1976) Tear pH and the hard contact lens patient. *Int Contact Lens Clin* **3**: 27.

27 Hill RM, Carney LG (1977) Tear pH and the soft contact lens patient. *Int Contact Lens Clin* **4**: 68.

28 Andrés S, Garcia ML, Espina M (1990) Tear pH, air pollution, and contact lenses. *Am J Optom Physiol Opt* **65**: 627.

29 Carney LG, Mauger TF, Hill RM (1990) Tear buffering in contact lens wearers. *Acta Ophthalmol* **68**: 75.

30 Vinding T, Eriksen JS, Nielsen NV (1987) The concentration of lysozyme and secretory IgA in tears from healthy persons with and without contact lens use. *Acta Ophthalmol* **65**: 23.

31 Fullard RJ, Carney LG (1986) Use of tear enzyme activities to assess the corneal response to contact lens wear. *Acta Ophthalmol* **64**: 216.

32 Imayasu M, Petroll M, Jester JV (1994) The relationship between contact lens oxygen transmissibility and binding of pseudomonas aeruginosa to the cornea after overnight wear. *Ophthalmology* **101**: 371.

33 Golding TR, Brennan NA (1989) The basis of tear ferning. *Clin Exp Optom* **72**: 102.

34 Kogbe O, Liotet S (1987) An interesting use of the study of tear ferning patterns in contactology. *Ophthalmologica* **194**: 150.

35 Morgan PB, Tullo AB, Efron N (1995) Infrared thermography of the tear film in dry eye. *Eye* **9**: 615.

36 Soh MP (1994) Infrared thermography of the anterior eye during contact lens wear. PhD thesis, University of Manchester.

37 Martin D, Fatt I (1986) The presence of a contact lens induces a very small increase in the anterior corneal surface temperature. *Acta Ophthalmol* **64**: 512.

38 Puffer MJ, Neault RW, Brubaker RF (1980) Precorneal tear turnover in the human eye. *Am J Ophthalmol* **89**: 369.

39 Tomlinson A, Cedarstaff TH (1982) Tear evaporation from the human eye: the effects of contact lens wear. *J Br Contact Lens Assoc* **5**: 141.

40 Holly FJ (1973) Formation and rupture of the tear film. *Exp Eye Res* **15**: 515.

41 Sharma A, Ruckenstein E (1985) Mechanism of tear film rupture and its implications for contact lens tolerance. *Am J Optom Physiol Opt* **62**: 246.

42 Liotet S (1987) A new hypothesis on tear film stability. *Ophthalmologica* **195**: 119.

43 Efron N, Brennan NA (1988) A survey of wearers of low water content hydrogel contact lenses. *Clin Exp Optom* **71**: 86.

44 Brennan NA, Efron N (1987) Hydrogel lens dehydration: a material dependent phenomenon? *Contact Lens Forum* **12**: 28.

45 Golding TR, Brennan NA, Efron N (1990) Soft lens lubricants and prelens tear film stability. *Optom Vis Sci* **67**: 461.

46 Efron N, Golding TR, Brennan NA (1991) The effect of soft lens lubricants on symptoms and lens dehydration. *Contact Lens Assoc Ophthalmol J* **17**: 114.

47 Caffrey BE, Josephson JE (1990) Is there a better 'comfort drop'? *J Am Optom Assoc* **61**: 178.

48 Lowther GE (1997) *Dryness, Tears and Contact Lens Wear*. Boston, Butterworth–Heinemann, p. 56.

49 Caffrey BE (1991) Influence of diet on tear function. *Optom Vis Sci* **68**: 58.

50 Patel S, Ferrier C, Plaskow J (1994) Effect of systemic ingestion of vitamin and trace element dietary supplements on the stability of the pre-corneal tear film in normal subjects. In: *Lacrimal Gland, Tear Flim and Dry Eye Syndromes* (ed. DA Sullivan). New York: Plenum Press.

51 Fatt I, Rocher P (1994) Contact lens performance in different climates. *Optom Today* **34**: 26.

52 Lowther GE, Semes L (1995) Effect of absorbable intracanalicular collagen implants in hydrogel contact lens patients with drying symptoms. *Int Contact Lens Clin* **22**: 238.

53 Giovagnoli D, Graham SJ (1992) Inferior punctal occlusion with removable punctal plugs in treatment of dry-eye related contact lens discomfort. *J Am Optom Asso* **63**: 481.

54 Bron A, Hornby S, Tiffany J (1997) The management of dry eye. *Optician* **214** (5613): 13.

55 Dohlman CH, Bouchoff SA, Mobilia EE (1973) Complications in use of soft contact lenses in corneal disease. *Arch Ophthalmol*, **90**: 367.

56 Kline LN, DeLuca TJ (1975) Effect of gel lens wear on the precorneal tear film. *Int Contact Lens Clin* **2**: 56.

57 Faber E, Golding TR, Lowe R (1991) Effect of hydrogel lens wear on tear film stability. *Optom Vis Sci* **68**: 380.

58 Albietz JM, Golding TR (1994) Differential diagnosis and management of common dry eye subtypes. *Clin Exp Optom* **77**: 244.

# Part IV
# Corneal Epithelium

# 9
# Staining

Prevalence
Signs and symptoms
Pathology
Aetiology
Observation and grading
Management and treatment
Prognosis
Differential diagnosis

The use of fluorescein in the examination of corneal integrity was introduced by Pflüger[1] in 1882, just six years before the first fitting of contact lenses to humans was reported by Fick.[2] However, it is only in the past 25 years that fluorescein has been used routinely by clinicians for this purpose.[3]

Corneal staining is probably the most familiar of all potential contact lens complications since its clinical importance is well established and it is easily observed.

Strictly speaking, corneal staining is not a condition in itself – rather, it is a general term that refers to the appearance of tissue disruption and other pathophysiological changes in the anterior eye as revealed with the aid of one or more of a number of dyes, such as fluorescein, rose bengal or alcian blue. These dyes are sometimes referred to as 'vital stains', which suggests that they stain living things; however, this is a misleading term because such stains can be taken up by dead cells and even inorganic material.[4]

It has become a convention among clinicians to use the term 'corneal staining' or 'epithelial staining' to describe the appearance of bright areas of fluorescence in the

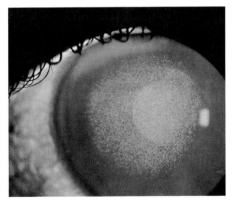

**Figure 9.1**
*Superficial punctate epithelial keratopathy*

epithelium following instillation of the dye fluorescein and illumination with cobalt blue light (Figure 9.1). Throughout this chapter, 'staining' refers to staining with fluorescein, unless otherwise stated.

## Prevalence

The prevalence of corneal staining of any

degree of severity in a population of contact lens wearers is thought to be as high as 60 per cent,[5] but often staining is of a low level and generally clinically insignificant. Indeed, corneal staining is frequently observed in non-lens wearers.[5,6]

In perhaps the largest survey ever undertaken of the ocular response to contact lens wear (66, 218 patients), Hamano *et al*[7] determined the prevalence of clinically significant staining (corneal erosion or superficial punctate keratitis greater than grade 2; see below) to be 0.9 per cent in soft lens wearers, 0.5 per cent in RGP lens wearers, and 1.3 per cent in PMMA lens wearers.

## Signs and symptoms

### Use of fluorescein
Fluorescein is combined with sodium salt to make it more soluble in water.[8] Although it is available as a 2 per cent solution, fluorescein is rarely used in this form because it supports the growth of bacteria that are potentially pathogenic to the eye, such as *Pseudomonas aeruginosa*.[9] Therefore, paper strips impregnated with fluorescein are

preferred; these strips have an orange-yellow colour. Fluorescein can be instilled by wetting the strip with two drops of sterile unpreserved saline, having the patient look up, and gently touching the strip on the inferior bulbar conjunctiva.

When examining a fluorescein-stained eye, it is important to prompt the patient to blink frequently. If the patient blinks infrequently, the tear film will break up leaving large dark areas of non-fluorescence which could mask true staining, or be misinterpreted as non-staining background fluorescence. Fluorescein break-up in the absence of blinking is the basis of an important test of tear film stability.[10]

Because fluorescein has a molecular weight of 376 it is smaller than the pore size of many hydrogels and can be absorbed into the lens, resulting in a yellow stain. Therefore, as a precaution, the eye should be irrigated with sterile saline prior to inserting a soft lens following examination of the eye with fluorescein. If a lens does become stained with fluorescein, it usually washes out following the next disinfection cycle.

High molecular weight fluorescein known as fluorexon[11] (molecular weight 710) is available but not used widely because it has relatively low fluorescent properties and causes discomfort and stinging in some patients.[12]

### Sequential fluorescein staining
Sequential staining refers to the repeated application of fluorescein over a period of minutes followed by observation with the slit-lamp biomicroscope in the usual way.[13] This has been suggested as a more sensitive technique that is predictive of epithelial complications of contact lens wear, although this link has not been proven. It is likely that sequential staining merely results in high concentrations of fluorescein in the eye that cause a toxic epithelial response. The value of this technique is therefore questionable.

### Use of rose bengal
Rose bengal is a mildly toxic, bright red stain that is adsorbed to and absorbed by compromised epithelial cells, mucus and fibrous tissue (Figure 9.2).[4] It is available as a one per cent solution or as impregnated filter strips. Bennett and Davis[12] suggest that much better results are obtained if the solution form is used. Following instillation, the eye is observed in white light.

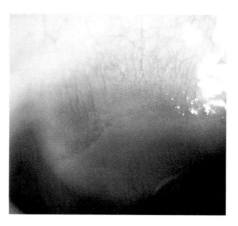

**Figure 9.2**
*Rose bengal staining leading edge of fibrovascular pannus*

In the absence of a complete tear film – and especially in the case of mucus deficiency – rose bengal is taken up by healthy epithelial cells.[4] Accordingly, this stain is especially useful for investigating dry-eye conditions; that is, a dry eye may display extensive staining with rose bengal, especially if there is a mucus deficiency.

### Slit-lamp biomicroscope appearance
Corneal staining following instillation of fluorescein is observed as a bright green fluorescence and may present in an infinite combination of shapes, locations, depths and intensities. A large number of terms have been used to describe the various forms of appearance of staining. Perhaps the most often noted form of disturbance is punctate staining, whereby small superficial discrete dots are observed on the corneal surface (see Figure 9.1). This is also referred to as micropunctate staining, superficial punctate erosion (SPE), or superficial punctate keratitis (SPK). Intense punctate staining is sometimes called 'stipple staining'.

A vast array of closely separated punctate spots gives rise to a diffuse appearance. The terms SPE and SPK are also used to describe this appearance. The overall pattern of fluorescence may be so diffuse as to obscure the constituent elements of staining, resulting in an appearance described as confluent or coalescent staining (Figure 9.3).

Other terms used to describe staining include arcuate stains, linear abrasions and dimple stains. The position is generally noted as superior, inferior, temporal, nasal or central. The depth of staining is noted as

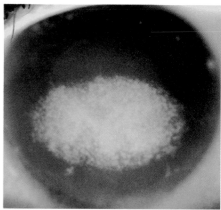

**Figure 9.3**
*Coalescent superficial corneal staining*

deep or superficial. Various syndromes have been suggested based on frequently observed characteristic staining patterns such as 'inferior epithelial arcuate lesion' ('smile stain'; Figure 9.4)[14], 'superior epithelial arcuate lesion' (SEAL; otherwise known as 'epithelial splitting' and depicted in Figure 9.5)[15] or exposure keratitis. Perhaps the most devastating form of staining that can be observed is the 'epithelial plug', which refers to a large discrete area (typically round in shape) of full-thickness epithelial loss (Figure 9.6).

Severe staining (grades 3 and 4) may be accompanied by bulbar conjunctival hyperaemia and chemosis, limbal hyperaemia, excessive lacrimation and in some cases stromal infiltrates, depending on the cause of the problem.

### Vision
Visual acuity is generally unaffected by corneal staining although a slight loss might

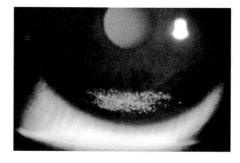

**Figure 9.4**
*Inferior epithelial arcuate lesion, or 'smile stain'*

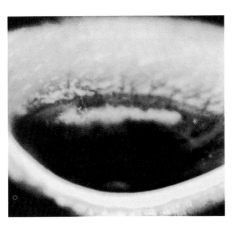

**Figure 9.5**
*Superior epithelial arcuate lesion (SEAL), or 'epithelial splitting'*

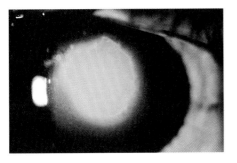

**Figure 9.6**
*Focal area of full-thickness epithelial loss, known as an 'epithelial plug'*

be expected in extreme cases (such as grade 4 staining as depicted in Figure 9.6).

As will be described below, epithelial recovery is generally rapid so any vision loss will also be quickly restored.

**Comfort**

A paradox of the corneal staining response is that there is no clear relationship between the severity of staining and the degree of ocular discomfort. For example, an exposure keratitis in the form of an extensive inferior arcuate diffuse staining pattern can be virtually asymptomatic, whereas a small tracking stain caused by a foreign body trapped beneath a rigid lens can be excruciatingly painful. Photophobia may be present in the case of an infection.

**Pathology**

The 'conventional wisdom' is that fluorescence indicates one of three phenomena:

- fluorescein entering damaged cells
- fluorescein entering intercellular spaces
- fluorescein filling gaps in the epithelial surface that are created when epithelial cells are displaced.

To determine precisely what it is that fluorescein stains, Wilson *et al*[16] examined rabbit corneas stained with fluorescein with the biomicroscope and later with a higher magnification epifluorescent microscope following excision. They determined that fluorescein primarily reveals cells that have taken up fluorescein optimally. Typically, this means degenerated or devitalised cells; however, this is not always the case. The bright fluorescent appearance is concentration-dependent, whereby concentrations greater or lesser than an optimum level will produce a lower level of fluorescence. Thus, cells with a dull fluorescence could actually contain a higher or lower concentration of fluorescein than a cell displaying bright fluorescence.

In many of their preparations, Wilson *et al*[16] observed a dull background fluorescence which indicates that fluorescein enters intercellular spaces, presumably in low concentrations, and on occasions enters the anterior stroma. This background fluorescence can result in a 'salt and pepper' appearance, whereby the 'salt' indicates cells that have filled with an optimum concentration of fluorescein, and the 'pepper' indicates cells that are filled with a higher or lower fluorescein concentration that 'blend in' with the background fluorescence.

More controversially, Wilson *et al*[16] suggested that bright fluorescence is unlikely to represent pooling of fluorescein due to missing cells because repeated irrigation did not change the bright fluorescent appearance

(indicating that such fluorescence must come from within the cell). Certainly, in cases of gross epithelial detachment, such as occurs with an epithelial plug (Figure 9.6), fluorescein clearly fills the void.

Figure 9.7 is a schematic representation of the way in which the corneal epithelium is stained by fluorescein and rose bengal.

**Aetiology**

There are numerous contact lens-related causes of epithelial staining which can be broadly classified into six aetiological categories: mechanical, exposure, metabolic, toxic, allergic and infectious. In many cases the pattern of staining can provide a clue to the cause. Each of these aetiological factors is considered below.

**Mechanical**

Sources of mechanical staining include lens defects, poor lens finish (e.g. rough edge),[17] lens binding (e.g. as can occur with overnight RGP extended wear lenses),[18] excessive lens bearing (e.g. tight rigid lens fit; bearing of a poorly blended optic zone junction; or decentred lens as depicted in Figure 9.8), foreign bodies beneath the lens, deposits on the posterior lens surface, or abrasion occurring during lens insertion or removal.

Staining induced by lens defects or posterior lens deposits usually takes the form of discrete areas of fluorescence corresponding to the location of the defect or deposit.[17] The staining may be arcuate as a result of natural lens rotation during wear. Staining due to lens binding appears as an arc corresponding to the lens edge, whereas

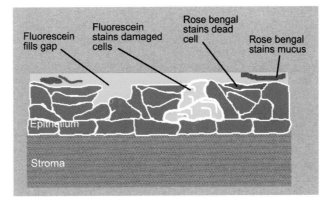

**Figure 9.7**
*Mechanism of fluorescein and rose bengal staining of corneal epithelium*

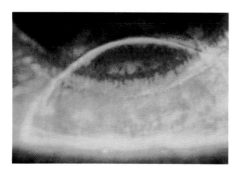

**Figure 9.8**
*Corneal and conjunctival imprint of edge of decentred rigid lens as revealed by fluorescein*

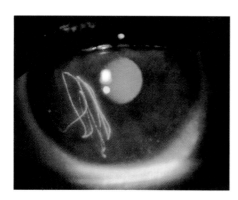

**Figure 9.9**
*Foreign-body track in rigid lens wearer*

excessive lens bearing can result in a more diffuse form of staining.

A foreign body often leaves a zig-zag track indicating the path it has taken across the corneal surface as a result of blinking (Figure 9.9). This phenomenon is rarely observed in soft lens wearers. Staining incurred during lens insertion or removal is often of a linear form. Since such staining is characteristically a 'chance occurrence', it is typically unilateral.

### Exposure

In soft lens wearers, exposure keratitis manifests typically as a band of inferior arcuate staining. This is due to epithelial disruption as a result of drying of the corneal surface. Such staining patterns are observed when soft lenses decentre superiorly, leaving an inferior band of exposed cornea that is not properly wetted because of less frequent blinking.[19]

The classic form of exposure keratitis in rigid lens wearers is known as 3 and 9 o'clock staining, which refers to a triangu-

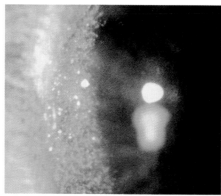

**Figure 9.10**
*Intense 9 o'clock staining in the left eye of a rigid lens wearer*

lar area of staining (apex away from the central cornea) at the nasal and temporal cornea outside the lens periphery (Figure 9.10).[20] Although this condition may be in part due to incomplete or infrequent blinking, it occurs primarily as a result of corneal non-wetting caused by the lids being bridged away from the cornea by the lens edge.

Desiccation staining with soft lenses can be categorised as a form of exposure keratitis.[21] This condition appears as a central stipple stain. It occurs when high water content lenses are made too thin, causing water to be drawn out of the cornea when the lens dehydrates during wear. All forms of exposure keratitis are typically bilateral.

### Metabolic

Contact lenses are known to induce various levels of epithelial hypoxia (oxygen deprivation) and hypercapnia (excessive carbon dioxide),[22] resulting in the production of metabolites (e.g. lactic acid) that can adversely affect epithelial structure and function and lead to tissue acidosis.

In the case of lenses of low oxygen transmissibility and/or lens overwear, such changes can be exacerbated, and the epithelial decompensation is observed as a generalised, diffuse staining encompassing most of the cornea; it is typically bilateral. The spontaneous focal loss of epithelium depicted in Figure 9.6 was attributed to the effects of severe hypoxia in a soft lens patient wearing −9.00D low water content (38 per cent) soft lenses.

Fine punctate staining can be observed

when epithelial microcysts break through the anterior epithelial surface.

### Toxic

Preservatives used in contact lens disinfection systems are generally formulated in low concentrations so that direct application to the eye is non-toxic. A dilemma facing contact lens solution manufacturers is that the relatively recent introduction of single-bottle multiple-purpose solutions that contain surfactant elements has resulted in formulations that are closer to the threshold for ocular toxicity.

Some preservatives such as chlorhexidine can bind strongly and reversibly to many hydrogel polymers or to protein deposits on the lens surface;[23] such preservatives can become concentrated in this way and eventually lead to a toxic reaction, which presents as an intense, diffuse staining across the whole cornea (Figure 9.11). Hydrogen peroxide, when introduced directly into the eye, can result in a severe and painful toxic reaction.[24]

### Allergic

An allergic reaction can take the form of a delayed or immediate hypersensitivity response. This is an acquired cell-mediated (antibody) immunological reaction that generally requires previous exposure and sensitisation to the offending antigen. In the immediate form, it may resemble a toxic response. Delayed hypersensitivity can manifest months or years following continued use of an apparently harmless product.

Thimerosal, benzalkonium chloride and chlorhexidine have all been implicated in

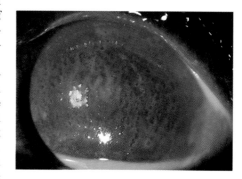

**Figure 9.11**
*Severe toxicity staining in a patient who inadvertently used a contact lens cleaner as a wetting solution*

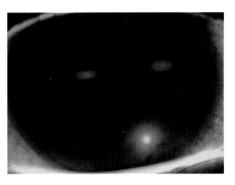

**Figure 9.12**
*Staining of a sterile peripheral ulcer revealing involvement of epithelium (central intense fluorescence) and stroma (diffuse background glow)*

the aetiology of allergic reactions to contact lens solutions. Fortunately, these substances are becoming obsolete, and sophisticated preservatives such as polyaminopropyl biguanide (Dymed), which are essentially non-toxic and non-allergenic, now dominate the market. Chlorine-based disinfection systems are also largely non-toxic and non-allergenic, although concerns have been expressed about the disinfection capacity of some formulations of these solutions.[25]

### Infectious

Infection by a variety of pathogens can result in corneal staining. Indeed, an infectious corneal ulcer is only defined as such if the affected region of stromal degradation is accompanied by an overlying epithelial defect and the ulcer is culture-positive. In such cases, staining is usually confined to the region of ulceration, which, in the early stages, can be quite small (Figure 9.12). Fluorescein may also diffuse into the stroma, resulting in a dull background fluorescence.

## Observation and grading

In many cases, epithelial defects can be observed using the slit-lamp biomicroscope under white light without the aid of fluorescein. As a general rule, observation in white light should always precede observation with fluorescein.

Once the fluorescein is instilled, the cornea should be examined with a broad beam

### Table 9.1   Grading scale for fluorescein staining

| Grade | Clinical interpretation |
|-------|-------------------------|
| 0 | No staining visible |
| 1 | Trace staining: such as very light, superficial, punctate staining (fewer than 10 dots); regional superficial stippling. Does not require clinical action |
| 2 | Mild staining: such as regional or diffuse punctate staining and moderate stipple staining. Does not normally require clinical action |
| 3 | Moderate staining: such as heavy stipple staining and dense coalescent staining. Normally requires clinical action |
| 4 | Severe staining: such as pan-corneal heavy stipple or coalescent staining; full-thickness epithelial plug loss. Requires clinical action |

at low magnification (×10, giving a full view of the cornea) under cobalt blue light in order to determine the overall level of staining. This is the preferred technique, for example, for assessing pan-corneal conditions such as 3 and 9 o'clock staining or desiccation staining. Closer examination using a 1 mm beam at higher magnification (×40) is required to detect more subtle forms of staining (such as fine foreign-body tracks) as well as to determine the depth of staining.

Fluorescein has a maximum absorption spectrum at 460 to 490 nm, with a maximum emission spectrum at 520 nm.[8] Based on this knowledge, filters can be interposed in the observation and illumination system of a slit-lamp biomicroscope to enhance conditions for viewing corneal staining.[26] Specifically, a Wratten #47B excitation filter should be placed in the illumination system; this has a peak transmission between 400 and 500 nm. A Wratten #12 filter (which absorbs all wavelengths below 500 nm and provides maximum transmission at 530 nm and beyond) placed in the observation system further enhances the observed fluorescence.

The general principle of the clinical severity scale from grades 0 to 4 can be applied to corneal staining.[27] Begley *et al*[28] have described a modified grading scale that

is consistent with this approach; this schema is described in Table 9.1 (see also Appendix A).

## Management and treatment

Unlike various other forms of ocular compromise with contact lens wear, it is often possible to identify the cause of corneal staining from the patient history, knowledge of the lenses worn and maintenance system used, inspection of the lens and analysis of the form of staining. Low level staining (grade 0–2) does not necessarily require action to be taken.

Minor staining is commonly observed in contact lens wearers; it is typically transient and in a daily lens wearer will have disappeared by the following morning, but persistent minor staining forming a characteristic pattern, as well as grade 3 or 4 staining, may require intervention.

It is of course not possible to detail all of the available strategies for alleviating staining that is deemed to be clinically excessive, but the general principles outlined below according to probable aetiology should provide some guidance. Whatever strategy is adopted, lens wear need only be ceased for 1 or 2 days for low level (grade 0–2) staining, and perhaps 4 or 5 days for more intense (grade 3 or 4) staining.

### Mechanical

Strategies for resolving staining of a mechanical aetiology are generally self-evident. In the case of lens defects, poor lens finish, or posterior lens deposits, the lens should be replaced. With rigid lenses, light polishing may solve the problem.

Numerous and often conflicting strategies have been advocated for alleviating lens binding following overnight RGP extended wear lenses; Woods and Efron[29] have recently demonstrated that regular rigid lens replacement (say, every 6 months) will significantly reduce the incidence of binding. Excessive rigid lens bearing is alleviated by modifying the lens fit. Foreign bodies are dealt with by rinsing the lens and sometimes also the eye. Abrasion occurring during lens insertion or removal may necessitate re-education of the patient with respect to lens insertion and removal techniques.

### Exposure

Exposure keratitis in soft lens wearers is usually due to a lens decentring superiorly.

This is managed by fitting a larger diameter lens or perhaps a lens of different design that centres better. In rigid lens wearers, the general principle to be followed in attempting to alleviate 3 and 9 o'clock staining is to ensure that the stained region is wetted properly. Strategies include adopting a lens design that allows for greater movement (typically a smaller, looser lens fit), blinking instructions, use of in-eye lubricants, or changing to soft lenses.

Desiccation staining, which is generally observed in association with the wearing of thin high water soft lenses, is prevented by designing lenses with greater average thickness according to the guidelines provided by McNally *et al*,[30] and/or using a lower water content material.

### Metabolic

Corneal staining attributed to epithelial hypoxia and hypercapnia is alleviated by following the general guidelines for alleviating metabolic stress as described in Chapter 11. In general, treatment options include refitting a lens of higher gas transmissibility, reducing wearing time, or changing from extended wear to daily wear.

### Toxic

The obvious strategy for treating corneal staining due to solution toxicity is to change to a solution that is non-toxic for that patient. Corneal burns due to instillation of hydrogen peroxide may require patient re-education in the use of peroxide systems or the prescription of a different system. Associated strategies include more frequent lens replacement to avoid a build-up of deposits that can absorb and concentrate preservatives, and the use of a lens made from a different polymer that is again less likely to absorb and concentrate the offending preservatives.

### Allergic

Similar strategies to those described above for treating toxicity staining are applied to the treatment of corneal staining due to solution allergy; that is, change to a solution that is non-allergenic for that patient, replace lenses more frequently and prescribe lenses made from a different polymer. Certainly, early-generation preservatives such as thimerosal, benzalkonium chloride and chlorhexidine should be avoided.

Atopic patients who are prone to suffer a reaction to a variety of preservatives are best fitted with daily disposable lenses so as to avoid contact with solutions altogether.

### Infectious

It is essential that the infectious agent is killed as quickly as possible to avoid widespread corneal damage. Resolution of the infection will generally result in the re-establishment of a normal epithelium. The issue of contact lens-related corneal infection and ulceration is considered in Chapter 14.

## Prognosis

Recovery from epithelial staining is generally quite rapid following removal of the causative agent. Light staining (grade 0–2) can recover within a few hours, and certainly overnight, assuming that lens wear has ceased. The foreign-body track depicted in Figure 9.9 completely resolved in 24 hours. More severe cases of corneal staining (grade 3 or 4) may take up to 4 or 5 days to disappear.

Resolution of epithelial staining is slower if lenses are worn during the recovery period because the lenses will inevitably induce a certain measure of anterior corneal hypoxia, providing a sub-optimal environment for epithelial growth and repair.

## Differential diagnosis

There are two main issues concerning the differential diagnosis of corneal staining; both issues relate to determining the aetiology of various forms of staining (rather than to differentiating corneal staining from other phenomena that could theoretically take on a similar appearance). The first issue is the clinical interpretation of different patterns of staining – a topic that has already been dealt with in some detail in this chapter. The distribution, depth and intensity of staining, whether the staining is unilateral or bilateral, and the associated history, can provide strong clues as to the cause of the condition.

Secondly, differentiation of the aetiology of corneal staining can be aided by the application of other vital stains – the most common being rose bengal. Dead cells, fibrotic tissue and excess mucus will stain heavily with rose bengal, making this stain especially useful for identifying degenerative conditions and dry eye.

## REFERENCES

1 Pflüger (1882) Zur Ernehrung der Cornea. *Klin Monatsbl Augenhelkd* **20**: 69.

2 Efron N, Pearson RM (1988) Centenary celebration of Fick's Eine Contactbrille. *Arch Ophthalmol* **106**: 1370.

3 Korb DR, Korb JME (1970) Corneal staining prior to contact lens wearing. *J Am Optom Assoc* **41**: 228.

4 Feenstra RPG, Tseng SCG (1992) Comparison of fluorescein and rose bengal staining. *Ophthalmology* **99**: 605.

5 Guillon JP, Guillon M, Malgouyres S (1990) Corneal desiccation staining with hydrogel lenses: tear film and contact lens factors. *Ophthal Physiol Opt* **10**: 343.

6 Norn MS (1970) Micropunctate fluorescein vital staining of the cornea. *Acta Ophthalmol* **48**: 108.

7 Hamano H, Kitano J, Mitsunaga (1985) Adverse effects of contact lens wear in a large Japanese population. *Contact Lens Assoc Ophthalmol J* **11**: 141.

8 Romanchuk KG (1982) Fluorescein: Physicochemical factors affecting its fluorescence. *Surv Ophthalmol* **26**: 269.

9 Vaughan DG (1955) The contamination of fluorescein solutions – with special reference to *Pseudomonas aeruginosa*. *Am J Ophthalmol* **39**: 55.

10 Lemp MA, Hamill JR (1973) Factors affecting tear film breakup in normal eyes. *Arch Ophthalmol* **89**: 103.

11 Refojo MF, Korb DR, Silverman HI (1972) Clinical evaluation of a new fluorescent dye for hydrogel lenses. *J Am Optom Assoc* **43**: 321.

12 Bennett ES, Davis LJ (1994) Noninfectious corneal staining. In: *Anterior Segment Complications of Contact Lens Wear* (ed. JA Silbert). New York. Churchill Livingstone, p. 43.

13 Korb DR, Herman JP (1979) Corneal staining subsequent to sequential fluorescein instillations. *J Am Optom Assoc* **50**: 316.

14 Zadnik K, Mutti DO (1985) Inferior arcuate staining in soft contact lens wearers. *Int Contact Lens Clin* **12**: 110.

15 Malinovsky V, Pole JJ, Pence NA (1989) Epithelial splits of the superior cornea in hydrogel contact lens patients. *Int Contact Lens Clin* **16**: 252.

16 Wilson G, Ren H, Laurent J (1995) Corneal epithelial fluorescein staining. *J Am Optom Assoc* **66**: 435.

17 Efron N, Veys J (1992) Defects in disposable contact lenses can compromise ocular integrity. *Int Contact Lens Clin* **19**: 8.

18 Swarbrick HA, Holden BA (1987) Rigid gas permeable lens binding; significance and contributing factors. *Am J Optom Physiol Opt* **64**: 815.

19 Barr JT (1985) Peripheral corneal desiccation staining – lens materials and designs. *Int Contact Lens Clin* **12**: 139.

20 Korb DR, Korb JME (1970) A study of three and nine staining after unilateral lens removal. *J Am Optom Assoc* **41**: 7.

21 Holden BA, Sweeney DF, Seger RG (1986) Epithelial erosions caused by thin high water content lenses. *Clin Exp Optom* **69**: 103.

22 Efron N, Ang JHB (1990) Corneal hypoxia and hypercapnia during contact lens wear. *Optom Vis Sci* **67**: 512.

23 Refojo MF (1976) Reversible binding of chlorhexidine gluconate to hydrogel contact lenses. *Contact Intraoc Lens Med J* **2**: 47.

24 Paugh JP, Brennan NA, Efron N (1988) Ocular response to hydrogen peroxide. *Am J Optom Physiol Opt* **65**: 91.

25 Lowe R, Vallas V, Brennan NA (1992) Comparative efficacy of contact lens disinfection solutions. *Contact Lens Assoc Ophthalmol J* **18**: 34.

26 Courtney RC, Lee JM (1982) Predicting ocular intolerance of a contact lens solution by use of a filter system enhancing fluorescein staining detection. *Int Contact Lens Clin* **9**: 302.

27 Woods R (1989) Quantitative slit-lamp observations in contact lens practice. *J Br Contact Lens Assoc (Scientific Meetings)*: 42.

28 Begley CG, Edrington TB, Chalmers RL (1994) Effect of lens care systems on corneal fluorescein staining and subjective comfort in hydrogel lens wearers. *Int Contact Lens Clin* **21**: 7.

29 Woods CA, Efron N (1996) Regular replacement of rigid contact lenses alleviates binding to the cornea. *Int Contact Lens Clin* **23**: 13.

30 McNally JJ, Chalmers R, Payor R (1987) Corneal desiccation staining with thin high water contact lenses. *Clin Exp Optom* **70**: 106.

# 10
# Microcysts

Prevalence
Signs and symptoms
Pathology
Aetiology
Observation and grading
Management and treatment
Prognosis
Differential diagnosis

The first report of the appearance of corneal epithelial microcysts in association with contact lens wear was published in 1976 by Ruben and co-workers.[1] These authors were correct in surmising that 'Corneal microcysts are evidence of chronic changes in the . . . epithelium . . .'.

This observation was confirmed in 1978 by Zantos and Holden,[2] who used the term 'microvesicles' in a report of a clinical trial, and in 1979 by Josephson[3] in a case report. Numerous scientific papers since then have carefully documented the appearance of microcysts in contact lens wearers so that a fairly complete account of their clinical manifestation can now be presented.

Epithelial microcysts can be readily observed with the slit-lamp biomicroscope (Figure 10.1). This sign is considered to be the most important indicator of chronic metabolic stress in the corneal epithelium.

## Prevalence

According to Holden et al[4] a small number of microcysts – typically fewer than 10 – can be observed in the eyes of non-contact lens

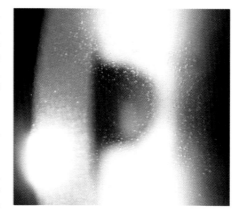

**Figure 10.1**
*Extensive formation of epithelial microcysts which can be clearly seen against the background of the pupil margin*

wearers. Thus, the appearance of a small number of microcysts in a contact lens wearer should not be cause for alarm.

Estimates of the prevalence of microcysts in association with various types and modalities of lens wear[1,4–10] are summarised in Table 10.1. Bearing in mind the different methodologies, lens types and study dura-

tions employed by the various authors, the concordance of estimates of prevalence is remarkable. In general, a lower prevalence of microcysts is associated with daily wear of contact lenses, compared with extended lens wear.

The prevalence of microcysts associated with both hydrogel lens extended wear and low-Dk to medium-Dk rigid lens extended wear approaches 100 per cent.

## Signs and symptoms

### Slit-lamp biomicroscope appearance
Microcysts can be seen in the central and paracentral cornea at low magnification (×15). They appear as minute scattered grey opaque dots with focal illumination and as transparent refractile inclusions with indirect retroillumination (Figure 10.2). Microcysts are often said to be irregular in shape but all of the photomicrographs of microcysts examined by this author suggest that they are generally of a uniform spherical or ovoid shape. Zantos[11] suggested that they can vary in size from 15 to 50 μm.[3] However, microcysts as

**Table 10.1  Prevalence of contact lens-induced epithelial microcysts reported in the literature**

| Lens type | Mode of lens wear | Lens Dk | Reported prevalence of microcysts (%) |
|---|---|---|---|
| No lens wear | – | – | 26[4] |
| PMMA[a] | DW[b] | Zero | 29[4] |
| Rigid | DW | 'Low' | 29[5] |
| Rigid | EW[c] | 'Very low' | 97[4] |
| Rigid | EW | 'Low' | 23,[6] 93,[7] 100[4] |
| Rigid | EW | 'Medium' | 84[4] |
| Rigid | EW | 'High' | 29[4] |
| Soft | DW | 'Medium' | 26[1], 34[4] |
| Soft | EW | 'High' | 43–77,[8] 71,[7] 86,[4] 97,[4] 100,[5,9,10] |
| Soft | CW[d] | 'High' | 41[4] |

[a] Polymethyl methacrylate.
[b] Daily wear.
[c] Extended wear.
[d] Continuous wear.

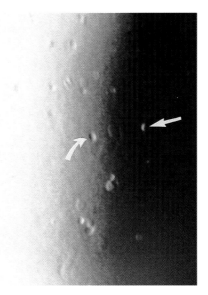

**Figure 10.3**
*High magnification slit-lamp photomicrograph showing microcysts (displaying reversed illumination; curved arrow) and fluid vacuoles (displaying unreversed illumination; straight arrow)*

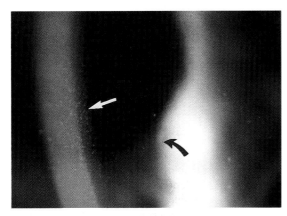

**Figure 10.2**
*Epithelial microcysts appear as grey dots in focal illumination (white arrow) and refractile inclusions in retroillumination (black arrow)*

large as the full thickness of the epithelium (50–75 μm) have not been reported, so it is likely that microcysts are in the order of 20 μm in diameter or less.

Careful observation at high magnification (×40) is required to differentiate epithelial microcysts from other epithelial inclusions such as fluid vacuoles or bullae which superficially take on a similar appearance. The preferred observation technique is marginal retroillumination. The observation and illumination arms should be set at least 45° apart. A 2 mm wide beam should be directed to one of the lateral margins of the pupil so that, when focused on the cornea, the background is evenly split between the illuminated iris and the black pupil. Microcysts are then readily observed in the region of the epithelium lying in front of the border of the iris and pupil. By slowly scanning laterally from side to side, an overall estimate of the number of microcysts can be derived.

The greater the number of microcysts, the greater is the probability of detecting slight superficial punctate staining, which represents a breaking open of the anterior epithelial surface as microcysts emerge from the deeper layers and are expunged from the cornea.

**Optical effects**

Epithelial microcysts display a characteristic optical phenomenon known as 'reversed illumination' when viewed using the above observation technique. That is, the distribution of light within the microcyst is opposite to the light distribution of the background[11] (Figure 10.3). Other inclusions such as vacuoles (also known as vesicles, bullae or microepithelial oedema), or mechanical epithelial defects such as dimple veiling (creating fluid-filled epithelial pits), display 'unreversed illumination' (Figure 10.3).

Simple optical principles can be used to demonstrate the significance of the optical appearance of microcysts and other epithelial inclusions (Figure 10.4). The 'reversed illumination' appearance indicates that the inclusion is acting as a converging refractor; therefore, it must consist of material that is of a higher refractive index than the surrounding epithelium.[12] Conversely, the 'unreversed illumination' appearance indicates that the inclusion is acting as a diverging refractor; therefore, it must consist of material that is of a lower refractive index than the surrounding epithelium.

The predominant inclusions which (a) are observed in association with all forms of contact lens wear, and (b) display characteristic patterns in terms of the time-course of onset and resolution, are those which display reversed illumination. These observations and features, together with our current understanding of the pathology and aetiology of the microcyst response, allow inclusions displaying

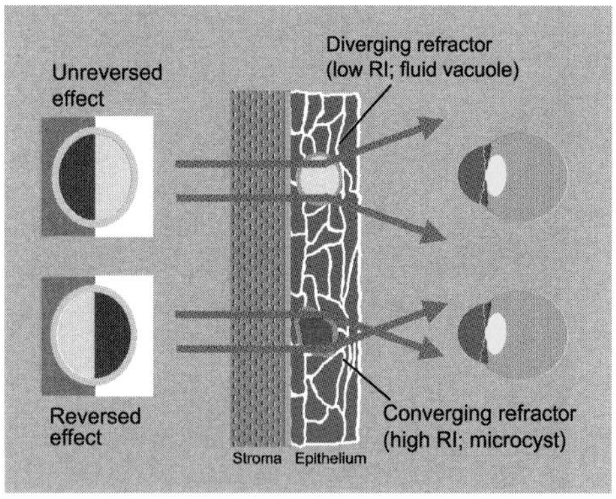

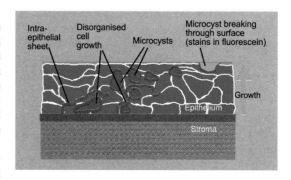

**Figure 10.4**
*Optical theory illustrating how (bottom) microcysts act as converging refractors and display reversed illumination, and (top) fluid vacuoles act as diverging refractors and display unreversed illumination (after Zantos[11])*

reversed illumination to be defined as 'microcysts'.

## Vision

Visual acuity is generally unaffected by microcysts although in extreme cases, when the number of microcysts approaches 200, there might be a slight loss of vision. Zantos and Holden[2] have reported a case where vision decreased by one line of acuity.

## Comfort

Microcysts are asymptomatic; patients are unaware that they have a microcyst response. Patients displaying an extensive microcystic response may experience some ocular discomfort and lens intolerance. However, this is likely to be the result of concurrent pathology. For example, a patient with a severe microcyst response may also have a mild anterior uveal reaction as part of an overall hypoxia-driven syndrome, which could cause ocular pain.

## Time course of onset

Microcysts can be detected as early as one week after commencing extended contact lens wear.[13] However, the rate of onset is generally slow and microcysts will not begin to appear in significant numbers until lenses have been worn for about 2 months. The number of microcysts will then increase at a more rapid rate over the next 2–4 months.[14]

Fonn and Holden[7] reported that the prevalence of microcysts in new patients fitted with extended wear lenses was 5 per cent after 5 weeks, 33 per cent after eight weeks and 71 per cent after 13 weeks.

The number of microcysts will eventually reach a steady state level, although cyclic patterns of microcysts have been reported in some patients.[14]

## Pathology

The optical phenomenon of reversed illumination, which microcysts display, suggests that they contain material of a higher refractive index than the surrounding tissue.[12] Bergmanson[15] postulated that microcysts represent an extracellular accumulation of broken-down cellular material trapped in the basal epithelial layers. In a process similar to that which occurs in Cogan's microcystic dystrophy,[16] the epithelial basement membrane reduplicates and folds, forming intraepithelial sheets that eventually detach from the basement membrane and encapsulate the cellular debris.

Based on her findings of the effects of 15 months' soft lens extended wear in cats,

Madigan[17] suggested that microcysts were not an accumulation of extracellular debris, but rather represent apoptotic (dead) cells which either (a) become phagocytosed (ingested) by living neighbouring cells, or (b) remain involuted in the intercellular spaces.

Figure 10.5 is a schematic representation of the likely pathological process by which microcysts are produced. Microcysts are thought to originate in the deepest layers of the epithelium where they are difficult to observe because they are only partially formed. They are then carried to the surface of the epithelium, which is constantly growing in the anterior direction. Microcysts approaching the corneal surface are more easily observed because they are now fully formed. They eventually break through the epithelial surface, sometimes leaving a minute pit which stains with fluorescein.

## Aetiology

There now exists an abundance of evidence to suggest that microcysts primarily represent visible evidence of chronic tissue metabolic stress and altered cellular growth patterns caused by the direct and/or indirect (acidosis) effects of hypoxia and/or hypercapnia. The primary evidence supporting this theory is that the prevalence of microcysts, as well as the number of microcysts present, correlates with the modality of lens wear (more microcysts occur with extended versus daily wear),[4] length of lens wear (number of microcysts increases with length of wear)[1,7] and the gas transmissibility (Dk/L) of the lens (lenses of lower Dk/L induce more microcysts).[4]

Holden *et al*[9] demonstrated that, after 5

**Figure 10.5**
*Pathogenesis of epithelial microcysts, which are formed in the basal epithelium and transported anteriorly as the epithelium grows in that direction*

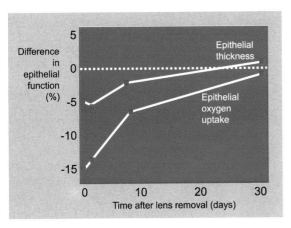

**Figure 10.6**
*Recovery of epithelial function upon lens removal following 5 years' extended wear of soft lenses (after Holden et al[9])*

years of soft lens extended wear, the epithelium suffers a 15 per cent reduction in oxygen uptake and a 6 per cent reduction in thickness (Figure 10.6). These findings concur with the observation of Hamano and Hori[18] that hydrogel lenses cause a 94 per cent suppression of mitosis after only 48 hours in rabbit cornea. Therefore, microcysts indicate that the corneal epithelium is not respiring or growing normally.

Other factors have been suggested as playing a role in the aetiology of microcysts. Efron and Veys[13] provided evidence that lens-induced mechanical trauma can induce microcysts. Dart[19] has suggested that microcysts are a toxic response to preservatives or other foreign substances in contact lens care solutions. However, this is unlikely because microcysts have been observed in patients using disposable lenses when no preservatives are used.

## Observation and grading

Once it has been established under high magnification (×40) that the inclusions being observed are indeed microcysts (see 'Differential diagnosis' below), the cornea should be observed at a low enough magnification so that the cornea fills the field of view (perhaps ×10 magnification). By scanning back and forth with a 1 mm vertical beam, it is possible to view the microcysts in direct focal illumination when they appear as minute grey dots.

Holden *et al*[4] counted the number of microcysts associated with the following modalities of lens wear:

- Soft lens daily wear – 5.
- Soft lens extended wear – 28.
- Very low Dk RGP extended wear – 23.
- Low Dk RGP extended wear – 17.
- Moderate Dk RGP extended wear – 3.
- High Dk RGP extended wear – 0.

Based on such accumulated evidence it is possible to devise a system of grading simply based upon the number of microcysts visible (Table 10.2) (see also Appendix A).

## Management and treatment

While the actual presence of microcysts is not thought to be dangerous, their existence in large numbers is worrying as this is representative of epithelial metabolic distress. Based on the working hypothesis that the severity of the microcyst response is related to the level of hypoxia/hypercapnia induced by contact lens wear, various strategies can be employed in an attempt to minimise the number of microcysts. Strategies that are both likely and unlikely to be successful are outlined below.

### Strategies likely to be successful

- *Increase Dk/L* – the number of microcysts will diminish if lenses of higher Dk/L are fitted.[4]
- *Decrease the frequency of overnight wear* – the number of microcysts will diminish if lenses are worn only one or two nights a week, instead of every night.[20]
- *Change from extended wear to daily wear* – the number of microcysts will diminish if lenses are not worn overnight.[4]
- *Change from soft to rigid lenses* – rigid lenses induce less microcysts than soft lenses of the same Dk/L because (a) corneal oxygenation beneath rigid lenses is enhanced by the blink-activated tear pump that does not function with soft lenses, and (b) rigid lenses leave a significant area of the cornea exposed directly to the atmosphere.[4,7]
- *Avoid defective lenses* – since lens defects are known to induce epithelial microcysts, the fitting of lenses that can induce

**Table 10.2   Microcyst grading scale**

| Grade | Number of microcysts | Clinical interpretation |
|---|---|---|
| 0 | 0 | No microcysts visible |
| 1 | 1–4 | This number of microcysts is commonly observed in wearers of all types of lenses as well as in normal non-lens wearers |
| 2 | 5–30 | This represents a mild microcystic response that warrants monitoring |
| 3 | 31–100 | This represents a moderate microcystic response that warrants close monitoring and generally requires clinical intervention. Some staining may be observed, vision may be reduced slightly, and the patient may be experiencing discomfort |
| 4 | >100 | This represents a severe microcystic response that demands immediate clinical intervention. Moderate staining will be observed, vision may be reduced slightly, and the patient may be experiencing discomfort |

mechanical trauma to the cornea should be avoided.[13]

### Strategies unlikely to be successful

- *Change from conventional to disposable extended wear* – the frequency of lens disposal has no effect on the cumulative hypoxia experienced by the cornea.[20]
- *Alter the extended wear overnight removal schedule* – Kenyon et al[5] demonstrated that the number of microcysts was unaffected by the wearing schedule (lens removal every 4, 7, 14 or 28 days).
- *Change solutions* – the number of microcysts is unaffected by the solutions used in conjunction with lens wear.

### Prognosis

The prognosis for eliminating microcysts is

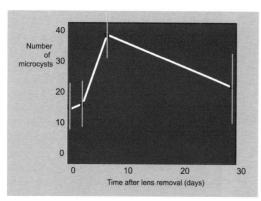

**Figure 10.7**
*Pattern of recovery of epithelial microcysts upon lens removal following 5 years' extended wear of soft lenses (after Holden et al[9])*

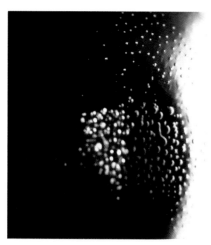

**Figure 10.8**
*Dimple veiling resulting from bubbles previously trapped beneath a rigid lens*

good, although the immediate post-lens wear response may alarm the unwary clinician. Holden et al[9] observed an average of 17 microcysts in the corneal epithelium of 27 patients who had worn high-water content soft lenses on an extended wear basis for 5 years. Following cessation of lens wear, the number of microcysts at first increased to a peak of 34 after 7 days. The number then decreased gradually towards total recovery within 3 months[3] (Figure 10.7). This phenomenon of an initial increase followed by a decrease in the microcyst response was noted earlier by Zantos.[11]

The initial increase and subsequent decrease in the number of microcysts following cessation of lens wear is thought to be due to the following mechanism. When the lens is removed, epithelial metabolism begins to return to normal, as evidenced by the recovery of epithelial oxygen consumption and thickness (refer again to Figure 10.6). Regular cell mitosis resumes.

This resurgence in epithelial metabolism and growth results in an accelerated removal of cellular debris (formation of microcysts) and a rapid movement of microcysts towards the surface. Because microcysts are more visible in the superficial epithelium (as a consequence of being fully formed), more microcysts are observed a few days after lens removal.

As the epithelium continues to function normally, the remaining microcysts are brought to the surface. In the absence of further microcystic development, the number of microcysts gradually decreases until they are completely eliminated from the cornea.

## Differential diagnosis

On casual observation, it is easy to overlook epithelial microcysts, which can take on the appearance of tear film debris. A differential diagnosis can be made following a blink – debris will be washed across the corneal surface whereas microcysts will remain in a fixed position.

The differentiation of microcysts from other epithelial inclusions has been discussed under 'Signs and symptoms'. Microcysts display reversed illumination, whereas other inclusions such as fluid vacuoles or gas bubbles display unreversed illumination.

Bubbles can become trapped beneath rigid lenses and create pits in the epithelium which fill with tear fluid. This phenomenon is known as 'dimple veiling' (Figure 10.8). Although these pits display reversed illumination, both in the presence and absence of lenses, they are much larger than epithelial microcysts and resolve within days compared with a 3 month resolution time for microcysts.

Approximately 50 per cent of patients who wear fluoro-silicone hydrogel lenses on an extended wear basis display a peculiar phenomenon known as 'mucus balls'. These formations can be observed in the post-lens tear film as small discrete particles, or 'plugs', and are similar in appearance to tear film debris. As many as 200 mucus balls can be seen at high magnification (×40) using the slit-lamp biomicroscope. They are typically seen in patients who sleep in fluoro-silicone hydrogel lenses; however, these formations are also observed in smaller numbers in patients who only wear these lenses during the daytime. Mucus balls are immovable beneath the lens and appear to be stuck to the epithelium. A higher number of mucus balls is associated with a looser lens fit. The number of mucus balls remains relatively consistent over time. They cause no discomfort or loss of vision, and appear to be of no consequence with respect to ocular health.

Mucus balls are composed primarily of collapsed mucin, as well as some lipid and tear proteins. The mechanism by which mucus balls form beneath the lens may in part be related to a physico-chemical phenomenon caused by the plasma-treated surface of fluoro-silicone hydrogel lenses. Specifically, the lipophilic surface of these lenses establishes a complex interfacial relationship with the tear film which creates a shearing force that has the effect of rolling up tear mucus into small spheres. The mechanical vehicles facilitating such events may be rapid eye movements during sleep and blink-induced lens movement upon awakening. Although fluoro-silicone hydrogel lenses are soft lenses, they are relatively stiff compared with conventional hydrogel lenses; this relative stiffness may also contribute to the above mechanism. In addition, the more viscous, mucus-rich nature of the closed-eye post-lens tear film is probably of aetiological significance in the formation of mucus balls.

Following lens removal, mucus balls are washed away with blinking but leave behind pits in the epithelial surface. These pits fill with tear fluid and thus give rise to the optical phenomenon of unreversed illumination, which is due to the fact that the fluid-filled pits have a lower refractive index than the surrounding tissue. This appearance is almost identical to dimple veiling caused by air bubbles trapped beneath rigid lenses (see Figure 10.8). Mucus ball-induced fluid-filled pits (displaying unreversed illumination), therefore, can be differentiated from epithelial microcysts (which display reversed illumination). This differential diagnosis can be confirmed by introducing fluorescein into the eye; mucus ball-induced fluid-filled pits will stain heavily and give the appearance of an extensive punctate keratitis, whereas epithelial microcysts do not stain except for a few small spots caused by some microcysts breaking through the epithelial surface.

Deposits on the endothelium, such as endothelial bedewing, also take on the reversed illumination appearance when viewed using retroillumination. However, these endothelial deposits can be differentiated from epithelial microcysts by determining, using an optic section, whether they are at the posterior (endothelial) or anterior (epithelial) surface of the cornea.

## REFERENCES

1 Ruben M, Brown N, Lobascher D (1976) Clinical manifestations secondary to soft contact lens wear. *Br J Ophthalmol* **60**: 529.

2 Zantos SG, Holden BA (1978) Ocular changes associated with continuous wear of contact lenses. *Aust J Optom* **61**: 418.

3 Josephson JE (1979) Coalescing microcysts after long-term use of extended wear lenses. *Int Contact Lens Clin* **6**: 24.

4 Holden BA, Grant T, Kotow M (1987) Epithelial microcysts with daily and extended wear of hydrogel and rigid gas permeable contact lenses. *Invest Ophthalmol Vis Sci* **28** (Suppl): 372.

5 Kenyon E, Polse KA, Seger RG (1986) Influence of wearing schedule on extended wear complications. *Ophthalmology* **93**: 231.

6 Polse KA, Rivera RK, Bonanno J (1988) Ocular effects of hard gas–permeable lens extended wear. *Am J Optom Physiol Opt* **65**: 358.

7 Fonn D, Holden BA (1988) Rigid gas-permeable vs hydrogel contact lenses for extended wear. *Am J Optom Physiol Opt* **65**: 536.

8 Fonn D, Gauthier C, Sorbara L (1990) Adverse response rates in concurrent short-term extended wear and daily wear clinical trials of hydrogel lenses. *Int Contact Lens Clin* **17**: 217.

9 Holden BA, Sweeney DF, Vannas A (1985) Effects of long-term extended contact lens wear on the human cornea. *Invest Ophthalmol Vis Sci* **26**: 1489.

10 Humphries JA, Larke JR, Parrish ST (1980) Microepithelial cysts observed in extended contact-lens wearing subjects. *Br J Ophthalmol* **64**: 888.

11 Zantos SG (1983) Cystic formations in the corneal epithelium during extended wear of contact lenses. *Int Contact Lens Clin* **10**: 128.

12 Bron AJ, Tripathi RC (1973) Cystic disorders of the corneal epithelium. I: Clinical aspects. *Br J Ophthalmol* **57**: 361.

13 Efron N, Veys J (1992) Defects in disposable contact lenses can compromise ocular integrity. *Int Contact Lens Clin* **19**: 8.

14 Holden BA, Sweeney DF (1991) The significance of the epithelial microcyst response: a review. *Optom Vis Sci* **68**: 703.

15 Bergmanson JPG (1987) Histopathological analysis of the corneal epithelium after contact lens wear. *J Am Optom Assoc* **58**: 812.

16 Cogan DG, Kuwabara T, Donaldson DD (1974) Microscopic dystrophy of the cornea. A partial explanation for its pathogenesis. *Arch Ophthalmol* **92**: 24.

17 Madigan M (1989) Cat and monkey as models for extended hydrogel contact lens wear in humans. PhD Thesis, University of New South Wales.

18 Hamano H, Hori M (1983) Effect of contact lens wear on the mitoses of corneal epithelial cells. *Contact Lens Assoc Ophthalmol J* **9**: 133.

19 Dart J (1986) Complications of extended wear hydrogel contact lenses. *Contax* March/April: 11.

20 Grant T, Chong MS, Holden BA (1988) Which is best for the eye: daily wear, two nights or six nights? *Am J Optom Physiol Opt* **65**: 40P.

# Part V
# Corneal Stroma

# 11
# Oedema

Definition of oedema
Demise of the 'CCC' criterion
Prevalence
Signs and symptoms
Pathology
Aetiology
Observation and grading
Management and treatment
Prognosis
Differential diagnosis

Contact lens-induced corneal oedema was recognised in the first two written accounts of the clinical application of contact lenses over a century ago. In his original treatise on contact lenses, published in 1888, AE Fick noted that the cornea became cloudy within hours of insertion of a glass haptic shell.[1]

Although Fick would not have been aware of the exact cause of this disturbing pathological change, it is clear that he was observing contact lens-induced corneal oedema. Even more remarkably, Fick observed that the onset of corneal clouding could be delayed by trapping an air bubble between the lens and cornea.

In his inaugural dissertation to the University of Kiel in Germany, A Müller provided a graphic subjective description of what was undoubtedly a marked contact lens-induced corneal oedema.[2] Müller correctly identified inadequate tear exchange beneath the lens as the cause, but was unable to find a solution at the time.

These pioneering works signalled the be-ginning of the battle against corneal oedema – yet despite numerous significant advances in lens materials, designs, fitting techniques and possible modalities of wear, we are still unable to claim an absolute victory over lens-induced oedema.

## Definition of oedema

Oedema refers to an increase in the fluid content of tissue. Since the cornea is only able to swell in the anterior–posterior direction as a result of the collagen fibre network in the stroma, the cornea can only increase in that dimension – that is, in thickness. For example, a cornea that swells from a thickness of 500 μm before lens wear to become 550 μm thick after lens wear has swollen 50 μm, or has experienced 10 per cent oedema.

Laboratory scientists have developed techniques for the precise measurement of corneal thickness and have noted that oe-dema is a reliable and repeatable index of the cornea's physiological integrity. Indeed, corneal oedema has become estab-lished as the reference against which to gauge other measures of corneal integrity.

## Demise of the 'CCC' criterion

Early textbook accounts describing the de-tection of corneal oedema associated with the wearing of contact lenses made from polymethyl methacrylate (PMMA) cited central corneal clouding (CCC) as the key diagnostic criterion indicating corneal compromise.[3] This condition occurred in patients wearing tightly fitted PMMA lenses that restricted tear exchange be-neath the lens and hence created hypoxic oedema of the central cornea. A discrete, round area of clouding could be observed clearly in the central cornea (Figure 11.1).

Central corneal clouding indicates a gross level of oedema that is rarely observed in modern contact lens practice. The as-tute observations made by contact lens

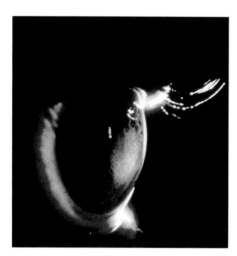

**Figure 11.1**
*Profile view of cornea, illuminated using sclerotic scatter technique, displaying marked central corneal clouding*

clinicians in recent years have revealed the existence of more subtle signs that can be used to predict the level of oedema in response to lens wear.

In this chapter, our understanding of the oedema response to contact lens wear will be reviewed, techniques available to the clinician for evaluating the extent of oedema will be described, and treatment alternatives for minimising the oedema response will be provided.

## Prevalence

Every human experiences corneal oedema during sleep. On awakening, the cornea immediately begins to reduce in thickness. A new steady-state thickness – representing a thinning of about 3 per cent – is reached after about 4 hours, indicating that the cornea has swollen about 3 per cent overnight.[4]

The prevalence of contact lens-induced oedema is essentially 100 per cent, since all contact lenses induce some level of oedema, with the possible exception of silicone elastomer lenses.[5] The amount of oedema is related primarily to the extent of corneal hypoxia that is induced by the lens. With current generation soft and rigid lenses, daytime corneal oedema typically varies between 1 and 6 per cent, and the level of overnight oedema measured upon waking up generally falls in the range 10–15 per cent.[6]

## Signs and symptoms

A variety of sophisticated clinical and laboratory techniques can be employed to measure precisely the extent of lens-induced corneal oedema, the most popular being optical pachometry and ultrasonic recording.[7] Specular microscopy, confocal microscopy, femtosecond laser ranging and interferometry have also been used to measure corneal thickness.

It is often necessary to use these techniques in clinical trials and laboratory research on contact lenses, or for the provision of baseline information before corneal surgery, but their clinical application is limited by the cost and inconvenience of the procedures.

Clinicians can estimate the magnitude of corneal oedema via careful observation with the slit-lamp biomicroscope, as a number of structural changes can be identified that correlate with various levels of oedema. These structural changes – striae, folds and haze – act as useful reference points or 'yardsticks' to form the basis of clinical decision-making.

### Striae

When viewed using direct focal illumination, striae appear as fine, wispy, white, vertically oriented lines (Figure 11.2), and are always located in the posterior stroma.[8] They can also appear as dark lines against

the orange fundus pupillary reflex when observed using retro-illumination. Striae are only seen when the level of oedema reaches about 5 per cent. As the level of oedema increases, striae become greyer and thicker, and increase in number.[9] Striae do not cause vision loss.

### Folds

Folds can be observed in the endothelial mosaic as a combination of depressed grooves or raised ridges, or as a general area of apparent buckling, when the level of oedema reaches about 8 per cent (Figure 11.2). They also increase in number as the level of oedema increases.[9] Folds are best observed using specular reflection. Vision is thought to be unaffected by folds.

### Haze

The stroma takes on a hazy, milky or granular appearance when the level of oedema reaches about 15 per cent (Figure 11.2). In essence, the stroma has suffered a loss of transparency. This can be viewed using a variety of observation techniques. The milky appearance is evident when the cornea is viewed against the pupil using indirect illumination – instead of the normal dark appearance, a fine grey haze is detected and fine iris detail is partially obscured. Sclerotic scatter technique will enhance this clinical picture. Contact lens-induced stromal haze can cause a slight

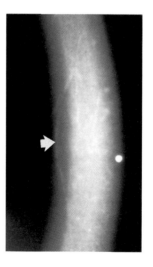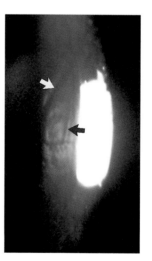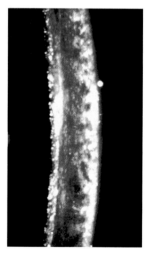

**Figure 11.2**
*Slit-lamp photographs depicting corneal signs of increasing oedema, from left to right. Left image: striae – a vertical striate line (arrow) can be observed in the posterior stroma in direct focal illumination. Centre image: folds – a depressed groove (white arrow) and raised ridge (black arrow) observed in specular reflection. Right image: haze – the stroma takes on a granular appearance at high levels of oedema as viewed in direct focal illumination*

degradation of vision when the level of oedema exceeds 20 per cent.

In a clinical setting, stromal haze indicates gross oedema and will often be associated with other signs and symptoms of ocular distress. It would perhaps be more appropriate to consider oedema of this level as a bullous keratopathy. Contact lens wear is more likely to be an exacerbating factor than the primary cause of the development of stromal haze, so other possible causes of this complication ought to be investigated.

## Pathology

The cornea is a sophisticated five-layered tissue of which 78 per cent is water. The stroma, which constitutes 90 per cent of the thickness of the cornea, has a constant tendency to imbibe water and swell. This tendency is counteracted by a fluid control mechanism (described as the 'pump–leak' model[10]) located in the endothelium, which acts to move water out of the stroma and back into the aqueous via a bicarbonate ion pump. If this mechanism is disrupted, or other physiological challenge is offered to the cornea, the demand on the endothelial pump to maintain deturgescence may become too great. Water will then enter the stroma, and the cornea will increase in thickness.

### Striae

Striae are thought to represent fluid separation of the predominantly vertically arranged collagen fibrils in the posterior stroma (Figure 11.3). This creates a local refractile optical effect whereby stromal transparency is reduced in the immediate vicinity of the separated fibrils. It was originally postulated that the vertical orientation of striae is an artefact of the vertical orientation of the slit beam of the biomicroscope; however, rotating the beam to a horizontal orientation does not alter this appearance (that is, horizontally oriented striae do not suddenly appear).

### Folds

It is thought that folds indicate a physical buckling of the posterior stromal layers in response to high levels of oedema (Figure 11.3). Because of the inherent transparency of the stroma, it is not possible directly to observe folding of stromal tissue. Instead, folding can be seen as altera-

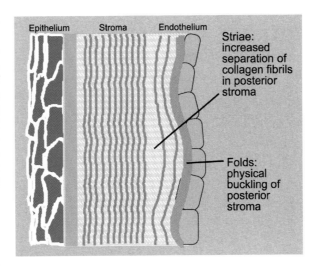

**Figure 11.3**
*Schematic representation of striae and folds*

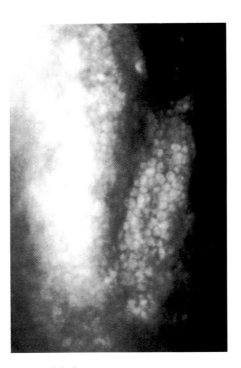

**Figure 11.4**
*High-magnification slit-lamp photomicrograph of deep folds in the endothelial mosaic, indicating buckling of the posterior stroma due to excessive oedema*

tions to the topography of the endothelial layer observed in specular reflection (Figure 11.4).

### Haze

Haze is essentially a more advanced form of striae, whereby there is a gross separation of collagen fibres throughout the full thickness of the stroma, which disrupts the regular geometry and orderly arrangement of the stromal lamellae. This causes a failure of the optical coherence of the stromal collagen layers and transparency is reduced.[10] The greater the oedema, the greater this disruption, and the greater is the extent of haze.

### Stromal thinning

Although low levels of oedema during the day may appear to be harmless, there is a growing body of evidence indicating that chronic oedema may compromise the physiological integrity of the cornea in the long term. It is now clear that long-term extended wear can induce a slight thinning of the stroma. Whereas stromal oedema is essentially an acute response to contact lens wear, stromal thinning is a chronic patho-physiological change observed in patients who have worn lenses for many years.

Stromal thinning was formally defined for the first time by Holden *et al*[11] although it had been reported anecdotally by earlier workers. Holden's group[11] detected stromal thinning by measuring the presenting corneal thickness of patients who had been wearing a lens in one eye only on an extended wear basis for an average of 5 years due to unilateral myopia or amblyopia. Upon ceasing lens wear, it was noted that corneal thickness in the lens-wearing eye decreased to a steady-state level that was

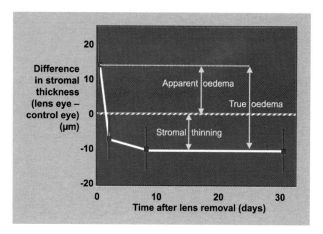

**Figure 11.5**
*Recovery of corneal oedema following cessation of lens wear for 1 month after 5 years of soft lens extended wear, illustrating the relationship between true oedema, apparent oedema and stromal thinning (adapted from Holden et al[11])*

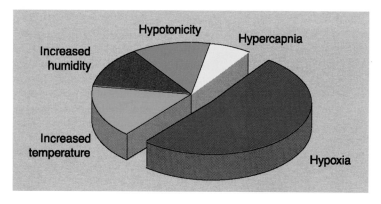

**Figure 11.6**
*Factors contributing to corneal oedema following sleep, revealing hypoxia to be the major cause*

effects, temperature changes, hypotonicity, inflammation and increased humidity. The extent to which these factors contribute to overnight corneal oedema[12] is indicated in Figure 11.6. While the factors contributing to contact lens-induced corneal oedema have not been investigated in this manner, it would seem reasonable to explain lens-induced oedema primarily in terms of the effects of epithelial hypoxia.

Contact lenses restrict corneal oxygen availability, creating a hypoxic environment at the anterior corneal surface. To conserve energy, the corneal epithelium begins to respire anaerobically. Lactate, a by-product of anaerobic metabolism, increases in concentration and moves posteriorly into the corneal stroma. This creates an osmotic load that is balanced by an increased movement of water into the stroma. The sudden influx of water cannot be matched by the removal of water from the stroma by the endothelial pump, resulting in corneal oedema[13] (Figure 11.7).

**Stromal thinning**
It is presumed that stromal thinning is due to the effects of chronic oedema.[11] Two mechanisms may be postulated. Firstly, stromal keratocytes may lose their ability to synthesise new stromal tissue due to (a) the direct effects of tissue hypoxia, and/or (b) the indirect effects of chronic lens-induced tissue acidosis due to an accumulation of lactic acid and carbonic acid. Secondly, constantly-elevated levels of lactic acid associated with chronic oedema may lead to some dissolution of the muco-

thinner than the fellow non-wearing eye (Figure 11.5).

It is important for clinicians to recognise that the phenomenon of contact lens-induced stromal thinning does not confound or invalidate interpretation of the clinical signs of oedema discussed above. Striae, folds and haze represent a given level of oedema irrespective of whether or not the stroma has thinned.

## Aetiology

### Stromal oedema
A number of possible mechanisms have been suggested as playing a role in lens-induced corneal oedema. These include hypoxia, retardation of carbon dioxide efflux (leading to tissue acidosis), mechanical

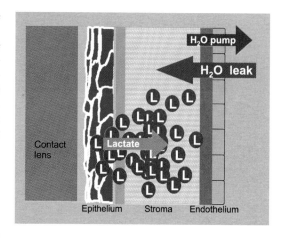

**Figure 11.7**
*Schematic representation of the aetiology of contact lens-induced stromal oedema. Excess lactate in the stroma resulting from anaerobic respiration of the epithelium draws water osmotically into the stroma*

polysaccharide ground substance of the stroma.

## Observation and grading

In the long-term interests of standardising the clinical grading of ocular complications of contact lens wear, an attempt is being made in this book to grade the severity of all conditions on a 0 to 4 scale, in accordance with the recommendation of Woods.[14] In the case of corneal oedema, it is possible to establish a grading scale that correlates directly with the extent of oedema (percentage swelling) and the observed number of striae and folds (Table 11.1). The construction of this table has been made possible by using equations established empirically by LaHood and Grant.[9]

The rationale provided by Woods[14] for the designation of each of the five grades (from 0 to 4) is that they confer the connotation of increasing clinical severity. In the context of this schema, the clinical interpretation of each grading as a descriptor of the severity of contact lens-induced stromal oedema is outlined below:

### Grade 0

This is the normal non-lens wearing situation of 0 per cent oed··· ··· during the day.

### Grade 1

This grade denotes slight ··· ···, up to 4 per cent oedema, which could include the normal 3 per cent oedema experienced by all humans overnight. Pachometric techniques must be employed to detect grade 1 oedema; this level of swelling cannot be measured using a slit-lamp biomicroscope.

### Grade 2

Observation of between one and three striae in the posterior stroma is designated as representing grade 2 oedema. This indicates 5–7 per cent swelling. In the clinic, grade 2 oedema will only be observed in patients who (a) are wearing contact lenses of extremely low-oxygen transmissibility, and/or (b) have slept in their lenses (that is, using contact lenses for extended wear).

Examples of the former case would include high hyperopic (over +8.00D) or high myopic (over −12.00D) corrections. With extended wear patients, striae will typically be observed only within 4 hours of awakening, because the cornea returns to steady-state thickness within this time-frame.[15] Patients using extended wear lenses should be scheduled for early morning appointments so that the full impact of overnight lens wear on the cornea can be assessed.

### Grade 3

If between one and 10 folds are detected, the oedema should be classified as grade 3. A significant number of striae (between 5 and 14) should also be observed. Practitioners will rarely observe folds in the normal clinical setting, since they only form at oedema levels of 8 per cent or greater. Because the cornea deswells at such a rapid rate upon eye opening, folds will only be observed within 1 hour of awakening in patients who have slept in lenses. Daily wear lenses are unlikely to induce oedema levels of 8 per cent or greater, even for the correction of high myopia.

### Grade 4

Corneal swelling of 15 per cent or greater is typically associated with the presence of at least 15 striae and 11 folds. The stroma takes on a hazy appearance, the degree of which increases with increasing oedema. The severe central corneal clouding viewed by sclerotic scatter depicted in Figure 11.8 would be classified as grade 4.

## Management and treatment

Since oxygen starvation is the primary cause of contact lens-induced oedema, strategies for reducing the oedema response

**Table 11.1  Oedema grading scale**

| Grade | % oedema | Number of striae | Number of folds | Extent of haze |
|---|---|---|---|---|
| 0 | 0 | 0 | 0 | None |
| 1 | 1 | 0 | 0 | None |
|  | 2 | 0 | 0 | None |
|  | 3 | 0 | 0 | None |
|  | 4 | 0 | 0 | None |
| 2 | 5 | 1 | 0 | None |
|  | 6 | 2 | 0 | None |
|  | 7 | 3 | 0 | None |
| 3 | 8 | 5 | 1 | None |
|  | 9 | 7 | 3 | None |
|  | 10 | 8 | 4 | None |
|  | 11 | 9 | 5 | None |
|  | 12 | 11 | 7 | None |
|  | 13 | 12 | 8 | None |
|  | 14 | 14 | 10 | None |
| 4 | 15 | 15 | 11 | Slight |
|  | 16 | 17 | 12 | Slight |
|  | 17 | 18 | 14 | Moderate |
|  | 18 | 20 | 15 | Moderate |
|  | 19 | 21 | 16 | Severe |
|  | 20 | 22 | 18 | Severe |

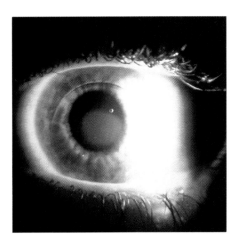

**Figure 11.8**
*Frontal view of severe central corneal clouding viewed by sclerotic scatter technique*

are generally directed towards mechanisms for increasing corneal oxygen availability during lens wear. There are some important differences between rigid and soft lenses in the way oxygen reaches the cornea. Thus, it is necessary to consider alternative oedema-reducing strategies for rigid and soft lenses separately, along with general strategies that apply equally to both types of lenses.

## Alleviating rigid lens oedema

- *Material Dk* – Materials of higher oxygen permeability (Dk) will allow greater levels of oxygen to reach the cornea. However, increasing Dk can have disadvantages such as increased lens flexibility (which reduces lens stability), reduced wettability, and lower deposit resistance.
- *Lens thickness* – A thinner lens will have a higher oxygen transmissibility (Dk/L) than a thicker lens made of the same material.[16] Again, there are some disadvantages to reducing lens thickness; a thinner lens will be more flexible (tending to reduce lens stability), mask less astigmatism and offer less resistance to breakage.
- *Base curve* – A flatter base curve will allow the lens to move more freely, resulting in a greater tear exchange and increased corneal oxygenation.
- *Edge lift* – Increasing the edge lift may enhance tear exchange by affording a larger reservoir of oxygenated tears at the lens periphery. However, increasing edge lift may also increase lens awareness.
- *Lens diameter* – A smaller lens, as well as covering a smaller area of the cornea, will allow greater lens movement and will enhance tear exchange.
- *Fenestrations* – It was originally thought that fenestrations in rigid lenses reduced oedema by providing additional avenues for oxygen passage to the cornea. However, this does not seem to be the case. Fenestrations are now thought to act by altering the fluid forces between lens and cornea. This serves to enhance lens movement, which in turn leads to an increased tear exchange and greater corneal oxygenation.

## Alleviating soft lens oedema

- *Material Dk* – With hydrogels, increasing material Dk essentially means increasing lens water content.[16] The potential drawback of higher water content hydrogels is that they are more fragile and lenses will

therefore need to be thicker, which can reduce comfort slightly.
- *Lens thickness* – Reducing lens thickness will increase Dk/L.[16] However, thinner lenses are more fragile and can lead to unacceptable corneal staining, particularly with higher water content materials.
- *Base curve* – There has been some debate as to whether flattening the base curve of hydrogel lenses results in an increased tear exchange, despite the observation that flatter lenses move more freely over the cornea. Nevertheless, flatter lenses allow tear film debris and desquamated epithelial cells to be flushed out more readily from beneath the lens, thus minimising metabolic disturbance to the cornea and reducing the potential for inducing oedema.
- *Lens diameter* – A smaller lens will move more freely over the cornea, which may allow more oxygen to reach the cornea via an increased tear pump.
- *Microfenestrations* – Conventional fenestrations (0.2 to 1.0 mm in diameter) in soft lenses can increase corneal oxygenation[17] and reduce oedema,[18] but fenestrated lenses are very uncomfortable.[19] A strategically positioned array of microfenestrations can reduce lens-induced corneal oedema significantly.[20] In particular, microfenestrations positioned in the lens periphery may be useful in reducing peripheral corneal oedema during the wearing of medium to high minus lenses (say, over −3.00D). However, the clinical viability of microfenestrations has yet to be established.

## General strategies for reducing oedema

- *Change from extended to daily wear* – Overnight lens wear is generally associated with increased levels of oedema, because corneal oxygen availability is significantly reduced when the eyelid is closed. Thus, converting a patient from extended wear to daily wear will reduce the overall oedema response.
- *Change from soft to rigid lenses* – For soft and rigid lenses of the same Dk/L, rigid lenses will generally deliver more oxygen to the cornea during open-eye wear because of the lid-activated tear pump. For the extended wear patient, converting from a hydrogel lens to a rigid lens will alleviate the physiological impact of lens wear by allowing a more rapid oedema reduction after awakening.
- *Reduce wearing time* – Following lens inser-

tion, oedema initially increases rapidly, then more gradually, over the first 6–8 hours of lens wear. Limiting the time that lenses may be worn each day will, therefore, reduce both the magnitude and the duration of corneal oedema.
- *Anti-inflammatory drugs* – A possible strategy for reducing lens-induced oedema is the use of non-steroid anti-inflammatory drugs. While it would not be feasible to use such drugs routinely, they could prove useful for the treatment of acute episodes of severe (grade 4) oedema. At present there is no conclusive evidence that contact lens-induced oedema can be modified by drug therapy.
- *Postpone lens wear* – It may be prudent to cease lens wear temporarily following an acute oedema episode, especially if associated with other pathological changes, such as limbal engorgement, infiltrates, or epithelial staining. Lens wear should be stopped until all pathological signs and associated symptoms have resolved.
- *Abandon lens wear* – Clearly a last resort, abandonment of lens wear must be considered if chronic oedema persists after all other possible treatment alternatives have failed.

The various strategies described for reducing lens-induced oedema should be employed in a systematic manner, with respect to (a) the severity of oedema as gauged biomicroscopically (based on the appearance of striae, folds and haze) and (b) the modality of lens wear (rigid vs soft; daily wear vs extended wear). Consideration should also be given to the time of day – morning or afternoon – that the observations of oedema are made.

Holden and Mertz[21] have provided criteria for the minimum contact lens Dk/L required to avoid excessive levels of oedema. These are $24 \times 10^{-9}$ (cm × mlO$_2$)/(sec × ml × mmHg) for daily lens wear and $87 \times 10^{-9}$ (cm × mlO$_2$)/(sec × ml × mmHg) for extended lens wear (Figure 11.9).

An overall schema for the management of contact lens-induced corneal oedema is presented in Table 11.2. A series of possible treatment alternatives are listed in approximate order of priority with respect to the slit-lamp signs and lens-wearing modality. This should not be considered as a firm set of rules. Rather, it is a flexible set of guidelines for oedema management based on our current understanding of the oedema response.

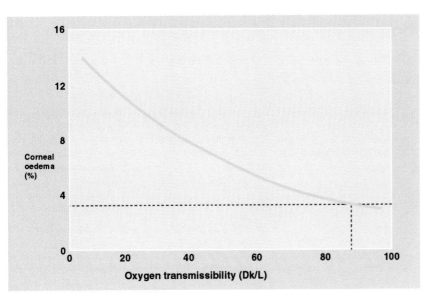

**Figure 11.9**
*Relationship between Dk/L versus oedema for extended wear (adapted from Holden and Mertz[21])*

## Prognosis

In general, the prognosis for recovery of the cornea from lens-induced oedema is excellent. In laboratory experiments, it can be demonstrated that the oedema induced when a patient wears a contact lens for the first time will resolve within four hours of lens removal.[15] Conversely, it was demonstrated by Holden *et al*[11] that oedema took 7 days to resolve following lens removal from patients who had worn extended wear lenses for 5 years.

The cases cited are likely to represent the two extremes (4 hours vs 7 days) of rate of recovery from lens-induced oedema. It may be that, within this range, the rate of recovery of oedema following lens wear is related to the total accumulated lens-wear experience. There do not appear to have been any reports of contact lens-induced oedema failing to resolve.

The rate at which the cornea recovers from lens-induced oedema has been suggested as a test of the health of the cornea. It is known, for example, that the corneas of patients suffering from Fuch's endothelial dystrophy[22] and of diabetic patients[23] have an impaired capacity to eliminate excess oedema. Specifically, the corneal deswelling rate is thought to reflect the integrity of the endothelium, which is responsible for corneal hydration control.

## Differential diagnosis

Striae can take on a similar appearance to ghost vessels and nerve fibres. The characteristics that allow these entities to be differentiated are discussed in Chapter 12. Fonn and Gauthier[24] have described the presence of fibrillary lines in both lens wearers and non-lens wearers; these seem to be similar to oedema-related striae, but are thought to be neural in origin and are apparently permanent.

Folds can occur naturally in a small proportion of normal patients and are often observed in diabetic patients.[25] It has recently been established that folds observed in diabetic daily lens wearers do not alter their appearance over a number of months.[26] Again, the capacity of lens-induced folds to resolve rapidly following lens removal is a key diagnostic criterion.

Various corneal dystrophies and diseases of the cornea and associated ocular structures, as well as iatrogenic interventions such as ophthalmic surgery or drug therapy, can result in stromal oedema. While it is beyond the scope of this chapter to review all of these possible causes of oedema, in most instances there will be associated signs and symptoms that cannot be reconciled with contact lens-induced oedema. For example, in addition to stromal oedema, Fuch's endothelial dystrophy is characterised by permanent and pronounced endothelial guttata, bullous keratopathy (large fluid vacuoles in the stroma), loss of vision and pain.

The key feature that distinguishes the signs of contact lens-induced corneal oedema – striae, folds and haze – from other clinical entities that take on a similar appearance is that lens-induced oedema will resolve soon after lens removal.

## REFERENCES

1 Efron N, Pearson RM (1988) Centenary celebration of Fick's *Eine Contactbrille*. *Arch Ophthalmol* **106**: 1370.

2 Pearson RM, Efron N (1989) Hundredth anniversary of August Muller's inaugural dissertation on contact lenses. *Surv Ophthalmol* **34**: 133.

3 Goldberg JB (1970) *Biomicroscopy for Contact Lens Practice: Clinical Procedures.* The Professional Press, Chicago.

4 Mandell RB, Fatt I (1965) Thinning of the human cornea on awakening. *Nature* **208**: 292.

5 LaHood D, Sweeney DF, Holden BA (1988) Overnight corneal oedema with hydrogel, rigid gas-permeable and silcone-elastomer contact lenses. *Int Contact Lens Clin* **15**: 149.

6 Holden BA, Mertz GW, McNally JJ (1983) Corneal swelling response to contact lenses worn under extended wear conditions. *Invest Ophthalmol Vis Sci* **24**: 218.

7 Chan-Ling T, Pye DC (1994) Pachometry: clinical and scientific applications. In: *Contact Lens Practice* (eds M Ruben and M Guillon). Chapman and Hall Medical, London.

8 Sarver MD (1971) Striate corneal lines among patients wearing hydrophilic contact lenses. *Am J Optom Physiol Opt* **48**: 762.

9 LaHood D, Grant T (1990) Striae and folds as indicators of corneal oedema. *Optom Vis Sci* **67**: 196.

10 Fatt I, Weissman BA (1992) *Physiology of the Eye. An Introduction to the Vegetative Functions* Butterworth–Heinemann, Boston, MA.

11 Holden BA, Sweeney DF, Vannas A (1985) Effects of long-term extended contact lens wear on the human cornea. *Invest Ophthalmol Vis Sci* **26**: 1489.

12 Sweeney DF, Holden BA (1991) The relative contributions of hypoxia,

**Table 11.2   Treatment strategies for contact lens-induced oedema**

| Observation | Daily wear patient | | Extended wear patient | |
|---|---|---|---|---|
| | Rigid | Soft | Rigid | Soft |
| Striae<br>(grade 2<br>5–7% oedema) | 1 Increase lens Dk<br>2 Looser fit<br>3 Reduce wearing time<br>4 Abandon lens wear | 1 Increase water content<br>2 Reduce thickness<br>3 Looser fit<br>4 Change to rigid lens | If < 4 h after waking:<br>'normal' finding<br>If > 4 h after waking:<br>1 Increase lens Dk<br>2 Looser fit<br>3 Change to daily wear | If < 4 h after waking:<br>'normal' finding<br>If > 4 h after waking:<br>1 Increase water content<br>2 Reduce thickness<br>3 Looser fit<br>4 Change to rigid lens<br>5 Change to daily wear |
| Folds<br>(grade 3<br>8–14% oedema) | 1 Cease wear: 1 week<br>2 Increase lens Dk<br>3 Looser fit<br>4 Reduce wearing time<br>5 Abandon lens wear | 1 Cease wear: 1 week<br>2 Increase water content<br>3 Reduce thickness<br>4 Looser fit<br>5 Change to rigid lens | If < 1 h after waking:<br>'normal' finding<br>If > 1 h after waking:<br>1 Increase lens Dk<br>2 Looser fit<br>3 Change to daily wear | If < 1 h after waking:<br>'normal' finding<br>If > 1 h after waking:<br>1 Increase water content<br>2 Reduce thickness<br>3 Looser fit<br>4 Change to rigid lens<br>5 Change to daily wear |
| Haze<br>(grade 4<br>>15% oedema) | 1 Initially: non-steroid anti-inflammatory drugs<br>2 Cease wear: 1 month<br>3 Increase lens Dk<br>4 Looser fit<br>5 Reduce wearing time<br>6 Abandon lens wear | 1 Initially: non-steroid anti-inflammatory drugs<br>2 Cease wear: 1 month<br>3 Increase water content<br>4 Reduce thickness<br>5 Looser fit<br>6 Change to rigid lens | If < 1 h after waking:<br>unacceptable<br>1 Initially: non-steroid anti-inflammatory drugs<br>2 Cease wear: 1 month<br>3 Increase lens Dk<br>4 Looser fit<br>5 Change to daily wear<br><br>If > 1 h after waking:<br>1 Initially: non-steroid anti-inflammatory drugs<br>2 Cease wear: 1 month<br>3 Change to daily wear | If < 1 h after waking:<br>unacceptable<br>1 Initially: non-steroid anti-inflammatory drugs<br>2 Cease wear: 1 month<br>3 Increase water content<br>4 Reduce thickness<br>5 Looser fit<br>6 Change to rigid lens<br>7 Change to daily wear<br><br>If > 1 h after waking:<br>1 Initially: non-steroid anti-inflammatory drugs<br>2 Cease wear: 1 month<br>3 Change to rigid lens<br>4 Change to daily wear |

osmolality, temperature and humidity to corneal oedema with eye closure. *Invest Ophthalmol Vis Sci* **32**: 739.

13 Klyce SD (1981) Stromal lactate accumulation can account for corneal oedema osmotically following epithelial hypoxia in the rabbit. *J Physiol* **332**: 49.

14 Woods R (1989) Quantitative slit-lamp observations in contact lens practice. *J Br Contact Lens Assoc (Scientific Meetings)*: 42–5.

15 O'Neal MR, Polse KA (1985) In vivo assessment of mechanisms controlling corneal hydration. *Invest Ophthalmol Vis Sci* **26**: 849.

16 Efron N (1991) Understanding oxygen: Dk/L, EOP, Oedema. *Trans Br Contact Lens Assoc* **14**: 65.

17 Efron N, Carney LG (1983) The effect of fenestrating soft contact lenses on corneal oxygen availability. *Am J Optom Physiol Opt* **60**: 503.

18 Brennan NA, Efron N, Carney LG (1986) The effects of fenestrating soft contact lenses on corneal swelling: a re-examination. *Clin Exp Optom* **69**: 120.

19 Ang JHB, Efron N (1987) Comfort of fenestrated hydrogel lenses. *Clin Exp Optom* **70**: 117.

20 Efron N (1992) Microfenestration of soft contact lenses. *Optician* **204**: 27.

21 Holden BA, Mertz GW (1984) Critical oxygen levels to avoid corneal oedema for daily and extended wear contact lenses. *Invest Ophthalmol Vis Sci* **25**:

22 Mandell RB, Polse KA, Brand RJ (1989) Corneal hydration control in Fuch's dystrophy. *Invest Ophthalmol Vis Sci* **30**: 845.

23 Weston BC, Bourne WM, Polse KA (1995) Corneal hydration control in diabetes mellitus. *Invest Ophthalmol Vis Sci* **36**: 586.

24 Fonn D, Gauthier C (1991) Prevalence of superficial fibrillary lines of the cornea in contact lens wearers. *Cornea* **10**: 507.

25 Henkind P, Wise GN (1961) Descemet's wrinkles in diabetes. *Am J Ophthalmol* **52**: 371.

26 O'Donnell C, Efron N (1995) Corneal endothelial folds in diabetes. *Optom Vis Sci* **72**: 57s.

# 12
# Neovascularisation

Prevalance
Signs and symptoms
Pathology
Aetiology
Observation and grading
Management and treatment
Prognosis
Differential diagosis

Although reports of contact lens-induced corneal neovascularisation can be traced back as far as 1929,[1] it is only in the past two decades that this problem has attracted the attention of contact lens practitioners.

Previously, practitioners have had to rely on conflicting and somewhat anecdotal guidelines about the limits of normal vascularisation, such as:

- '... a millimetre is about as far into the cornea as neovascularisation should be allowed to go...'[2]
- '... vessels extending in from the limbus for a distance of l.5 mm...'[3]
- '... superficial vessels to the extent of 2 mm or 3 mm must be considered abnormal'.[4]

A variety of terms can be used to describe the vascular response of the cornea to lens wear. This has unfortunately resulted in some ambiguity in the literature, with various authors using different terms to describe the same phenomenon or using the same term to describe different phenomena. Some of the more commonly used terms to define the presence of blood vessels in the cornea are:

- *Vascularisation.* The normal existence of vascular capillaries in the cornea (encroaching no more than 0.2 mm into the cornea from the limbus).
- *Neovascularisation.* The formation and extension of vascular capillaries in and into previously unvascularised regions of the cornea.
- *Limbal hyperaemia.* Increased blood flow, resulting in distension of the limbal blood vessels. Hyperaemia may be active when due to dilatation of blood vessels, or passive when the drainage is hindered. (It is also termed limbal injection or engorgement.)
- *Vessel penetration.* Apparent ingrowth of vessels, typically towards the corneal apex, measured from an arbitrary reference at the corneoscleral junction.
- *Vasoproliferation.* Increase in the number of vessels.
- *Vascular pannus.* Vascularisation and connective-tissue deposition beneath the epithelium, usually in the superior limbal region.
- *Vascular response.* A general term encompassing any alteration to the normal vasculature, including those entities described above.

## Prevalence

The original haptic lenses were capable of inducing corneal neovascularisation, although there is little data on the magnitude of the problem, apart from isolated case reports.[1,5–7] Certainly, the prevalence of corneal neovascularisation among wearers of polymethyl methacrylate (PMMA) lenses was very low.[8]

Reports of the prevalence of corneal neovascularisation among patients wearing hydrogel lenses on an extended wear basis for cosmetic reasons are inconsistent, with retrospective studies indicating substantially fewer cases of abnormal vascularisation than in prospective studies. The prevalence of neovascularisation during rigid (gas permeable) lens wear appears to be extremely low.

Corneal neovascularisation has a greater prevalence in patients using extended wear hydrogel lenses for aphakic correction

**Table 12.1 Prevalence of contact lens-induced stromal neovascularisation reported in the literature**

| Lens type | Mode of lens wear | Patient type | Reported prevalence of vascularisation (%) |
|---|---|---|---|
| PMMA[a] | DW[c] | Cosmetic | 0.03[8] |
| Rigid[b] | DW | Cosmetic | 0.0[10] |
| Rigid | EW[d] | Cosmetic | 0.0[10,11] |
| Soft | DW | Cosmetic | 0.64,[12] 1.25[13] |
| Soft | DEW[3] | Cosmetic | 0.86[12] |
| Soft | EW | Cosmetic | 0.0,[14] 0.2,[15] 1.75,[12] 7.0,[16] 8.7[3] |
| Soft | EW | Aphakic | 14.2[17] |
| Soft | EW | Therapeutic | 2.88,[18] 35.0[19] |

[a] Polymethyl methacrylate
[b] Rigid gas-permeable
[c] Daily wear
[d] Extended wear
[e] Disposable extended wear

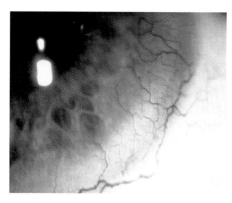

**Figure 12.1**
*Extensive superficial neovascularisation extending approximately 2.5 mm into the cornea*

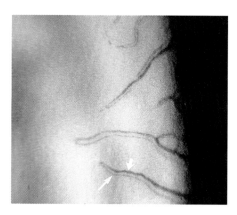

**Figure 12.2**
*At high magnification, it is possible to distinguish arteriolar (thick arrow) and venular (thin arrow) components of a capillary spike*

than in cosmetic lens wearers. Such a finding is not unexpected in view of the surgical trauma that the cornea has endured, the compromised physiological status of the cornea as a result of surgery[9] and the necessarily thick lenses that must be worn to provide optical correction for an aphakic eye.

The reported prevalence of corneal neovascularisation in patients wearing soft lenses for therapeutic reasons varies markedly. The extent of neovascularisation in such patients might be related to the underlying corneal pathology being treated, the type of lens fitted and the mode and duration of lens wear.

Published estimates[3,10–19] of the prevalence of len-induced neovascularisation are presented in Table 12.1. When considering the data presented, it is important to remember that there are significant differences in sample sizes, experimental protocols, patient characteristics and criteria chosen for considering a vascular response as being normal versus abnormal between studies.

## Signs and symptoms

### 'Normal' vascular response to lens wear

Using the limit of the visible iris as a reference point, McMonnies and co-workers[20] found the mean linear extent of limbal vessel filling, measured inferiorly, to be 0.13 mm in non-wearers, 0.22 mm in rigid lens wearers and 0.47 mm in soft lens wearers (daily wear). Stark and Martin[3] and Holden *et al*[21] reported an increased vascular response of 0.52 mm and 0.50 mm, respectively, associated with soft extended lens wear.

Whether reports of vascular responses represent the filling of capillaries that were empty, dilatation of fine vessels that were barely visible, true penetration of vessels into the stroma or a combination of the above is often unclear. Nevertheless, the fact that a number of authors[3,20,21] have independently established that various modes of lens wear can alter the appearance of the limbal vasculature provides support for the concept of a normal (although undesirable) lens-induced vascular response.

### 'Abnormal' vascular response to lens wear

Adjacent to the limbus, there is a vascular plexus at all levels, from which ingrowing vessels typically emerge. A variety of neovascularisation patterns can occur, which are considered under three headings.

*Superficial neovascularisation*
This is the most common form of contact lens-induced vascular response.[4] In the undisturbed eye, episcleral branches of the anterior ciliary artery form a plexus around the limbus known as the superficial marginal arcade. Minute branches form at right-angles to this plexus, encroaching into the cornea and looping inward towards the corneal apex (Figure 12.1). The resultant vascular loops or arcades are typically semi-circular; they tend to anastomose, with each successive arc becoming smaller, ultimately forming a rich vascular plexus around the limbus.[4]

Vessels encroaching into the cornea form arterioles and then capillaries. Arterial and venous capillaries may lie close together, giving the appearance of a single capillary spike when viewed under low magnification;[22] at high magnification, however, the two capillary components can be distinguished (Figure 12.2). Venous capillaries often return along a deeper and more tortuous course and appear finer.

Vision loss in superficial neovascularisation is rare and will only occur if vessels encroach onto the pupillary axis.

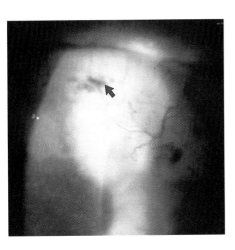

**Figure 12.3**
*Haemorrhaging of a deep stromal vessel*

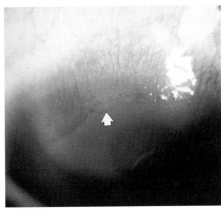

**Figure 12.4**
*Fibrovascular pannus, with an even leading edge of fibrous tissue stained with rose bengal*

*Deep stromal neovascularisation*
Contact lenses can induce neovascularisation at all levels of the stroma, from just beneath the anterior limiting lamina down to the posterior limiting lamina.[4] The condition develops insidiously and may progress in the absence of acute symptoms.[23] The typical appearance is a large feeding vessel emerging sharply from the limbus, usually in the mid-stroma, rapidly developing into finer, wildly tortuous branches and ending in buds with numerous small vessel anastomoses. This irregular pattern is thought to be due to a breakdown in the structure of the stroma.[22]

Loss of vision can occur when there has been leakage of lipid into the stroma.[24] Donnenfeld et al[24] documented five cases of haemorrhaging of deep corneal vessels that were induced by contact lens wear (Figure 12.3); in one of these cases, a penetrating keratoplasty was required for visual rehabilitation.

*Vascular pannus*
A pannus is an extensive ingrowth of tissue from the limbus onto the peripheral cornea. The penetration occurs between the epithelium and anterior limiting lamina, resulting in a separation of these layers and often leading to a destruction of the anterior limiting lamina.[23] The term 'micropannus' is used when the extent of invasion is less than 2.0 mm from the limbus.[25]

There are two forms of pannus – active (inflammatory) and fibrovascular (degenerative); both types may be observed in contact lens wearers. An active pannus is avascular and is composed of sub-epithelial inflammatory cells. In the latter stages, it may be associated with secondary scarring of the stroma.

A fibrovascular pannus consists of an ingrowth of collagen and vessels and often contains fatty plaques.[23] The clinical appearance of a fibrovascular pannus is a congested band of vessels penetrating in an orderly fashion into the cornea, with the limit of penetration remaining even across its width. The invading end of the pannus often contains a considerable amount of fibrotic tissue, which stains brightly with rose bengal (Figure 12.4). This condition is observed in contact lens patients in association with superior limbic kerato-conjunctivitis.[26] As this name suggests, the pannus is observed at the superior limbus (see Chapter 7).

## Pathology

The ultrastructural tissue changes observed in contact lens-induced corneal neovascularisation have been described by Madigan et al[27] in a primate model. Vessel lumina were approximately 15 μm to 80 μm in diameter and contained erythrocytes and, sometimes, leucocytes. Numerous extravascular leucocytes were observed around blood vessels, and the surrounding stromal lamellae were disorganised and separated, with lines of keratocytes lying between them (Figure 12.5).

The overlying corneal epithelium was often affected, with general oedema, cell loss and the presence of large fluid-filled vesicles. The underlying Descemet's layer and endothelium were apparently unaffected.

The likely sequelae of events in the development of a vascular response can be predicted, based on general vascular response studies in lower animals. In particular, detailed investigations of corneal neovascularisation in the rat[28] following focal injury caused by chemical cautery have allowed three distinct phases of vessel formation to be defined – the prevascular latent period, neovascularisation and vascular regression.

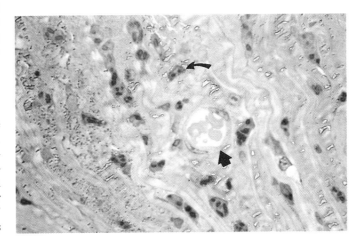

**Figure 12.5**
*Light micrograph of single blood vessel (thick arrow) induced by contact lens wear in primate stroma. Note the erythrocytes in the vessel lumen, the single endothelial cell wall, distorted stromal lamellae and keratocytes (curved arrow)*

# Aetiology

Numerous theories have been advanced to explain why corneal neovascularisation occurs, all of which are potentially relevant to the contact lens-induced vascular response. These theories are summarised below.

## Metabolic theory

### Hypoxia

Lack of oxygen is known to induce neovascularisation in other body tissues; naturally, similar mechanisms could also occur in the cornea.[29] Contact lenses are known to cause corneal hypoxia.[30]

Imre,[31] however, points out that some hypoxic tissues do not vascularise. In addition, Michaelson and co-workers[32] found that the development of neovascularisation following chemical burns in rabbits was unaffected by the ambient oxygen tension.

### Lactic acid

Lactic acid could be implicated in lens-induced corneal neovascularisation in two ways: first, contact lenses can create hypoxia in the cornea, leading to lactic acid production,[33] and, second, tightly fitting soft lenses may indent the conjunctiva and restrict venous drainage, causing lactic acid to accumulate in the peripheral cornea.[34]

### Oedema

The presence of excess fluid in the cornea (oedema) is thought by Cogan[35] to be sufficient to induce neovascularisation. This is supported by the finding of Thoft and co-workers[36] that oedema facilitates anterior stromal neovascularisation in rabbits. Clinically, corneal oedema is frequently present prior to neovascularisation,[37] and some authors believe that corneal neovascularisation does not occur in the absence of swelling.[38] Certainly, contact lenses can induce significant levels of oedema, particularly during extended wear.[39] The aetiological role of oedema can be challenged given the absence of neovascularisation in conditions where there is permanent oedema (i.e. congenital endothelial dystrophy and long-term extended lens wear). Baum and Martola[40] suggest that stromal oedema alone is insufficient stimulus for corneal neovascularisation.

### Stromal softening

Chronic oedema as a result of contact lens

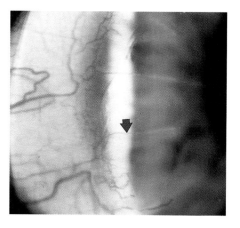

**Figure 12.6**

*Ingrowth of vessels (arrow) from the limbus along radial keratotomy scars*

wear may cause a breakdown of stromal ground substance or individual collagen fibrils, resulting in stromal thinning.[41] Oedema could also cause the stroma to soften or lose compactness, thus reducing the physical barrier to vessel penetration. Sholley and co-workers[42] have suggested that infiltrating neutrophils could release collagenases, proteases and elastases, which degrade the stroma and facilitate the ingrowth of vascular endothelial cells. While this theory could have some relevance to the normal vascular response to contact lens wear described earlier, experimental verification of a physical degradation or softening of stromal tissue in response to contact lens wear has not been produced.

The growth of vessels from the limbus along radial keratotomy scars (Figure 12.6) lends support to the 'stromal softening' theory because disorganised scar tissue can be considered a weakness in the normally compact stroma, equivalent to a softened stroma.

## Angiogenic suppression theory

According to this theory, there is a factor in the cornea that restrains cell division and migration of vascular cells of the pericorneal plexus.[43] Corneal fibroblasts and lymphocytes are thought to be involved in this process.[44] For corneal neovascularisation to occur, substances that inactivate the normally-present angiogenic inhibitors are required. Such substances could be, for example, any of the vasogenic agents described below. But this theory lacks solid experimental support, and Fromer and

Klintworth[45] argue that positive chemotaxis towards a vasostimulating factor is a more suitable explanation of observed patterns of corneal neovascularisation.

## Vasostimulation theory

This theory, which has most support, suggests that corneal neovascularisation is produced by locally generated or introduced vasostimulatory factors.[25] There are numerous candidates for this vasostimulatory activity, such as free cellular elements, humoral components, epithelial cell factors and extrinsic substances.

## Neural control theory

Cassel and Groden[46] suggest that there may be a neural influence on corneal vascularisation. They have provided experimental support for this theory by examining the limbal vascular response to a cautery burn in a central trephined area of cornea in rabbits. Limbal vessel growth was more advanced in the trephined corneas compared with matched controlled corneas that were not trephined. Since trephination produces denervation in the trephined zone,[47] the impaired limbal vascular response in the trephinated cornea could be attributed to an absence of neural influence. The effects of contact lenses on corneal neurology and sensitivity have been well documented.[48] If the neural control theory of Cassel and Groden is accepted,[46] it could be argued that the vascular response to lens wear is mediated by lens-induced changes to corneal neurology.

## A model of contact lens-induced neovascularisation

No single theory can account for corneal neovascularisation in response to contact lens wear. Indeed, virtually all the mechanisms discussed above can be triggered by some aspect of contact lens usage. Many of these theories can be incorporated into a model of lens-induced neovascularisation. In Figure 12.7 two main aetiological factors are presented. First, the contact lens creates tissue hypoxia, leading to corneal oedema and stromal softening. Second, the contact lens has contributed to a mechanical injury to the epithelium, resulting in a release of enzymes. Inflammatory cells migrate to this site and release

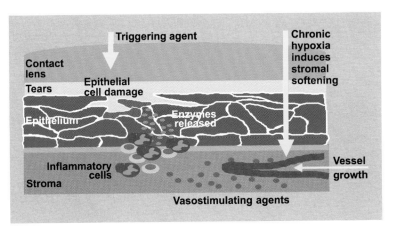

**Figure 12.7**
*Dual aetiology model of contact lens-induced neovascularisation, depicting chronic hypoxia leading to stromal softening as a precursor; and epithelial irritation acting as a stimulus to vessel growth*

derived from published data of the extent of vessel penetration with the various modalities of lens wear. Calculation of the mean plus one standard deviation gives the range within which approximately 85 per cent of the population will fall, which would be an acceptable criterion to adopt for 'normality'. Thus, the limits of 'normal' vascular ingrowth, measured from the limit of visible iris, should be (rounded upwards) 0.2 mm, 0.4 mm, 0.6 mm and 1.4 mm for no wear, daily wear rigid, daily wear soft and extended wear soft regimes respectively. Taking these values as a reference, the various grades of vascularisation can be denoted in the context of the 'clinical severity' scale of Woods[40] as described in Table 12.2 and illustrated in Appendix A.

Figure 12.9 is a schematic representation of the various patterns of contact lens-induced corneal neovascularisation. Vessel formations are depicted in different degrees of severity, which can be categorised using the grading system described.

vasostimulating agents that cause vessels to grow in that direction. As is obvious from the preceding discussion, this is only one of a number of possible models that could be proposed to explain stromal neovascularisation in response to contact lens wear.

## Observation and grading

The distinguishing characteristic of superficial vessels is that they can be seen to be continuous with the superficial marginal arcade. They can be observed using direct focal illumination, but are best viewed using either direct or indirect retro-illumination (Figure 12.8). High magnification (×40) is often required to trace the path of the returning venules deeper in the cornea. Individual blood corpuscles can usually be observed at this magnification. Fine vessels associated with cellular infiltration can be viewed more easily under red-free illumination.[22]

It is essential that a grading system incorporates a designation pertaining to the normal vascular response to lens wear described earlier. Such a criterion can be

## Management and treatment

Needless to say, the best form of treatment of corneal neovascularisation is prevention. Adherence to this maxim could be achieved by fitting a lens that does not touch the cornea, provides no resistance to the passage of oxygen or carbon dioxide (therefore creating no oedema or tissue

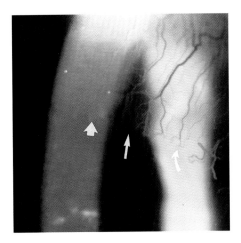

**Figure 12.8**
*Extensive superficial neovascularisation at the level of the anterior stroma, viewed by direct focal illumination (thick arrow), direct retro-illumination (curved arrow) and indirect retro-illumination (thin arrow)*

**Table 12.2  Neovascularisation grading scale**

| Grade | Clinical interpretation |
|---|---|
| 0 | No neovascularisation; that is, the presence of vessels up to 0.2 mm in from the limbus (as observed in non-lens wearers) |
| 1 | Superficial neovascularisation greater than 0.2 mm but less that the 'limits of normality' (0.4 mm for daily wear rigid; 0.6 mm for daily wear soft; and 1.4 mm for extended wear soft) |
| 2 | Superficial neovascularisation considerably greater than the 'limits of normality' (0.4 mm for daily wear rigid; 0.6 mm for daily wear soft; and 1.4 mm for extended wear soft) |
| 3 | Superficial neovascularisation considerably greater than the 'limits of normality' (0.4 mm for daily wear rigid; 0.6 mm for daily wear soft; and 1.4 mm for extended wear soft); vessels approaching the pupil margin (under typical 'lights on' consulting room conditions) |
| 4 | Extensive superficial neovascularisation; vessels encroaching into the pupillary zone (under typical 'lights on' consulting room conditions). Any extent of deep stromal neovascularisation |

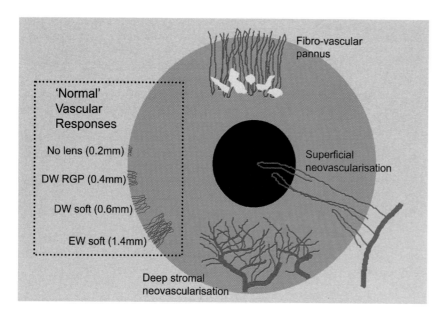

**Figure 12.9**
*Schematic representation of the various patterns of contact lens-induced stromal neovascularisation*

acidosis) and does not involve the use of any form of chemical.

As such a lens does not exist, practitioners are faced with a compromise situation. If corneal neovascularisation is a primary concern, lens design features known to provide minimal interference with corneal physiology are required, namely high-oxygen transmissibility (to minimise hypoxic oedema and hypercapnic acidosis), minimal mechanical effect (as judged by patient comfort[50]) and good movement (to avoid venous stasis resulting from limbal compression in soft lenses[34]). Care systems likely to induce toxic or allergic responses should be avoided, and regular aftercare visits are essential.

If neovascularisation of grade 2 or more develops, the practitioner should take action to arrest and hopefully reverse the vascular ingrowth. Since it is rarely possible to identify the specific cause of the vascular response, a systematic trial and error approach must be adopted. If an epithelial injury and/or localised keratitis is present, lens wear should be ceased until the condition resolves. In the absence of obvious concurrent pathology, the most prudent action would be to replace the lens with one likely to provide an optimal physiological response. It may also be advisable to change to a lens type (such as daily disposable lenses) or a care system that will provide minimal exposure of the lens, and thus the eye, to chemicals.

Other options to be considered include changing from extended wear to daily wear, using frequent replacement or disposable lenses, reducing wearing time or even ceasing lens wear. In view of the extremely low prevalence of corneal neovascularisation in patients wearing rigid contact lenses, a change to rigid lenses should be considered if the problem persists with soft lenses.

Certain drugs can control or reduce corneal neovascularisation. Duffin and co-workers,[51] for example, demonstrated that topical administration of a non-corticosteroid anti-inflammatory agent (flurbiprofen; a prostaglandin inhibitor) significantly suppressed contact lens-induced corneal neovascularisation in rabbits wearing rigid lenses. Topical corticosteroids can also prevent vascular ingrowth of the cornea.[52] Ruben,[4] however, warns that the use of such drugs is not without danger; for example, the use of steroids in patients with dry-eye syndrome can result in viral and fungal infections.

Grade 3 or 4 neovascularisation indicates that there may be a serious threat to vision and immediate action is required. Lens wear should be ceased for an extended period – at least until the vessels no longer lie in the pupillary area. Patients should be monitored carefully if lens wear is recommenced, as ghost vessels may refill rapidly and the neovascularisation process may recur. If vessels remain in the pupillary area, the patient should be counselled about the possibility of abandoning lens wear permanently.

In extreme cases, surgical intervention may be required, such as diathermy, bipolar galvanic electrolysis, or laser or microcautery occlusion of the vessels.[4] Where vision loss due to secondary fibrosis has occurred, keratoplasty may be necessary to restore useful vision.

## Prognosis

Published evidence suggests that the normal form of peripheral vascular ingrowth (grade 1) may undergo regression when contact lens wear is ceased. Holden and co-workers[21] observed that, one month following the removal of extended wear hydrogel lenses that had been worn for an average of 5 years, the extent of limbal vessel penetration appeared to decrease. Holden's group,[21] however, was unable to provide statistical verification of this observation (Figure 12.10).

Klintworth and Burger[28] noted that large vessels that invaded the rat cornea following chemical cautery injury persisted for as long as 2 months. Ausprunk and co-workers[53] observed complete regression of vessels in rabbit corneas 10 weeks after the vascularising stimulus was removed. Madigan *et al*[27] reported a gradual decrease in the visibility of vessels after cessation of lens wear in vascularised monkey corneas; larger vessels emptied, leaving 'ghost vessels' of reduced diameter (10 μm to 25 μm), while the smaller, superficial vessels apparently regressed (Figure 12.11). Only a few ghost vessels were observed 14 months after lens removal. McMonnies[22] has noted that fully established corneal vessels do not seem to regress in human eyes and can persist indefinitely, remaining as ghost vessels.

While the rate of vascular regression in humans is still open to debate, practitioners should note that cessation of lens wear will at least halt the progression of vessel infiltration into the cornea. Madigan *et al*[27] reinserted lenses into monkey eyes that had suffered contact lens-induced neovascularisation 9 months previously. Within 36 hours, the existing 'ghost vessels' had refilled and the overall appearance, including asso-

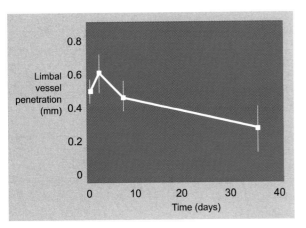

**Figure 12.10**
*Apparent regression of neovascularisation following cessation of lens wear for one month after 5 years of soft lens extended wear (adapted from Holden et al[41])*

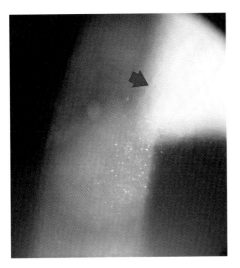

**Figure 12.11**
*Ghost vessels (arrow) in primate cornea 3 months after lens wear ceased*

ciated epithelial oedema, was similar to that observed during the original phase of neovascularisation.

Resumption of lens wear must be treated with extreme caution and be accompanied by a rigorous and frequent aftercare protocol, since it is evident from the primate model of Madigan *et al*[27] that ghost vessels will refill rapidly if a stimulus to neovascularisation – which may simply be lens wear – is reintroduced.

## Differential diagnosis

Stromal neovascularisation has a distinct appearance, so it is unlikely that this con-

dition will be confused with other complications of contact lens wear. It is perhaps more important to distinguish between the various forms of vascular response, with a view to determining the aetiology of the

condition. This is not always straightforward; for example, the only difference between neovascularisation induced by contact lens wear versus that which may be occurring coincidentally as part of an unrelated pathological process may be the extent of the reaction.

Grohe and Lebow[54] have described a chronic inflammatory complication of rigid lens wear called vascularised limbal keratitis (VLK), whereby vessels can grow into the cornea beyond the 'normal' limits. This condition is characterised by adjacent conjunctival neovascularisation and hyperaemia, a local raised epithelial mass and corneal staining (Figure 12.12). An additional clue to differential diagnosis is that VLK may be associated with symptoms of discomfort, photophobia and increased lacrimation, whereas the insidious form of lens-induced neovascularisation described throughout this chapter is asymptomatic.

Ghost vessels have a similar appearance to nerve fibres, but are less like striae. The

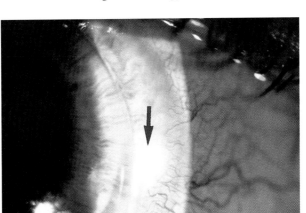

**Figure 12.12**
*Active stage of vascular limbal keratitis with raised limbal-epithelial mass and prominent vascular leash observed after 6 days of rigid extended wear*

**Table 12.3   Differential diagnosis of ghost vessels**

|  | Ghost vessels | Nerve fibres | Striae |
|---|---|---|---|
| Connection to limbus | Yes | Yes | No |
| Colour | Grey/white | Grey/white | Grey/white |
| Bifurcations | Yes | Yes | No |
| Stromal depth | Any | Any | Deep |
| Orientation | Radial | Radial | Vertical |
| Form | Discrete: abrupt end | Discrete: can be long | 'Feathery': faded ends |
| Diameter | 10–12 μm | 0.1–0.25 μm | 5 μm |
| Permanence | Resolution in months | Permanent | Resolution in minutes |

distinguishing features of these three structures are compared in Table 12.3.

## REFERENCES

1 Lauber H (1929) Praktische durchfurung von myopiekorrektion mit kontaktglasern. *Klin Monatsbl Augenheilkd* **82**: 535.

2 Allansmith MR (1984) Neovascularisation – how much and how far? *J Am Optom Assoc* **55**: 199.

3 Stark WJ, Martin NF (1981) Extended-wear contact lenses for myopic correction. *Arch Ophthalmol* **99**: 1963.

4 Ruben M (1981) Corneal vascularisation. In: *Complications of Contact Lenses* (eds D Miller, PF White), Little, Brown and Co., Boston, MA, p. 27.

5 Strebel J (1937) Objektive nachweise der orthopadischen heilwirkung der haftglasser beim hornhautkegel. *Klin Monatsbl Augenheilkd* **99**: 30.

6 Dixon WS and Bron AJ (1973) Fluorescein angiographic demonstration of corneal vascularisation in contact lens wearers. *Am J Ophthalmol* **75**: 1010.

7 Dixon JM, Lawaczek E (1963) Corneal vascularisation due to contact lenses. *Arch Ophthalmol* **69**: 72.

8 Dixon JM (1967) Corneal vascularisation due to corneal lenses: the clinical picture. *Trans Am Ophthalmol Soc* **65**: 333.

9 Holden BA, Polse KA, Fonn D (1982) Effects of cataract surgery on corneal function. *Invest Ophthalmol Vis Sci* **22**: 343.

10 Levy B (1985) Rigid gas-permeable lenses for extended wear: a one–year clinical evaluation. *Am J Optom Physiol Opt* **62**: 889.

11 Kamiya C (1986) Cosmetic extended wear of oxygen permeable hard contact lenses: one-year follow-up. *J Am Optom Assoc* **57**: 182.

12 Poggio EC, Abelson M (1993) Complications and symptoms in disposable extended wear lenses compared with conventional soft daily wear and soft extended wear lenses. *Contact Lens Assoc Ophthalmol J* **19**: 31.

13 Roth HW (1978) The etiology of ocular irritation in soft lens wearers: distribution in a large clinical sample. *Contact Intraoc Lens Med J* **4**: 38.

14 Maguen E, Nesburn AB, Verity SM (1984) Myopic extended wear contact lenses in 100 patients: a retrospective study. *Contact Lens Assoc Ophthalmol J* **10**: 335.

15 Lamar L (1983) Extended wear contact lenses for myopes: a follow-up study of 400 cases. *Ophthalmology* **90**: 156.

16 Binder PS (1983) Myopic extended wear with Hydrocurve II soft contact lenses. *Ophthalmology* **90**: 623.

17 Spoor TC, Hartel WC, Wynn P (1984) Complications of continuous-wear soft contact lenses in a non-referral population. *Arch Ophthalmol* **102**: 1312.

18 Dohlman CH, Boruchoff MD, Mobilia EF (1973) Complications in use of soft contact lenses in corneal disease. *Arch Ophthalmol* **90**: 367.

19 Schecter DR, Emery JM, Soper JW (1975) Corneal vascularisation in therapeutic soft-lens wear. *Contact Intraoc Lens Med J* **1**: 141.

20 McMonnies CW, Chapman-Davies A, Holden BA (1982) The vascular response to contact lens wear. *Am J Optom Physiol Opt* **19**: 795.

21 Holden BA, Sweeney DF, Swarbrick HA (1986) The vascular response to long-term extended contact lens wear. *Clin Exp Optom* **69**: 112.

22 McMonnies CW (1983) Contact lens-induced corneal vascularisation. *Int Contact Lens Clin* **10**: 12.

23 Apple DJ, Rabb MF (1978) *Clinicopathologic Correlation of Ocular Disease: a Text and Stereoscopic Atlas*, 2nd edn. Mosby, St Louis, p. 80.

24 Donnenfeld ED, Ingraham H, Perry HD (1991) Contact lens-related deep stromal intracorneal haemorrhage. *Ophthalmology* **98**: 1793.

25 Grayson M (1983) *Diseases of the Cornea*, 2nd edn. CV Mosby, St Louis, p. 336.

26 Sendele DD, Kenyon KR, Mobilia EF (1983) Superior limbic keratoconjunctivitis in contact lens wearers. *Ophthalmology* **90**: 616.

27 Madigan MC, Penfold PL, Holden BA (1990) Ultrastructural features of contact lens-induced deep corneal neovascularisation and associated stromal leucocytes. *Cornea* **9**: 144.

28 Klintworth GK, Burger PC (1983) Neovascularisation of the cornea. Current concepts of its pathogenesis. In: *Non-infectious Inflammation of the Anterior Segment* (ed. GN Foulkes). Little, Brown and Co, Boston, MA, p. 27.

29 Ashton N, Cook C (1983) Mechanisms of corneal vascularisation. *Br J Ophthalmol* **37**: 193.

30 Efron N, Carney LG (1981) Models of oxygen performance for the static, dynamic and closed-lid wear of hydrogel contact lenses. *Aust J Optom* **64**: 223.

31 lmre G (1972) Neovascularisation of the eye. In: *Contemporary Ophthalmology* (ed JG Bellows). Williams and Wilkins, Baltimore, MD, p. 88.

32 Michaelson IC, Herz N, Kertesz R (1954) Effect of increased oxygen concentration on new vessel growth in the adult cornea. *Br J Ophthalmol* **38**: 588.

33 Hamano H, Hori M, Kawabe H (1983) Effects of contact lens wear on mitosis of corneal epithelium and lactate content in aqueous humor of rabbit. *Jpn J Ophthalmol* **27**: 451.

34 McMonnies CW (1984) Risk factors in the etiology of contact lens induced corneal vascularisation. *Int Contact Lens Clin* **5**: 286.

35 Cogan DG (1949) Vascularisation of the cornea. *Arch Ophthalmol* **41**: 406–16.

36 Thoft RA, Friend J, Murphy HS (1979) Ocular surface epithelium and corneal vascularisation in rabbits: the role of wounding. *Invest Ophthalmol Vis Sci* **18**: 85.

37 Arentsen JJ (1986) Corneal neovascularisation in contact lens wearers. In: *Contact Lenses and External Disease* (ed. EJ Cohen). Boston, MA, p. 15.

38 Berggren L, Lempberg R (1973) Neovascularisation in the rabbit cornea after intracorneal injection of cartilage extracts. *Exp Eye Res* **17**: 261.

39 Holden BA, Mertz GW, McNally JJ (1983) Corneal swelling response to contact lenses worn under extended-wear conditions. *Invest Ophthalmol Vis Sci* **24**: 218.

40 Baum JL, Martola EL (1968) Corneal edema and corneal vascularisation. *Am J Ophthalmol* **65**: 881.

41 Holden BA, Sweeney DF, Vannas A (1985) Effects of long-term extended contact lens wear on the human cornea. *Invest Ophthalmol Vis Sci* **26**: 1489.

42 Sholley MM, Grimbrone MA, Coltran RS (1978) The effects of leukocyte depletion on corneal neovascularisation. *Lab Invest* **38**: 32.

43 Maurice DM, Zauberman H, Michaelson IC (1966) The stimulus to neovas-

cularisation in the cornea. *Exp Eye Res* **5**: 168.

44 Kaminiski M, Kaminska G (1978) Inhibition of lymphocyte-induced angiogenesis by enzymatically isolated rabbit cornea cells. *Arch Immunol Theor Exp* **26**: 1079.

45 Fromer CH, Klintworth GK (1976) An evaluation of the role of leukocytes in the pathogenesis of experimentally induced corneal vascularization: studies related to the vasoproliferative capability of polymorphonuclear leukocytes and lymphocytes. *Am J Path* **82**: 157.

46 Cassel G, Groden LR (1984) New thoughts on ocular neovascularisation:

a neurally controlled regenerative process? *Ann Ophthalmol* **16**: 138.

47 Rozsa AJ, Guss RB, Beuerman RW (1983) Neural remodelling following experimental surgery of the rabbit cornea. *Invest Ophthalmol Vis Sci* **24**: 1033.

48 Millodot M (1984) A review of research on the sensitivity of the cornea. *Ophthal Physiol Opt* **4**: 305.

49 Woods R (1989) Quantitative slit lamp observations in contact lens practice. *J Br Contact Lens Assoc (Scientific Meetings)*: 42.

50 Efron N, Brennan NA, Currie JM (1986) Determinants of the initial comfort of

hydrogel contact lenses. *Am J Optom Physiol Opt* **63**: 819.

51 Duffin RM, Weissman B, Ueda J (1982) Complications of extended wear hard contact lenses in rabbits. *Int Contact Lens Clin* **9**: 101.

52 Olson CL (1966) Subconjunctival steroids and corneal hypersensitivity. *Arch Ophthalmol* **75**: 651.

53 Ausprunk DH, Falterman K, Folkman J (1978) The sequence of events in the regression of corneal capillaries. *Lab Invest* **38**: 284.

54 Grohe RM, Lebow KA (1989) Vascularised limbal keratitis. *Int Contact Lens Clin* **7** and **8**: 197.

# 13
# Sterile infiltrative keratitis

Terminology
Prevalence
Signs and symptoms
Pathology
Aetiology
Patient management
Prognosis
Differential diagnosis

Few of the contact lens-induced ocular complications discussed in this book lead to a permanent loss of sight; indeed, many of these conditions (e.g. corneal staining, epithelial microcysts, stromal oedema) will resolve if lens wear is ceased. Stromal infiltrates, in the absence of significant epithelial compromise or associated pathology, are usually benign.[1] However, they can also be a key sign of infectious keratitis, which is potentially sight-threatening and often must be dealt with as a medical emergency.

This chapter will concentrate on contact lens-induced sterile infiltrative keratitis (CL-SIK); that is, the appearance of stromal infiltrates in the absence of microbial infection (Figure 13.1).

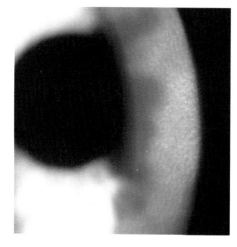

**Figure 13.1**
*CL-SIK in the form of a broad band of circumcorneal haziness*

## Terminology

A variety of terms are used to describe conditions in which corneal infiltrates are observed:

- *Infiltrate* – material that has passed into

tissue spaces or cells, which may include fluids, cells or other substances. The 'other substances' may be natural to the part or cell (but in excess) or foreign to the part or cell.[2]
- *Infiltrative keratitis* – an inflammation of

corneal tissue characterised in part (or in whole) by the presence of infiltrates.
- *Ulcerative keratitis* – an inflammation of corneal tissue characterised in part (or in whole) by extensive epithelial compromise and underlying epithelial and/or stromal infiltrates, and possible stromal melting.
- *Microbial keratitis* – an inflammation of corneal tissue due to direct infection by a microbial agent such as a bacteria, virus, fungus or amoeba.
- *Infectious keratitis* – an inflammation of corneal tissue attributable to the processes of microbial infection.
- *Sterile keratitis* – an inflammation of corneal tissue attributable to processes other than microbial infection.
- *Culture-positive* – micro-organisms were positively identified following a culture of the affected tissue.
- *Culture-negative* – no micro-organisms were identified following a culture of the affected tissue.
- *Intra-epithelial infiltrates* – infiltrates (predominantly inflammatory cells) within the epithelium.
- *Sub-epithelial infiltrates* – infiltrates (predominantly inflammatory cells) lying be-

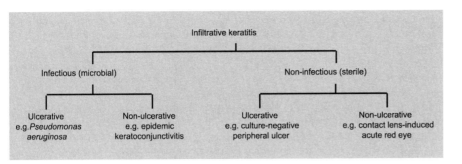

**Figure 13.2**
*A schema for the classification of infiltrative keratitis*

tween the epithelial basement membrane and Bowman's membrane and/or in the anterior stroma.

- *Stromal infiltrates* – infiltrates (predominantly inflammatory cells) in any part of the stroma.

Figure 13.2 is a flow diagram of a schema for classification of infiltrative keratitis. An infectious keratitis can be ulcerative (e.g. *Pseudomonas aeruginosa* keratitis) or non-ulcerative (e.g. epidemic keratoconjunctivitis). A positive culture result will provide strong evidence that the keratitis is infectious (microbial), but a negative culture result simply means that microbial agents could not be detected in the tissue. In the latter case, a keratitis may still be classified clinically as 'infectious' based upon the size of the ulcer and associated signs and symptoms.[3]

A non-infectious (sterile) infiltrative keratitis will typically be culture-negative. Any ulceration in such cases can be due to a variety of non-infectious mechanisms, such as toxicity (e.g. solution toxicity or endotoxins from bacteria harbouring on a contact lens), immunological reaction, trauma, metabolic disturbance etc. An example of this type of reaction is the so-called 'culture-negative peripheral ulcer' (CNPU).[4] Various non-ulcerative clinical manifestations of CL-SIK have been described in the literature; these include 'contact lens-induced acute red eye' (CLARE) and 'asymptomatic infiltrates' (AI).[4] Bacteria have been isolated at the time of a CLARE event; however, it is likely that these bacteria have exerted their pathogenicity via endotoxicity from a remote site to the injury (e.g. colonisation on a contact lens) rather than direct invasion of corneal tissue.

## Prevalence

In what was one of the first properly controlled studies of continuous wear contact lenses, Zantos[5] reported that 41 per cent of 34 patients developed corneal infiltrates over a 2-year period. In a retrospective evaluation of the records of 500 extended wear soft lens patients examined between 1977 and 1983, 10 per cent of patients were found by Gordon and Kracher[6] to have suffered from an episode of CL-SIK. Josephson and Caffery[1] reported that 4 per cent of all of their soft lens patients developed CL-SIK, but they did not report the lens wear modality.

Hamano *et al*[7] reported the incidence of CL-SIK in patients wearing various lens types and modalities to be as follows: PMMA lenses 0.4 per cent; RGP lenses 0.2 per cent; silicone elastomer lenses 0.8 per cent; HEMA lenses 0.4 per cent; high water content soft lenses < 0.1 per cent; weekly disposable soft lenses 0.1 per cent; and daily disposable soft lenses 0.1 per cent. Vajdic *et al*[8] reported much higher incidence figures: disposable daily wear soft lenses 15 per cent; disposable extended wear soft lenses 7 per cent; daily wear RGP lenses 3 per cent; and extended wear RGP lenses 2 per cent.

Stapleton *et al*[9] established the following estimates of relative risk of developing CL-SIK with different lens types and modalities: daily wear RGP lenses (referent) 1.0; PMMA lenses 1.0; daily wear soft lenses 2.1; and extended wear soft lenses 2.4.

The incidence of CLARE in patients wearing extended wear soft lenses was found by Grant to be 30 per cent per patient-year with high water content lenses and 15 per cent per patient-year with low water content lenses.[10] The incidence reduced to about 6 per cent when lenses were replaced regularly. The incidence of CNPU is ap-

proximately 3 per cent per patient-year among hydrogel extended wear patients.[4]

Much of the data discussed above relate to retrospective studies. In such studies, episodes of CL-SIK would only have been recorded if the attending practitioner deemed the appearance of infiltrates to be clinically significant and worthy of noting on the record card. Indeed, retrospective analyses are known generally to underestimate the prevalence of subtle clinical phenomena. Sweeney *et al*[11] demonstrated that if one looks carefully enough, mild disturbances to corneal transparency that could reasonably be interpreted as mild stromal infiltration will frequently be observed, although most of these occurrences are clinically insignificant.

## Signs and symptoms

According to Zantos,[12] infiltrates appear as a diffuse band of haziness near the limbus (see Figure 13.1), focal spots of haziness in any region of the cornea (Figure 13.3), or a combination of the two. In most cases the infiltrates are 'sub-epithelial'; that is, beneath the epithelium but almost always in the anterior half of the stroma. Less frequently, intra-epithelial infiltrates can be observed. On slit-lamp examination, the areas of infiltration appear as hazy, grey areas giving a dull, grainy appearance. Infiltrates are usually best examined under diffuse illumination at low magnification. Small feint focal infiltrates can be more difficult to see and are perhaps best observed using indirect illumination. Infiltrates are often located in the proximity of local bul-

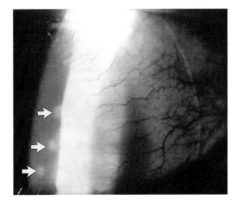

**Figure 13.3**
*Infiltrates in the corneal mid-periphery (arrows) in association with soft lens-induced stromal neovascularisation*

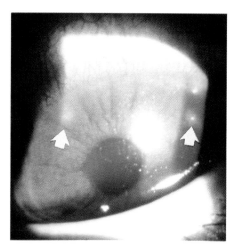

**Figure 13.4**
*Infiltrates (arrows) near a region of limbal hyperaemia in the case of a patient suffering from CL-SIK*

bar conjunctival and limbal hyperaemia (Figure 13.4). There is a general tendency for episodes of CL-SIK to be uniocular, with the exception of a toxic reaction to solution preservatives used for the first time, where a bilateral reaction is generally observed.

The dilemma that clinicians face in managing patients presenting with corneal infiltrates is that there is considerable overlap in the clinical presentation of infected versus sterile infiltrates. Stein *et al*[13] reported that increased pain, discharge, epithelial staining and anterior chamber reaction were associated with infected ulcers. In CL-SIK, infiltrates were usually smaller, forming a multiple or arcuate pattern, and without significant pain, epithelial staining or anterior chamber reaction.

However, these are only general guidelines. Stein *et al*[13] reported that although most sterile infiltrates were small – with 70 per cent measuring less than 1.0 mm in diameter – 35 per cent of infected infiltrates were also less than 1.0 mm in diameter. This agrees with the findings of Mertz *et al*[14] in patients wearing disposable soft extended wear lenses; in nine reported cases of presumed CL-SIK (with a negative result reported in all six cases that were cultured), the infiltrates ranged widely in diameter: from less than 1.0 mm in five patients, to 1.5 mm in three patients and 3.5 mm in one patient.

In the studies of Stein *et al*[13] and Mertz *et al*,[14] epithelial defects were noted in about half of the patients who were diagnosed as having CL-SIK. Both groups noted a mild

anterior chamber reaction in some CL-SIK patients, but no cases of hypopyon. Mertz *et al*[14] reported that pain and photophobia were the most common initial symptoms in CL-SIK; in their series, discomfort was mild to moderate in six patients and severe in three, with six patients noting the onset of symptoms upon waking. These findings highlight the considerable difficulty that clinicians often encounter when trying to differentially diagnose between CL-SIK and infectious keratitis.

### Contact lens-induced acute red eye (CLARE)

Previously referred to as 'acute red-eye reaction' and 'tight lens syndrome', CLARE is an acute complication of extended soft lens wear. In its mild form, the patient notices problems upon waking naturally; when severe, the patient may be awakened by the symptoms, which include ocular pain, tearing and photophobia. The patient then quickly discovers that he or she has a red eye (Figure 13.5). Clinical signs include conjunctival and limbal hyperaemia, and small corneal infiltrates near the limbus.[4]

The lens may display little or no movement upon initial examination of a patient suffering from CLARE, and debris can sometimes be seen trapped beneath the lens. Epithelial staining may be detected following lens removal. Other transient clinical signs include anterior chamber flare, endothelial bedewing and guttata, low-grade corneal neovascularisation, foci of swollen epithelium, and small non-staining areas on the corneal surface (dry spots).[12]

Sweeney *et al*[15] reported that 10 per cent of 49 consecutive presenting cases of CLARE were bilateral and the mean time to the first

occurrence of CLARE after being fitted with extended wear soft lenses was $8.8 \pm 10.3$ months.

### Culture-negative peripheral ulcer (CNPU)

This condition, which is typically seen in hydrogel extended wear patients, is characterised by the presence of one or two small, round, full-thickness epithelial lesions (without raised edges) in the peripheral or paracentral cornea. The patient may experience mild to moderate ocular discomfort or foreign-body sensation, mild photophobia and increased tearing. Associated signs may include conjunctival and limbal hyperaemia, and infiltrates beneath or surrounding the epithelial lesion.[4]

According to Sweeney *et al*,[15] all 12 consecutive presenting cases of CNPU were uniocular and the mean time to the first occurrence of CNPU after being fitted with extended wear soft lenses was $25.8 \pm 22.3$ months.

### Asymptomatic infiltrates (AI)

This condition merely refers to the presence of infiltrates in the cornea in the absence of significant patient symptoms or epithelial compromise. In some cases AI may be a precursor to CNPU.

Suchecki *et al*[16] reported 52 cases of CL-SIK that appear to meet the definition of either CNPU or AI. Ocular discomfort, conjunctival hyperaemia and anterior chamber reaction were minimal or absent. Of the 52 patients, 62 per cent were wearing extended wear soft lenses, 33 per cent were wearing daily wear soft lenses, and 5 per cent were wearing RGP lenses. Approximately half of these patients displayed punctate staining or

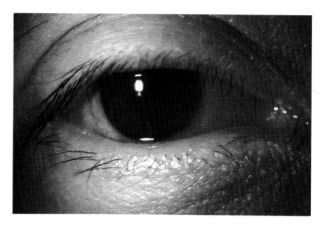

**Figure 13.5**
*Clinical presentation of CLARE in an extended wear patient, with a bound lens still in place*

a frank epithelial defect overlying the lesion; patients displaying these signs would be diagnosed as suffering from CNPU. The remaining patients probably suffered from AI.

## Pathology

The hazy region of infiltration observed clinically is presumed to comprise primarily inflammatory cells, but it may also include bacterial endotoxins (often the cause of the problem), and serum and proteins that may leak from the limbal vessels. Sankaridurg *et al*[17] have developed an animal model (guinea pig) of endotoxin-mediated stromal infiltration. Histopathological examination of the affected regions of the stroma revealed focal or diffuse infiltration of polymorphonuclear leucocytes.

In an extraordinary experiment, Holden *et al*[18] obtained a biopsy of the cornea and conjunctiva of four human patients suffering from CNPU. All four patients were wearing extended wear soft contact lenses. Histopathological examination of the corneal sections revealed a focal area of epithelial loss surrounded by a severely attenuated epithelium. Bowman's layer appeared to be intact and of normal thickness – an observation to which the authors attached great significance. The anterior corneal stroma was infiltrated with numerous polymorphonuclear leucocytes beneath the area of epithelial compromise. The conjunctival epithelium appeared normal and diffuse inflammatory cell infiltration, predominantly with mononuclear cells, was observed in the conjunctival stroma

## Aetiology

By definition, CL-SIK is an inflammatory reaction, and as such, the following aetiological factors may be involved.

### Bacterial contamination
It is recognised that in CL-SIK there is no direct bacterial infection; that is, bacteria do not enter and replicate within the cornea. Instead, bacteria can indirectly exert a pathogenic effect on tissue through toxin or enzyme production, which can activate the immune system leading to an inflammatory tissue response. Dead or dying bacteria can also release toxins; in particular, endotoxins from Gram-negative bacteria have been implicated as a major cause of

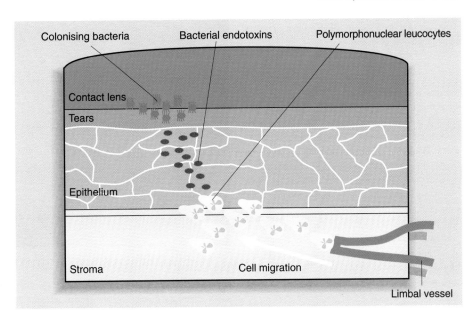

**Figure 13.6**
*Schematic representation of the aetiology of infiltrates caused by bacterial endotoxins*

tissue damage. Endotoxin is comprised of lipopolysaccharide. It is a component of the outer membrane of Gram-negative organisms and imparts its pathogenicity by causing antibody and cytokine production, neutrophil migration and complement activation.[19] The endotoxins cause inflammatory cells – typically polymorphonuclear leucocytes – to migrate from the limbal vessels to the site of the injury (Figure 13.6), creating stromal haze.

Baleriola-Lucus *et al*[20] found that 36 per cent of lenses taken from asymptomatic patients versus 100 per cent of lenses taken from patients suffering from CLARE were contaminated with Gram-negative bacteria, thus implicating such bacteria in the aetiology of CL-SIK. A similar experiment was conducted on patients suffering from CNPU by Wilcox *et al*,[21] who concluded that those patients whose lenses harboured high levels of Gram-positive bacteria were more likely to develop CNPU than other patients.

The aetiological role of Gram-negative bacteria in CLARE has been further reinforced in a study using an animal eye model (guinea pig).[22] Single or multiple small focal corneal infiltrates could be induced within 24 hours by inserting lenses contaminated with live Gram-negative bacteria into the guinea pig eyes.

### The closed eye
The fact that CL-SIK has a high prevalence in extended wear patients suggests that there may be something about the closed lid environment that is of aetiological significance. The stagnating tear layer beneath the closed lid is associated with raised levels of IgA and albumin, activation of complement and plasminogen and recruitment of large numbers of polymorphonuclear leucocytes.[4] These changes represent a sub-clinical inflammatory state which could develop into an overt inflammation in the presence of a stimulus such as bacterial endotoxins.

### Tight lens
A tight, non-moving lens is problematic because potentially pathogenic agents such as decaying debris or colonising bacteria on the posterior lens surface are trapped in close and constant apposition with a fixed location on the corneal surface. With a mobile lens, the probability of compromise is minimised because the pathogenic agents are constantly moved around and are dispersed or expelled from beneath the lens.

### Hypoxia
The level of oxygen beneath contact lenses under the closed eyelid is generally very low.[23] Blood vessels tend to dilate under the influence of hypoxia. Since infiltrates are derived from the limbal vasculature, hypoxia-induced vasodilatation could be viewed as a potentially significant predisposing factor. That is, inflammatory cells will be able to escape more easily through

the wall of a dilated vessel should a suitable stimulus present itself.

## Mechanical trauma

Two cases of peripheral infiltrates were observed by Efron and Veys[24] in the eyes of patients wearing lenses containing edge defects. The likely mode of pathogenesis is that the defective lens edge abrades the epithelium. Enzymes are released from decaying epithelial cells and act as a chemotaxic stimulus to inflammatory cell migration from the limbal capillaries. It is possible that trauma induced by defective lens edges could be partly responsible for infiltrates observed in patients wearing certain types of moulded lenses with imperfect edges.[14]

## Lens deposits

Contact lenses are known to coat with proteins, lipids, calcium and other forms of organic and inorganic matter. If such substances denature and are interpreted as being foreign by the immune system of the body, they can act as an antigenic stimulus to the recruitment of tissue antibodies, such as polymorphonuclear leucocytes – hence an infiltrative response. Lens deposits may also be implicated in the development of infiltrates by their direct mechanical abrasion of the corneal surface (see 'Mechanical trauma' above).

Indirect evidence that lens deposits are involved in infiltrate formation comes from clinical studies which show that the incidence of CLARE in patients wearing conventional extended wear lenses can be reduced from between 15 per cent to 30 per cent per patient-year to less than 6 per cent per patient-year by changing to frequent replacement or disposable lenses.[10]

## Solution toxicity

Focal or diffuse infiltrates near the limbus are a classic sign of solution toxicity. A toxic reaction can occur due to exposure to noxious preservatives, buffers, enzymes, chelating agents or other chemical agents that are incorporated into contact lens solutions. In particular, solutions containing thimerosal and chlorhexidine can induce a severe toxic reaction which includes the appearance of infiltrates (Figure 13.7). Such substances become absorbed into the lens matrix during lens storage, and later diffuse back into the eye in toxic concentrations.

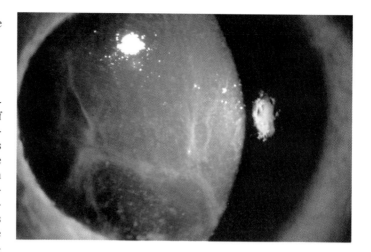

**Figure 13.7**

*A severe case of CL-SIK due to solution toxicity. In this case, the patient was wearing soft lenses in association with solutions containing thimerosal and chlorhexidine*

## Poor hygiene

The finding of Vajdic *et al*[8] of a higher incidence of CL-SIK in patients wearing disposable daily wear soft lenses (15 per cent) versus those wearing disposable extended wear soft lenses (7 per cent) suggests that lens handling and/or the characteristics of lens care products are implicated in the aetiology of CL-SIK. Furthermore, Bates *et al*[25] reported a significant association between the occurrence of CL-SIK and the level of contact lens hygiene and case contamination in patients wearing daily wear soft contact lenses. The above findings concur with the established link (discussed previously) between the development of CLARE and CNPU with bacterial contamination of lenses.

# Patient management

The management strategy adopted for a patient suffering from an episode of CL-SIK will depend upon the way in which the condition presents clinically.

## General advice

All contact lens patients, in particular those wearing lenses on an extended wear basis, should be advised that sleeping in lenses carries a greater risk of developing an adverse reaction compared with daily lens wear. Furthermore, patients should be advised to remove their lenses if they develop eye redness and/or discomfort. They should be advised to consult their eye care practi-

tioner, especially if the redness and discomfort are noticed upon awakening.

## Lens removal

Severe ocular discomfort is alleviated immediately upon lens removal, although photophobia may persist for some hours. Infiltrates remain for weeks or months (see 'Prognosis'). The patient should be examined as a matter of urgency and a decision must be made as to whether the patient should be referred for medical treatment in case the keratitis is infectious. One or more of the following signs/symptoms necessitate urgent referral: severe ocular pain that persists following lens removal, extensive and/or intensive epithelial staining overlying the infiltrates, extensive anterior chamber flare, hypopyon, extreme conjunctival hyperaemia that persists following lens removal, or significant loss of vision.

In mild cases of CL-SIK such as CLARE, CNPU or AI, where none of the criteria for urgent referral are met, the patient must cease lens wear and be examined later the same day and daily thereafter for at least a week to verify that all signs and symptoms are resolving. During this period, the patient may notice a continuance of mild irritation, photophobia and excess tearing. Logistic or geographical factors may make it difficult for the patient to obtain immediate medical attention; that being the case, topical antibiotic therapy is indicated as a prophylactic measure.

If the signs and symptoms do not appear to be resolving after 3 or 4 days, or if there is a worsening of any aspect of the condition, the patient should be referred immediately for medical treatment. If there is a progressive recovery, lens wear should not be resumed until there has been a 75 per cent resolution of infiltrates and a complete resolution of all other signs and symptoms.

### Medical treatment

A corneal scraping will typically be performed to determine if the condition is infectious and possibly to identify the offending micro-organism. Broad-spectrum antibiotics will then be instilled pending the result of the corneal scraping because such episodes are best presumed to be infectious unless proved otherwise. Steroids may be prescribed subsequently if the result is culture-negative and the epithelium is intact. Mydriatics may also be prescribed to prevent the formation of posterior synechiae. The patient may be given analgesics to alleviate the pain.

### Apply cold compress

Swarbrick and Holden[4] recommend the application of a cold compress to the eye in the case of a patient suffering from CLARE. This procedure is said to be helpful in relieving ocular discomfort.

### Fit disposable lenses

As revealed earlier, regular lens replacement lessens the risk of developing CL-SIK. This is primarily attributable to the avoidance of lens deposition and consequent inability of bacteria to colonise on the lens. Daily disposable lenses are indicated for patients deemed to be susceptible to episodes of CL-SIK.

### Alleviate mechanical trauma

If the source of the trauma is lens deposits, then regular lens replacement should solve the problem. If certain features of the lens – such as a disagreeable physical design or a poor edge finish – are thought to be the cause of CL-SIK, then a different lens type should be prescribed.

### Improve care system

A bilateral occurrence of CL-SIK soon after commencing use of a new care solution generally indicates a toxic reaction to one or more of the components of that solution. As stated previously, the preservatives thimerosal and chlorhexidine have often been connected with such episodes. Changing to modern lens care solutions containing new-generation, high molecular weight preservatives, or non-preserved hydrogen peroxide disinfection solutions, will usually solve the problem.

Heat disinfection should generally be avoided in view of the finding of Kotow *et al*[26] of a high incidence of CLARE in extended wear patients using heat to disinfect their high water content lenses.

### Improve hygiene

It is vital to stress to all patients, and in particular extended wear patients, the importance of strict attention to all aspects of hygiene. Thorough hand washing prior to lens handling (*in vivo* and *in vitro*) and scrupulous attention to lens case care are key aspects to reinforce.

### Loosen lens fit

Most disposable lenses are available in a choice of base curves. As a general rule, the flattest base curve should be prescribed unless of course the fit is totally unacceptable. A loose fit facilitates a more effective exchange of debris and allows some degree of tear mixing beneath the lens so as to avoid prolonged apposition of colonising bacteria against a fixed location on the cornea.

### Change to daily wear

If a relatively loose fit is not achievable, the risks of developing CL-SIK during sleep may outweigh the benefits of extended wear, and the patient should be advised that daily wear would be safer.

### Fit RGP lenses

It is now well established that the incidence of virtually all forms of adverse physiological events is lower in RGP lenses versus soft lenses.[9] Certainly, this is the case in respect of CL-SIK.[7-9] The reasons for the relative safety of RGP lenses are as follows: inert materials (generally resistant to long-term deposit build-up), relatively high oxygen performance,[27] small size (not covering the limbus), greater lens movement and consequent tear exchange and mixing, and greater post-lens tear film.

### Fit low water content lenses

According to Swarbrick and Holden,[4] the incidence of CLARE is generally greater with higher water content lenses. This may be due to the greater capacity for such lenses to absorb and re-release contaminants into the eye, the more rapid ageing of such lenses, and the greater propensity for spoliation, compared with lower water content lenses.

### Improve oxygen performance

This generally means fitting silicone-hydrogel lenses, or higher water content and/or thinner lenses.[28] The fitting of lenses of higher water content poses a dilemma because this strategy contradicts the advice that CLARE is less likely to occur with lower water content lenses. Perhaps the answer lies in the choice of material ionicity; ionic materials tend to attract high levels of proteins and low levels of lipids, whereas the opposite is true for non-ionic lenses.[29] Thus, practitioners have some control over deposit formation, although considerable intersubject variability in deposition characteristics may in reality preclude material type as a variable in attempting to avoid or minimise occurrences of CL-SIK.[30]

## Prognosis

In general, the prognosis for recovery from episodes of CL-SIK is excellent. All symptoms and signs other than infiltrates generally resolve rapidly over the first 48 hours following lens removal. Resolution occurs more slowly over the next two weeks, by which time only infiltrates are present. Josephson and Caffery[1] noted that the greater the severity of infiltrates, the longer is the time course of recovery. In the most severe cases they recorded, infiltrates fully resolved within 3 months.

Sweeney *et al*[15] reported that patients who have experienced a CLARE reaction have as much as a 50 per cent chance of recurrence if they continue to use extended wear lenses. After an initial occurrence, the mean time to the second occurrence is $12.0 \pm 11.9$ months. The mean time to a third occurrence is $16.5 \pm 16.4$ months. Patients did not suffer a recurrence of CNPU over a 45-month follow-up period.

In exceptional cases infiltrates can take years to resolve. Kremer and Cohen[31] described the case of a 36-year-old female wearing extended wear soft lenses who presented with irritation and redness of the left eye, superficial stromal infiltrates and overlying epithelial defects. Cultures were negative and, despite treatment, partial ring infiltrates developed and minimal scarring could still be observed two years later. The authors concluded that this was probably an atypical case of an immunological reaction to bacteria.

## Differential diagnosis

The most critical diagnoses when evaluating a case of stromal infiltrates is to determine whether the condition is infective or sterile – an issue addressed previously in this chapter.

Epidemic keratoconjunctivitis can take on a similar appearance to CL-SIK – with eye redness, foreign-body sensation, tearing and photophobia (Figure 13.8).[32] This condition is usually bilateral and associated with the formation of focal subepithelial infiltrates scattered over the whole cornea. Tiny pits in the overlying epithelium stain with fluorescein. The infiltrates typically have a distinctive appearance of 'fluffy' edges (Figure 13.9), and take much longer to resolve than infiltrates seen in CL-SIK. In addition, patients suffering from epidemic keratoconjunctivitis may have an associated upper respiratory tract infection, regional lymphadenopathy and follicular conjunctivitis.

It is often difficult to differentiate stromal infiltrates from stromal opacities. Pimenides *et al*[33] reported four cases of deep stromal opacities in long-term soft lens wearers. They appeared to be either white, grey or

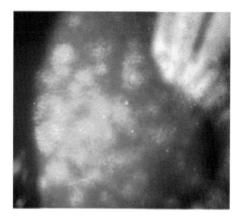

**Figure 13.9**
*High-magnification photomicrograph of focal infiltrates with characteristic 'fluffy' edges in a patient with epidemic keratoconjunctivitis*

brown, but could be distinguished from infiltrates because these opacities were located deep in the stroma (infiltrates associated with CL-SIK reside in the anterior half of the stroma). Similar posterior stromal opacities were reported by Remeijer *et al*[34] and Holland *et al*.[35] All of the above authors[33–35] attributed their observations to the effects of chronic hypoxia and associated endothelial dysfunction. Figure 13.10 shows a bizarre case of a defined, bilateral and symmetrical ring of stromal haze in the mid-peripheral stroma; the rings had been present for eight years and the cause is unknown.

Stromal scars are usually more white in colour (compared with the typical dull grey appearance of infiltrates) and more dense than infiltrates. The key feature distinguishing scars from infiltrates is that scars are usually observed in an otherwise completely quiet eye without any associated pathology, and they generally do not resolve over time.

## REFERENCES

1 Josephson JE, Caffery BE (1979) Infiltrative keratitis in hydrogel lens wearers. *Int Contact Lens Clin* **6**: 223.

2 *Blakiston's Pocket Medical Dictionary* (1973) (edn. A Osol), 3rd edn. McGraw-Hill, New York.

3 Guillon M, Guillon JP, Bansal M (1994) Incidence of ulcers with conventional and disposable daily wear soft contact lenses. *J Br Contact Lens Assoc* **17**: 69.

4 Swarbrick HA, Holden BA (1997) Extended wear lenses. In: *Contact Lenses* (eds AJ Phillips and L Speedwell), 4th edn. Butterworth–Heinemann, Oxford, ch. 15.

5 Zantos SG (1981) The ocular response to continuous wear of contact lenses. PhD Thesis, University of New South Wales, Sydney.

6 Gordon A, Kracher GP (1985) Corneal infiltrates and extended wear contact lenses. *J Am Optom Assoc* **56**: 198.

7 Hamano H, Watanabe K, Hamano T (1994) A study of the complications induced by conventional and disposable contact lenses. *Contact Lens Assoc Ophthalmol J* **20**: 103.

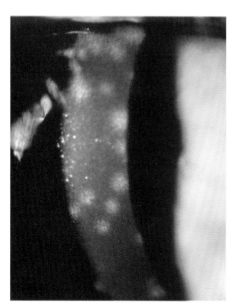

**Figure 13.8**
*Focal infiltrates in a patient suffering from epidemic keratoconjunctivitis*

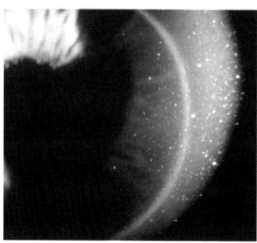

**Figure 13.10**
*Idiopathic ring of stromal haze in the mid-peripheral stroma*

8  Vajdic CM, Sweeney DF, Cornish R (1995) The incidence of idiopathic corneal infiltrates with disposable and rigid gas-permeable daily and extended wear. *Invest Ophthalmol Vis Sci* **36**: S151.

9  Stapleton F, Dart J, Minassian D (1992) Nonulcerative complications of contact lens wear. *Arch Ophthalmol* **110**: 1601–1606.

10  Grant T (1991) Clinical aspects of planned replacement and disposable lenses. In: *The Contact Lens Yearbook 1991* (ed. C Kerr). Medical and Scientific Publishing, Hythe.

11  Sweeney DF, Terry RL, Papas E (1996) The prevalence of 'infiltrates' in a non contact lens wearing population. *Invest Ophthalmol Vis Sci* **37**: S71.

12  Zantos SC (1984) Management of corneal infiltrates in extended-wear contact lens patients. *Int Contact Lens Clin* **11**: 604.

13  Stein RM, Clinch TE, Cohen EJ (1988) Infected vs sterile corneal infiltrates in contact lens wearers. *Am J Ophthalmol* **105**: 632.

14  Mertz PHV, Bouchard CS, Mathers WD (1990) Corneal infiltrates associated with soft contact lenses: a report of nine cases. *Contact Lens Assoc Ophthalmol J* **16**: 269.

15  Sweeney DF, Grant T, Chong MS (1993) Recurrence of acute inflammatory conditions with hydrogel extended wear. *Invest Ophthalmol Vis Sci* **34**: S1008.

16  Suchecki JK, Ehlers WH, Donshik PC (1996) Peripheral corneal infiltrates associated with contact lens wear. *Contact Lens Assoc Ophthalmol J* **22**: 41.

17  Sankaridurg PR, Sharma S, Rajeev B (1996) An animal model for contact lens induced corneal inflammation. *Invest Ophthalmol Vis Sci* **37**: S872.

18  Holden BA, Reddy MK, Sankaridurg PR (1997) The histopathology of contact lens induced peripheral corneal ulcer. *Invest Ophthalmol Vis Sci* **38**: S201.

19  Stapleton F, Phillips AJ, Hopkins GA (1997) Drugs and solutions in contact lens practice and related microbiology. In: *Contact Lenses* (eds AJ Phillips and L Speedwell), 4th edn. Butterworth–Heinemann, Oxford, ch. 4.

20  Baleriola-Lucus C, Grant T, Newton-Howes J (1991) Enumeration and identification of bacteria on hydrogel lenses from asymptomatic patients and those experiencing adverse responses with extended wear. *Invest Ophthalmol Vis Sci* **32**: S739.

21  Wilcox MDP, Sweeney DF, Sharma S (1995) Culture-negative peripheral ulcers are associated with bacterial contamination of contact lenses. *Invest Ophthalmol Vis Sci* **36**: S152.

22  Sankaridurg PR, Rao GN, Sharma S (1997) Production of corneal infiltrates in a guinea pig model using contact lenses soaked in live Gram-negative bacteria. *Invest Ophthalmol Vis Sci* **38**: S137.

23  Efron N, Ang JHB (1990) Corneal hypoxia and hypercapnia during contact lens wear. *Optom Vis Sci* **67**: 512.

24  Efron N, Veys J (1992) Defects in disposable contact lenses can compromise ocular integrity. *Int Contact Lens Clin* **19**: 8.

25  Bates AK, Morris RJ, Stapleton F (1989) 'Sterile' corneal infiltrates in contact lens wearers. *Eye* **3**: 803.

26  Kotow M, Grant T, Holden BA (1987) Avoiding ocular complications during hydrogel extended wear. *Int Contact Lens Clin* **14**: 95.

27  Tranoudis I, Efron N (1995) Oxygen permeability of rigid contact lens materials. *J Br Contact Lens Assoc* **18**: 49.

28  Efron N (1991) Understanding oxygen: Dk/L, EOP, oedema. *Trans Br Contact Lens Assoc* **14**: 65.

29  Jones L, Evans K, Sariri K (1997) Lipid and protein deposition of N-vinyl pyrrolidone-containing group II and group IV frequent replacement contact lenses. *Contact Lens Assoc Ophthalmol J* **23**: 122.

30  Tighe B (1997) Patient-dependence and material-dependence in contact lens deposition. Paper presented at the Annual Clinical Conference and Exhibition of the British Contact Lens Association, Bournemouth, 6–8 June.

31  Kremer I, Cohen EJ (1993) Ring infiltrates associated with contact lens wear. *Contact Lens Assoc Ophthalmol J* **19**: 191.

32  Kaufman HE, Rayfield MA (1988) Viral conjunctivitis and keratitis. In: *The Cornea* (eds HE Kaufman, BA Barron, MB McDonald). Churchill Livingstone, New York, ch. 12.

33  Pimenides D, Steele CF, McGhee CNJ (1996) Deep corneal stromal opacities associated with long term contact lens wear. *Br J Ophthalmol* **80**: 21.

34  Remeijer L, Van Ril G, Beekhuis WH (1990) Deep corneal stromal opacities in long-term contact lens wear. *Ophthalmology* **97**: 281.

35  Holland EJ, Lee RM, Bucci FA (1995) Mottled cyan opacification of the posterior cornea in contact lens wearers. *Am J Ophthalmol* **119**: 620.

# 14
# Microbial infiltrative keratitis

Incidence
Relative risk
Signs and symptoms
Pathology
Aetiology
Patient management
Prognosis
Differential diagnosis

The formation of infiltrates in the stroma can be due to a variety of factors such as solution toxicity, hypoxia, mechanical trauma, lens deposits and endotoxin release from bacterial contamination. In virtually all of these cases, the infiltration is self-limiting; however, stromal infiltrates may be associated with a microbial infection, which is often progressive and potentially devastating to the cornea. This chapter will concentrate on contact lens-induced microbial infiltrative keratitis (CL-MIK); that is, the appearance of stromal infiltrates in the presence of microbial infection.

Certainly, CL-MIK is the most severe reaction that can occur in response to contact lens wear. At best, the patient suffers from considerable pain and must incur the discomfort, cost and inconvenience associated with the acute management of this condition. At worst, the patient may suffer from a partial or complete loss of sight. The most severe case of MIK recorded resulted in bilateral large deep corneal ulcers and hypopyon; the right eye perforated spontaneously, the patient developed secondary glaucoma and bilateral optic atrophy,

which resulted in total bilateral blindness (Figure 14.1).[1]

The various terms that have been used to describe conditions in which corneal infiltrates are observed were defined in chapter 13 together with a schema for classifying the various forms of infiltrative keratitis (see Figure 13.2), so these will not be repeated in

detail here. By definition, all cases of microbial keratitis are 'infiltrative' because, at the very least, micro-organisms have entered and destroyed tissue. Other infiltrative elements such as inflammatory cells and excess fluid are usually also present.[2]

Microbial keratitis is defined as an inflammation of corneal tissue due to direct

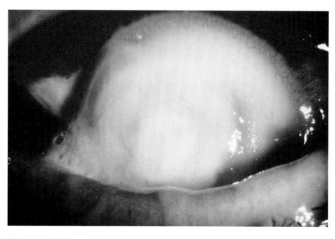

**Figure 14.1**
*Severe case of CL-MIK which eventually resulted in perforation, optic atrophy and permanent blindness*

infection by a microbial agent such as a bacterium, virus, fungus or amoeba; the term 'infectious keratitis' is essentially synonymous with this. The term 'ulcerative keratitis' has also been used as a synonym for microbial keratitis; however, this usage is not always correct because a given case of microbial keratitis may not necessarily be ulcerative, and an ulcerative keratitis may not necessarily be microbial.

## Incidence

Numerous papers have been published which have attempted to define the incidence of CL-MIK, and the relative risk associated with various types of lenses and modalities of lens wear. It is pertinent to note that the results of these studies are generally in good agreement.

Determination of the incidence of CL-MIK among contact lens wearers is problematic for a number of reasons:

- The total number of lens wearers in the population from which patients suffering from CL-MIK are derived is difficult to determine.
- It is not always clear as to whether the reported keratitis cases were microbial or sterile.
- It is difficult logistically to identify all cases of CL-MIK that occur within a defined population.

Notwithstanding these difficulties, Poggio et al[3] conducted a large prospective study in the New England area of the USA and were able to determine the incidence of CL-MIK to be 4.1 per 10 000 patients per year for daily soft lens wear and 20.9 per 10 000 patients per year for extended soft lens wear. Similar results were subsequently obtained by MacRae et al,[4] who cited the incidence per 10 000 patients per year to be 5.2 for daily soft lens wear and 18.2 for extended soft lens wear. They also reported an incidence of 6.8 per 10 000 patients per year for daily wear of rigid gas-permeable lenses.

Nilsson and Montan[5] reported the annualised incidence of CL-MIK per 10 000 wearers in Sweden to be 2.2 and 13.3 for daily wear and extended wear of conventional soft lenses, 2.2 and 10.0 for daily wear and extended wear of disposable soft lenses, and 1.5 for daily wear of rigid gas permeable lenses.

It is interesting that Guillon et al[6] found a much higher incidence of CL-MIK per 10 000 daily soft lens wearers in the UK – 39 for conventional lenses and 18 for disposable lenses. The authors attributed these higher incidence figures to the fact that their study gathered data from primary care settings utilising a more encompassing definition of corneal ulceration, whereas other studies focused on medically diagnosed cases of confirmed and often severe keratitis.

Notwithstanding this qualification, the data of Guillon et al[6] indicate the likely frequency of suspected keratitis cases presenting to primary care contact lens practitioners in the UK. Simple calculation reveals that a practitioner examining 10 patients per week wearing conventional daily wear lenses should see approximately 2 cases of suspected CL-MIK per year. In his analysis of all data on contact lens-induced corneal ulceration in the US published up to 1992,[7] Benjamin concluded that US contact lens practitioners should each expect, on average, to see 1.7 cases of CL-MIK per year.

## Relative risk

An alternative approach to determining the incidence of CL-MIK is to establish the relative risk of developing the condition in response to different combinations of lens type and modality of wear. This form of analysis does not require knowledge of the total population of lens wearers; instead, the number of contact lens wearers with and without CL-MIK presenting to a given clinic over a defined time period needs to be determined.

Using this approach, Mathews et al[8] at Moorfields Eye Hospital in the UK found that, relative to daily wear rigid gas-permeable lenses (which are arbitrarily assigned a risk of developing CL-MIK of 1.0), the risk of developing CL-MIK with other types and modalities of lens wear is as follows: daily wear conventional soft lenses 1.1; extended wear conventional soft lenses 2.6; daily wear disposable soft lenses 4.1 and extended wear disposable soft lenses 8.1. In a similar study at the Johns Hopkins Chinic in the US, Buehler et al[9] reported the risk of developing CL-MIK to be as follows: daily wear conventional soft lenses 1.0; extended wear conventional soft lenses 2.8; and extended wear disposable soft lenses 3.9.

Thus, both of these studies,[8,9] conducted by different researchers on opposite sides of the Atlantic ocean, confirmed that there is a greater risk of developing CL-MIK with extended wear lenses. The data of Mathews et al[8] also suggest that there is a greater risk associated with the wear of disposable lenses – a notion that is highly controversial since the *raison d'être* of disposability is that disposable contact lens wear is associated with enhanced safety, not greater risk. Possible explanations for these findings are discussed under 'Aetiology'.

## Signs and symptoms

An early symptom of CL-MIK is a foreign-body sensation in the eye associated with an increasing desire to remove the lenses. In the case of an actual foreign body, or with other causes of lens-related ocular discomfort, lens removal leads to immediate relief. Continuing or worsening discomfort following lens removal should lead a clinician to suspect CL-MIK. Associated symptoms include pain, eye redness, swollen lids, increased lacrimation, photophobia, discharge and loss of vision (Figure 14.2).

Aside from the obvious signs of eye redness and lacrimation, an area of infiltration will typically be observed at the site of infection (Figure 14.3). In the early stages, infiltrates may be confined primarily to the epithelium. As the disease progresses, the stroma becomes increasingly hazy and the epithelium above the infiltration begins to break down, leading to corneal staining (Figure 14.4).

In the early stages of CL-MIK, conjuncti-

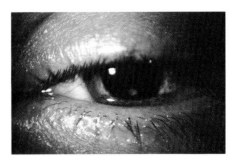

**Figure 14.2**
*Early stages of Pseudomonas keratitis, with limbal hyperaemia, increased lacrimation and swollen eyelids. A small white ulcer can be seen near the inferior pupil margin*

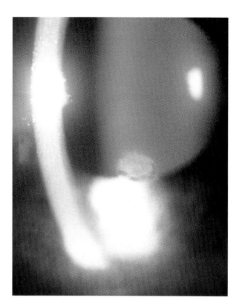

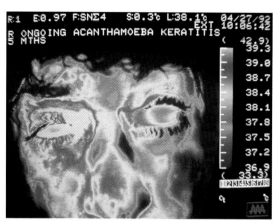

**Figure 14.5**
*Ocular thermogram of a patient with Acanthamoeba keratitis of the right eye, showing the increased temperature of the affected eye*

**Figure 14.3**
*High magnification slit-lamp photograph of the corneal ulcer depicted in Figure 14.2*

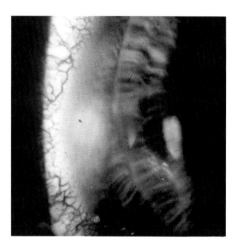

**Figure 14.4**
*Peripheral corneal ulcer in the early stages showing fluorescein staining of the ulcer and background fluorescence indicating diffusion into the stroma*

val redness may be confined to the limbal and bulbar region adjacent to the region of infection thus providing the clinician with an important clue as to its location. This clue is soon lost as the condition advances and the eye becomes more inflamed with circumlimbal conjunctival redness (Figure 14.5).

Bacterial keratitis can have a rapid and devastating time course, and be associated with anterior chamber flare, iritis and hy-

popyon. A mucopurulent discharge will be evident, although the discharge can sometimes be serous. If not properly treated, the stroma can melt away leading to corneal perforation in a matter of days (see Figure 14.1).

The time course of *Acanthamoeba* keratitis is not as rapid; typical signs include corneal staining, pseudodendrites, epithelial and anterior stromal infiltrates which may be focal or diffuse, and a classic radial keratoneuritis (Figure 14.6) – the last being a circular formation of opacification that becomes apparent relatively early in the disease process. A fully developed corneal ulcer may take weeks to form.

## Pathology

The high incidence of CL-MIK reported in recent years has lead to a renewed interest in the pathology of this condition and the mode of infection with various micro-organisms is now more fully understood. The two micro-organisms implicated in the vast majority of cases of CL-MIK are *Pseudomonas*, a Gram-negative bacteria, and *Acanthamoeba*, a free-living amoeba. Other Gram-negative bacteria have been cultured from infected corneas at the same time, such as *Serratia*, *Enterobacter*, *Escherichia coli* and *Klebsiella*. Gram-positive organisms such as *Staphylococcus aureus* and *Staphylococcus epi-*

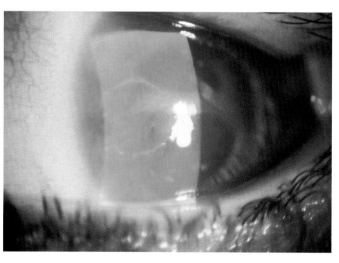

**Figure 14.6**
*Breakdown of the epithelium in the classic pattern of radial keratoneuritis in a patient with an Acanthamoeba infection*

*dermis* have less frequently been isolated from corneal ulcers.

Fungi are known to be capable of invading contact lens materials but there is no evidence that contact lens wear is a risk factor for fungal eye infection. Isolated cases of corneal fungal infection caused by *Fusarium* and *Curvularia* have been reported in contact lens wear,[10] although this association would appear to be casual rather than causal. Similarly, contact lens wearers may coincidentally contract viral infections such as epidemic keratoconjunctivitis (non-ulcerative) or herpes simplex keratitis (ulcerative), but again there is no reason to believe that contact lens wear itself has been a contributing factor in the development of the infection.

Contact lens wear can alter the flora of certain groups of contact lens wearers – including those who have used certain chemical disinfection systems, elderly contact lens wearers, and persons who have discontinued contact lens wear.[11,12] However, studies of the microbiological environment of the eyes of contact lens wearers suggest that there is little correlation between the types of bacteria that contaminate lens care paraphernalia and ocular flora in corresponding patients. Thus, contamination alone cannot explain changes to ocular flora that occur during contact lens wear.

In order for infection to occur, contact lens wear must somehow compromise corneal defences against infection.[13] Recent research has focused on the reasons that this compromise favours infection with *Pseudomonas*, and to a lesser extent, *Acanthamoeba*.

### Pseudomonas aeruginosa

Using cells removed from corneas by irrigation, Fleiszig *et al*[14] found that extended wear of hydrogel lenses increases *Pseudomonas* adherence to human corneal epithelial cells (Figure 14.7). It has also been demonstrated that *Pseudomonas* lipopolysaccharide is a major factor contributing to the ability of *Pseudomonas* to adhere to the cornea and to contact lenses,[15] and that bacterial pili, which were previously reported to be major factors in *Pseudomonas* adherence, play only a minor role.[16]

A key to understanding the pathology of *Pseudomonas* infection is to understand why this bacterium does not adhere to the healthy cornea, whereas it is known to

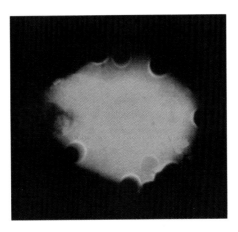

**Figure 14.7**
*In vitro preparation showing Pseudomonas bacteria (small, dark orange rods) adherent to a human epithelial cell (orange). The semicircles at the edge of the cells are an artefact of the preparation mount*

adhere readily to most surfaces, including inert surfaces, without the necessity for specific receptors. The answer lies in the natural protective layers of the corneal surface; specifically, the mucus layer of the tear film and the epithelial cell surface glycocalyx (which also contains mucin molecules) inhibit *Pseudomonas* adherence to the intact healthy corneal surface (Figure 14.8).[17,18] The precise mechanism involves *Pseudo-*

*monas* binding to mucin molecules and competitive inhibition of bacterial adherence to the cornea.

Epithelial cell polarity determines the susceptibility of epithelial cells to *Pseudomonas* invasion and cytotoxicity.[19] Specifically, the basolateral cell surfaces (the sides and the bottoms of cells) are much more susceptible to infection than the spiral cell membrane (the top surface of cells). This research indicates another way that the intact healthy cornea is able to resist infection and why corneal surface injury predisposes to infection.

It is now known that some strains of *Pseudomonas* invade corneal epithelial cells during corneal infection.[20] Previously it was thought that this bacterium was an extracellular pathogen; that is, *Pseudomonas* resided only in extracellular compartments during disease. The significance of bacterial invasion of epithelial cells is that once the bacterium is inside a cell it then has the potential to alter internally host cell function. Meanwhile it is protected from factors of the host immune system and from most forms of antibiotic therapy – neither of which can enter epithelial cells. This finding has led to a flurry of new research, in the ophthalmic field as well as in research related to cystic fibrosis and other lung infections caused by *Pseudomonas* (*Pseudomonas* pneumonia is the leading cause of death in cystic fibrosis, and

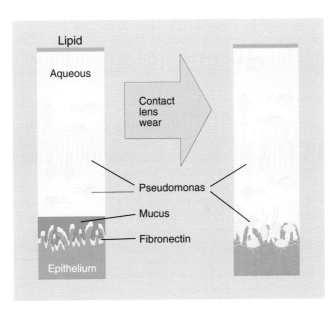

**Figure 14.8**
*Schematic diagram of the corneal surface. Left: Pseudomonas bacteria in the tear film are unable to attach to the epithelial surface due to the mucous and fibronectin layers. Right: contact lens wear depletes the protective layers and Pseudomonas attaches to the epithelium*

has become one of the leading causes of death in AIDS patients).

*In vitro* systems have been used to study *Pseudomonas* invasion of corneal epithelial cells, using whole cornea, cultured corneal cells, and epithelial cells washed from human corneas by irrigation.[21] Using these systems it has been demonstrated that bacterial uptake by cells is an active process involving the host cell cytoskeleton, that host cell signal transduction mechanisms are involved, and that there is rapid replication of bacteria inside host cells. The lipopolysaccharide outer core has been found to be a major bacterial factor in *Pseudomonas* invasion of epithelial cells.[22]

Another important recent discovery is that there are two types of *Pseudomonas* that cause clinical disease, and that the pathogenesis of the two types is entirely different.[23] One type invades corneal epithelial cells without killing the host cell, and probably causes disease largely via the host immune response (invasive strains). The other type is cytotoxic for corneal and other epithelial cells; that is, these bacteria kill the host cell (cytotoxic strains).

There are genetic differences between these two types of *Pseudomonas* that explain their different behaviour, and these differences lie in the *exsA* regulated pathway of the bacterial chromosome.[24] Using mutants that lack this pathway it has been demonstrated that strains that were previously cytotoxic changed the invasive phenotype. These results probably explain much of the contradictory information in the previous literature relating to pathogenesis and treatment of *Pseudomonas* eye infections. Clearly, these findings will also relate to the development of new strategies to reduce the risk of contact lens-related infections, and to the development of new forms of drug therapy.

### *Acanthamoeba*

*Acanthamoeba* has chameleon-like tendencies in that it is able to transform from a chemotherapeutically susceptible trophozoite to a resistant cystic form. The trophozoites are polygonal and can be up to 45 µm in diameter, and the cysts are double-walled and up to 16 µm in length. *Acanthamoeba* species are widely distributed in the natural environment and have been isolated from swimming pools, hot tubs, soil, dust, reservoirs, under ice, the nasopharyngeal mucosa in healthy humans and even the air we breathe.

## Aetiology

The question as to why a given patient develops CL-MIK is multifactorial, complex and controversial. The various factors that have been proposed as being of aetiological significance are discussed below.

### Adherence of micro-organisms to lenses

If micro-organisms can adhere to and colonise on the surface of a contact lens, that lens becomes a vector for ocular contamination when the lens is transferred to and from the storage medium, notwithstanding the antimicrobial efficacy of the storage solution which is discussed separately.

The tenacity with which bacteria adhere to lens surfaces depends on the lens material and whether or not the lens has been worn. In the case of unworn lenses, ionicity, hydrophobicity and water content are the key determinants of adherence; however, adherence is also probably species-dependent – a factor which may explain apparently contradictory published data on the subject.

Bacteria will adhere to worn lenses in accordance with the type of deposit on the lens. The general notion that a worn lens will adhere more bacteria is not always true. For example, mid-water content ionic lenses have a propensity for depositing charged protein such as lysozyme.

Paradoxically, lysozyme acts as a natural antibacterial agent in the eye. If the lysozyme does not become denatured on the lens surface, it can retain this antibacterial capacity and thus prevent adherence of live bacteria.[25]

### Solution inefficacy

It is generally believed that all contact lens disinfection systems on the market provide adequate antimicrobial efficacy during lens storage provided that the patient is totally compliant. However, numerous studies of compliance[26] (see below) have demonstrated that only 10–60 per cent of patients can be categorised as fully compliant. It is important, therefore, that a sufficient 'safety margin' is built into contact lens disinfection systems to allow for a degree of expected non-compliance.

Prior to the introduction of multipurpose chemical disinfection systems containing safe, large molecular weight preservatives such as Dymed and Polyquad, practitioners in the UK were largely prescribing chlor-

ine-based systems for their disposable lens patients. Efron *et al*[27] were the first to highlight a high incidence of CL-MIK in a cohort of patients wearing Etafilcon-A lenses using chlorine systems. In this cohort, patients were advised that surfactant cleaning prior to disinfection was not necessary.

In the above scenario, it could be said that patients were placed in 'double jeopardy'. Firstly, chlorine-based disinfection systems have only marginal efficacy;[28] that is, there is very little margin for error, and therefore there is a potentially greater risk of developing CL-MIK when using such systems. Secondly, by not surfactant cleaning lenses prior to disinfection, patients were 'overloading' the system by presenting the chlorine solution with a bioburden that was too great for antimicrobial efficacy to be guaranteed.

The initial findings of Efron *et al*[27] were subsequently confirmed by Radford *et al*[29] who demonstrated that, in patients using daily wear disposable lenses, the risk of *Acanthamoeba* keratitis when using a chlorine-based disinfection system was ×15 greater compared with the use of a hydrogen peroxide disinfection system (the referent). This finding assumed full compliance; the risk increased to ×41 with non-compliant patients using chlorine systems and to ×56 when patients used no disinfection system.

### The closed eye

There is clearly a greater incidence of CL-MIK in patients who sleep in lenses. The greater levels of hypoxia and hypercapnia compared to open-eye levels[30] coupled with tear stagnation beneath lenses in the closed-lid environment are factors that could lead to epithelial compromise. Organic debris such as desquamated epithelial cells, tear film debris and bacteria trapped beneath the lens, and the general subclinical inflammatory state under the closed lid, physically and metabolically compromise the epithelium and interfere with cellular defence mechanisms.

### Hypoxia

Prolonged hypoxia is known to have a number of adverse effects on the epithelium, such as loss of sensitivity, development of epithelial microcysts, reduced oxygen uptake rate, thinning, glycogen depletion, reduced mitosis, increased fragility and weakened attachments to the underlying stroma. It is not surprising, therefore, that Solomon *et al*[31] demonstrated a link between the level of hypoxia-induced corneal swelling (a good indication of the level of epithelial hypoxia) and the development of CL-MIK in the rabbit eye. Oedema of 20 per cent resulted in corneal ulcers in half the corneas tested and oedema of 43 per cent resulted in all corneas tested developing corneal ulcers.

## Mechanical trauma

Animal models of corneal infectivity have been used to demonstrate that a physical breakdown of the epithelial surface is a precursor to CL-MIK. Adherence of *Pseudomonas aeruginosa* is greater to traumatised corneas than non-traumatised corneas.[15,32] Furthermore, van Klink *et al*[33] concluded that 'corneal abrasion was absolutely necessary for the induction of *Acanthamoeba* keratitis in hamsters infected with contaminated lenses' (Figure 14.9).

Although more subtle forms of epithelial compromise such as metabolic disturbance may predispose the development of CL-MIK, the studies described above confirm that overt, clinically detectable epithelial trauma is a precursor to the development of CL-MIK. It is for this reason that lens-induced epithelial trauma – that can be induced by excessive lens deposition, poor insertion technique, poor lens designs, ill-fitting lenses, lens defects or foreign bodies – must be minimised in contact lens patients.

## Lens deposits

As discussed previously, the nature of deposition will govern the degree to which micro-organisms attach to the lens surface.

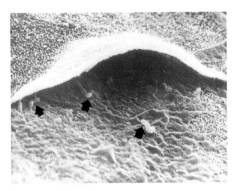

**Figure 14.9**
*Scanning electron micrograph of the cornea showing Pseudomonas bacteria (arrows) about to enter beneath an epithelial cell that has partially sloughed off*

A fresh coating of biologically active lysozyme is considered to be an advantage in that it is naturally antimicrobial. Other deposits may provide a nutrient-rich breeding ground for micro-organisms, which may form a glycocalyx and eventually a complete biofilm. Future research may be directed to developing strategies for encouraging selective deposition from the tear film of components that inhibit biofilm formation and microbial colonisation.

## Lens case care

It would seem obvious that lens case cleanliness is a key prerequisite for reducing the possibility of ocular contamination and thus the risk of CL-MIK; however, the proof of such an association is weak. Many patients with filthy lens cases have not suffered CL-MIK, and numerous patients who develop CL-MIK have been found to be scrupulous in their lens and case care. Fleiszig and Efron[12] found little correlation between the type and number of micro-organisms in the eye and case of soft lens wearers, indicating that in uncomplicated lens wear the eye is highly efficient at eradicating micro-organisms introduced into the eye.

## Patient hygiene

A fundamental source of lens contamination prior to insertion is the cleanliness or otherwise of the finger used to insert the lens. This raises the issue of personal hygiene. Compliance studies have shown that 16–50 per cent of patients do not pay proper attention to hand washing prior to lens insertion.[34]

Most patients execute their lens care routine in the bathroom, often adjacent to a toilet, which is perhaps not the most sterile environment available, but the most convenient. In the UK, the cold water supply to bathrooms is normally via a storage tank in the loft, which is known to be a common breeding environment for *Acanthamoeba*.

The finding of Schein *et al*[35] that there is a higher incidence of CL-MIK in patients who smoke may relate more to the poor hygiene one would naturally associate with smokers rather than the systemic or topical ocular pathophysiological effects of nicotine.

## Patient non-compliance

Patient non-compliance can contribute to the development of CL-MIK, but its importance tends to have been overstated. Mathews *et al*[8] reported cases of patients using:

- Chlorine-based systems without a surfactant cleaning step.
- Surfactant cleaners alone.
- Saline solution alone.

In many cases these patients were being fully compliant with instructions provided by their practitioners.

There are indeed countless ways in which patients can be erroneous or non-compliant in the execution of their lens care regimes,[26] and attempts at enhancing compliance by better education are largely unsuccessful.[36] A pragmatic approach to the question of patient non-compliance is to assume that all patients are potentially non-compliant to some degree; consequently, lens care systems should be designed with sufficient redundancy or safety margin to allow for this.[37]

## Diabetes

Schein *et al*[35] demonstrated that diabetic patients are at greater risk of developing CL-MIK than non-diabetic patients. This may relate to the known compromises in the diabetic patient in terms of corneal structure and function, such as altered metabolism and weakened epithelial attachments to the underlying basement membrane.

## Warm climate

Many cases of CL-MIK have been documented in which climate appears to have been a contributing factor; specifically, patients living in, or travelling to, warmer climates seem to have a greater risk of developing CL-MIK, presumably due to more favourable living conditions for micro-organisms. This link has not been proven but is worthy of note. Katz *et al*[38] reported a higher incidence of CL-MIK in the summer months. The relatively low incidence of CL-MIK in Sweden[5] could be attributed in part to the colder climate there.

## Disposable lens use

Radford *et al*[29] reported that a relatively small excess risk of developing CL-MIK is associated with the use of disposable lenses, independent of other risk factors; that is, in apparently compliant patients using efficacious care systems. These authors proposed a number of possible reasons for this increased risk that relate to the lenses used:

- Rapid *in vivo* lens dehydration.
- High levels of protein absorption.

- High prevalence of manufacturing defects in lenses.

An alternative explanation is that the apparently greater risk of CL-MIK relates to the way in which the lenses were prescribed at the time of the study of Radford *et al.*[29] Many practitioners in the UK were using disposable lenses as 'problem solvers'; thus, it is possible that disposable lenses were being worn by a cohort of patients who were in any case more likely to develop CL-MIK.

## Patient management

Because of the potentially devastating effects of CL-MIK, any case of contact lens related ocular discomfort that persists after lens removal should be treated with grave suspicion.

### General advice
There is now available abundant evidence on the risk of developing CL-MIK with various lens types and modalities of wear. The key risk factor is overnight lens wear. Patients should be advised that although sleeping in lenses carries a far greater risk of developing CL-MIK compared with daily wear, the incidence is still very small. It is up to the patient to weigh up the risk verses the benefits of extended lens wear. All patients should be advised to remove their lenses if they have a sore red eye and to see their practitioner or seek medical attention if the discomfort persists or worsens in the first few hours following lens removal.

Patients travelling to warm environments should be warned of the possible increased risk of developing CL-MIK and the importance of complying with a full care regimen must be emphasised. Diabetic patients should be warned of the increased risk of infection due to their metabolic condition,[35] but at the the same time they should be advised that the absolute chance of developing CL-MIK is still very low (based on low incidence figures).

### Ocular examination
A contact lens patient presenting with a sore red eye should be examined as a matter of urgency and a decision must be made as to whether to refer the patient for medical treatment in case the keratitis is infectious. One or more of the following signs/symptoms necessitate urgent referral: severe ocular pain that persists following lens removal, extensive and/or intensive epithelial staining overlying the infiltrates, extensive anterior chamber flare, hypopyon, extreme conjunctival hyperaemia that persists following lens removal, or significant loss of vision.

### Medical treatment
A corneal scraping will typically be performed to determine if the condition is infectious and possibly to identify the offending micro-organism. Broad-spectrum antibiotics will then be instilled pending the result of the corneal scraping because such episodes are best presumed to be infectious unless proved otherwise. The choice of antibiotic should take into account the range of likely causative bacteria as revealed by epidemiological studies. Unfortunately, the results of scrapings are often equivocal because:

- Antibiotics may have been instilled as a necessary precautionary measure prior to hospitalisation.
- Numerous organisms may be isolated making it difficult to identify the true culprit.
- The result may be falsely culture-negative by chance.

Specific fortified antibiotics may be prescribed if the causative organism is positively identified.

Antibiotics can also be delivered by subconjunctival injection or even intravenously if corneal perforation is a possibility. Numerous other medical therapies may be utilised depending on circumstances; in summary, these are:

- *Mydriatics* – to prevent posterior synechia.
- *Collagenase inhibitors* – to minimise stromal melting.
- *Non-steroidal anti-inflammatory agents* – to reduce inflammation and limit the infiltrative response.
- *Analgesics* – to alleviate pain.
- *Tissue adhesives* – are applied when the stroma has become extremely thin or perforated.
- *Debridement* – to enhance the penetration of drugs into the eye.
- *Bandage lens* – to assist in re-epithelialisation.
- *Collagen shield* – can be soaked in therapeutic drugs which are slowly released back into the eye during wear.

Surgical interventions include a penetrating graft, which may need to be performed in the case of large perforations or non-healing deep central ulceration, or possibly a lamellar graft.

During the early phase of the condition, steroids are generally not prescribed (especially if the ulcer is culture-positive) because these drugs inhibit epithelial metabolism and retard the re-epithelialisation and other tissue repair activity. Steroids may be prescribed with extreme caution in the late healing phase to dampen the host response.

### Alleviate mechanical trauma
The clinical strategies that can be adopted to minimise the possibility of mechanical trauma are self-evident. The causes, and their solutions, include:

- *Lens deposits* – use a more effective care system, have the patient adopt more effective care procedures and/or replace lenses more regularly.
- *Poor insertion technique* – re-educate the patient on insertion techniques and consider alternative methods of lens insertion.
- *Poorly designed lenses* – choose an alternative design, or change from soft to rigid lenses or *vice versa*.
- *Ill-fitting lenses* – alter lens fit as appropriate.
- *Lens defects*[39] – advise patients to study lenses carefully for the presence of defects and/or prescribe a lens type known to be of high cosmetic quality.
- *Foreign body-induced trauma* – locate and remove the foreign body, and replace the lens if it has become damaged.

### Improve care system
Lens care systems which are known to be efficacious against the key offending micro-organisms should be prescribed. In this regard, many authors have advised against the use of chlorine-based disinfection systems as these systems have been shown to carry increased risk for the development of *Pseudomonas* and *Acanthamoeba* keratitis.[8,27,29]

Whatever system is prescribed, it is vital that the patient adheres to the full care regimen specified by the manufacturer, including the use of surfactant cleaners and protein removal systems as required. This entails giving appropriate advice in the first instance, monitoring patient compliance with this advice at subsequent aftercare visits, and taking remedial action if required.

### Improve hygiene

All patients, and in particular extended wear patients, must be advised of the importance of strict attention to all aspects of hygiene. Thorough hand washing prior to lens handling or in-eye lens manipulation and scrupulous attention to lens case care are key aspects to reinforce.

### Avoid tap water

The risk of developing *Acanthamoeba* keratitis will be greatly reduced by avoiding the use of tap water and home-made saline, as *Acanthamoeba* is ubiquitous in water supplies and thrives in saline solution in the absence of preservatives.[40]

### Change to daily wear

Available epidemiological evidence suggests that the risk of developing CL-MIK is greater when patients sleep in lenses. Changing from extended wear to daily wear will therefore represent a safer option.

### Fit RGP lenses

Again, the epidemiological evidence suggests that the risk of developing CL-MIK is lowest with RGP lens wear. This is attributed to high levels of oxygen transmissibility,[41] superior tear exchange,[42] greater post-lens tear film thickness, small lens size (not impinging on the limbus) and generally lower levels of problematic deposition on such lenses. Fitting patients with RGP lenses will therefore represent a low-risk option for CL-MIK.

### Improve oxygen performance

In view of the link between hypoxia and the induction of CL-MIK,[31] any measure to increase corneal oxygen availability during lens wear will lessen the risk of developing CL-MIK. In the case of soft lenses, this generally means fitting higher water content and/or thinner lenses,[42] or silicone-hydrogel lenses. The cornea is also likely to receive high levels of oxygen with RGP lenses due to their smaller size and greater tear exchange.

## Prognosis

The prognosis for recovery from CL-MIK is variable and depends largely on the speed and efficacy of treatment. If a patient removes his/her lenses promptly, seeks immediate advice, a correct diagnosis is made, and prompt, appropriate and aggressive therapeutic measures are enforced, the prognosis is good and the patient may ultimately be left with only a minor scar that does not interfere with vision. A delay in treatment and the use of inappropriate medication can result in total vision loss.[1]

In the case of *Staphylococcus* and *Streptococcus*, improvement in the condition may not be apparent until 24–48 hours after therapy has commenced. The micro-organisms are generally eradicated from the cornea within seven to 10 days.

*Pseudomonas* infections may appear to worsen slightly during the first 24 hours after medication has commenced. The condition will gradually improve thereafter, with the micro-organism persisting for 14 days or longer.

*Acanthamoeba* keratitis has a slow time course of recovery. The condition may progress over many months with periods of apparent improvement followed by regression. Patients are inevitably left with superficial nebulae corresponding to the site of infection (Figure 14.10).

## Differential diagnosis

An important diagnosis to be made in the early stages of a suspected CL-MIK is the differentiation between a sterile versus infective keratitis. As Stein *et al*[2] have pointed out, the key difference between sterile versus infective infiltrative keratitis is the severity of the signs and symptoms. Infected ulcers produce moderate to severe pain, unilateral discharge, photophobia, large areas of infiltration, epithelial breakdown and an anterior chamber reaction. Sterile ulcers are associated with smaller regions of infiltration, no discharge, less likelihood of epithelial disruption, mild or absent pain, mild photophobia and no anterior chamber flare. However, these are only general guidelines and there is considerable overlap between the two conditions (Figure 14.11). In view of the potentially serious consequences of infectious corneal disease, practitioners are advised to consider cases of infiltrative keratitis to be microbial if unsure.

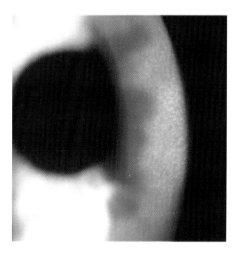

**Figure 14.11**
*Extensive infiltration in a case of sterile infiltrative keratitis, with the epithelium still intact*

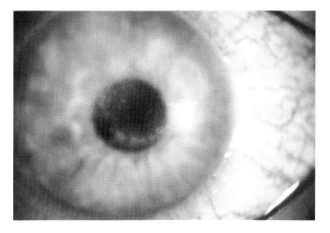

**Figure 14.10**
*Residual scar formation during the late healing phase of a patient suffering from Acanthamoeba keratitis*

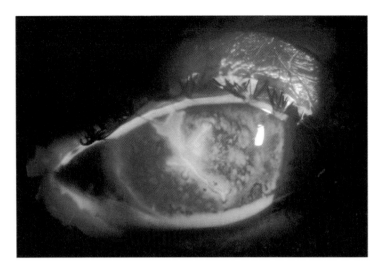

**Figure 14.12**
*Dendritic pattern of corneal ulceration in a contact lens wearer who had contracted herpes keratitis. The patient was an AIDS carrier*

*Acanthamoeba* keratitis can take on a similar clinical appearance to herpetic keratitis, and to a lesser extent *Pseudomonas* keratitis. In advanced stages of these conditions, the clinical geographical distribution of the ulcers across the corneas indicates the likely cause; a classic dendritic form of ulceration is evident in herpetic keratitis (Figure 14.12), whereas in *Acanthamoeba* the ulcer takes on a circular pattern.

The ultimate differential diagnosis will be provided by the results of cultures, smear tests and tissue staining, whereby the offending organism can be identified; however, the results of such tests cannot always be relied upon for reasons explained earlier. Judgements must often therefore be based on clinical evaluation of the presenting signs and symptoms, the pattern of disease progression, and the responsiveness of the condition to treatment alternatives.

Atypical patterns of infiltration may mimic the infiltrative response that accompanies CL-MIK, but these can usually be differentially diagnosed by the absence of both severe symptoms and associated pathology such as epithelial breakdown and aqueous flare (Figure 14.13).

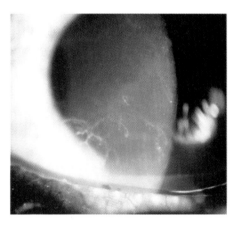

**Figure 14.13**
*Infiltrative pattern mimicking dendritic keratitis in a patient who had developed a reaction to a chemical disinfection system*

## REFERENCES

1 Chalupa E, Swarbrick HA, Holden BA (1987) Severe corneal infections associated with contact lens wear. *Ophthalmol* **94**: 17.

2 Stein RM, Clinch TE, Cohen EJ (1988) Infected vs sterile corneal infiltrates in contact lens wearers. *Am J Ophthalmol* **105**: 632.

3 Poggio EC, Glynn RJ, Schein OD (1989) The incidence of ulcerative keratitis among users of daily-wear and extended wear soft contact lenses. *N Engl J Med* **321**: 779.

4 MacRae S, Herman C, Stulting RD (1991) Corneal ulcer and adverse reaction rates in premarket contact lens studies. *Am J Ophthalmol* **111**: 457.

5 Nilsson SE, Montan PG (1994) The annualized incidence of contact lens-induced keratitis in Sweden and its relation to lens type and wear schedule: results of a three-month prospective study. *Contact Lens Assoc Ophthalmol J* **20**: 225.

6 Guillon M, Guillon JP, Bansal M (1994) Incidence of ulcers with conventional and disposable daily soft contact lenses. *J Br Contact Lens Assoc* **17**: 69.

7 Benjamin WJ (1992) Risks and incidences of 'ulcerative keratitis'. *J Br Contact Lens Assoc* **15**: 143.

8 Mathews TD, Frazer DG, Minassian DC (1992) Risks of keratitis and patterns of use with disposable contact lenses. *Arch Ophthalmol* **110**: 1559.

9 Buehler PO, Schein OD, Stamler JF (1992) The increased risks of ulcerative keratitis among disposable soft contact lens users. *Arch Ophthalmol* **110**: 1555.

10 Wilson LA, Ahearn DG (1986) Association of fungi with extended wear soft contact lenses. *Am J Ophthalmol* **101**: 434.

11 Fleiszig SMJ, Efron N (1992) Conjunctival flora in extended wear of rigid gas-permeable contact lenses. *Optom Vis Sci* **69**: 354.

12 Fleiszig SMJ, Efron N (1992) Microbial flora in current and former contact lens wearers. *J Clin Microbiol* **30**: 1156.

13 Fleiszig SMJ, Efron N (1988) Pathogenesis of contact lens-induced bacterial corneal ulcers. *Clin Exp Optom* **71**: 147.

14 Fleiszig SMJ, Efron N, Pier GB (1992) Extended wear enhances *Pseudomonas aeruginosa* adherence to human corneal epithelium. *Invest Ophthalmol Vis Sci* **33**: 2908.

15 Fletcher EL, Fleiszig SMJ, Brennan NA (1993) Lipopolysaccharide in adherence of *P. aeruginosa* to cornea and contact lenses. *Invest Ophthalmol Vis Sci* **34**: 1930.

16 Fletcher EL, Weissman BA, Efron N (1993) The role of pili in the attachment of *Pseudomonas aeruginosa* to unworn hydrogel contact lenses. *Curr Eye Res* **12**: 1067.

17 Fleiszig SMJ, Zaidi TS, Pier GB (1994) Ocular mucus and *Pseudomonas aeruginosa* adherence. *Adv Exp Med Biol* **350**: 359.

18 Fleiszig SMJ, Zaidi TS, Ramphal R (1994) Modulation of *P aeruginosa* adherence to the corneal surface by mucus. *Infect Immun* **62**: 1799.

19 Fleiszig SMJ, Evans DJ, Do N (1997) Epithelial cell polarity affects *Pseudomo-*

*nas aeruginosa* invasion and cytotoxicity. *Infect Immun* **65**: 2861.

20 Fleiszig SMJ, Zaidi TS, Fletcher EL (1994) *Pseudomonas aeruginosa* invades corneal epithelial cells during experimental infection. *Infect Immun* **62**: 3485.

21 Fleiszig SMJ, Zaidi TS, Pier GB (1995) *Pseudomonas aeruginosa* survival and multiplication within corneal epithelial cells *in vitro*. *Infect Immun* **63**: 4072.

22 Zaidi TS, Fleiszig SMJ, Preston MJ (1996) LPS outer core is a ligand for corneal cell binding and ingestion of *P. aeruginosa*. *Invest Ophthalmol Vis Sci* **37**: 976.

23 Fleiszig SMJ, Zaidi TS, Preston MJ (1996) The relationship between cytotoxicity and epithelial cell invasion by corneal isolates of *Pseudomonas aeruginosa*. *Infect Immun* **64**: 2288.

24 Fleiszig SMJ, Wiener-Kronish JP, Miyazaki H (1997) *Pseudomonas aeruginosa*-mediated cytotoxicity and invasion correlate to distinct genotypes at the loci encoding exoenzyme S. *Infect Immun* **65**: 579.

25 Lawin-Brussel CA, Refojo MF, Leong F-L (1991) *Pseudomonas* attachment to low-water and high-water, ionic and nonionic, new and rabbit-worn soft contact lenses. *Invest Ophthalmol Vis Sci* **32**: 657.

26 Claydon BE, Efron N (1994) Non-compliance in contact lens wear. *Ophthal Physiol Opt* **14**: 356.

27 Efron N, Wohl A, Toma N (1991) *Pseudomonas* corneal ulcers associated with daily wear of disposable hydrogel contact lenses. *Int Contact Lens Clin* **18**: 46.

28 Lowe R, Vallas V, Brennan NA (1992) Comparative efficacy of contact lens disinfection solutions. *Contact Lens Assoc Ophthalmol J* **18**: 34.

29 Radford CF, Bacon AS, Dart JKG (1995) Risk factors for *Acanthamoeba* keratitis in contact lens users: a case control study. *Br Med J* **310**: 1567.

30 Efron N, Ang JHB (1990) Corneal hypoxia and hypercapnia during contact lens wear. *Optom Vis Sci* **67**: 512.

31 Soloman OD, Loff H, Perla B (1994) Testing hypotheses for risk factors for contact lens-associated keratitis in an animal model. *Contact Lens Assoc Ophthalmol J* **20**: 109.

32 Klotz SA, Au Y, Misra RP (1989) A partial-thickness epithelial defect increases adherence of *Pseudomonas aeruginosa* to the cornea. *Invest Ophthalmol Vis Sci* **30**: 1069.

33 Van Klink F, Alizadeh H, He Y (1993) The role of contact lenses, trauma and Langerhans cells in a Chinese hamster model of *Acanthamoeba* keratitis. *Invest Ophthalmol Vis Sci* **34**:1937.

34 Claydon BE, Efron N, Woods C (1996) A prospective study of non-compliance in contact lens wear. *J Br Contact Lens Assoc* **19**: 133–140.

35 Schein OD, Glynn RJ, Poggio EC (1989) The relative risk of ulcerative keratitis among users of daily-wear and extended wear soft contact lenses. A case control study. *N Engl J Med* **321**: 773.

36 Claydon BE, Efron N, Woods C (1997) A prospective study of the effect of education on non-compliant behaviour in contact lens wear. *Ophthal Physiol Opt* **17**: 137.

37 Efron N. Guest editorial (1997) The truth about compliance. *Contact Lens Ant Eye* **20**: 79.

38 Katz HR, LaBorwit SE, Hirschbein MJ (1997) A retrospective study of seasonal influence on ulcerative keratitis. *Invest Ophthalmol Vis Sci* **38**: S136.

39 Efron N, Veys J (1992) Defects in disposable contact lenses can compromise ocular integrity. *Int Contact Lens Clin* **19**: 8.

40 Moore MB, McCulley JP, Luckenbach M (1985) *Acanthamoeba* keratitis associated with soft contact lenses. *Am J Ophthalmol* **100**: 396.

41 Tranoudis I, Efron N (1995) Oxygen permeability of rigid contact lens materials. *J Br Contact Lens Assoc* **18**: 49.

42 Efron N (1991) Understanding oxygen: Dk/L, EOP, oedema. *Trans Br Contact Lens Assoc* **14**: 65.

# Part VI
# Corneal Endothelium

# 15
# Bedewing

Incidence
Signs and symptoms
Pathology
Aetiology
Patient management
Prognosis
Differential diagnosis

Eye care practitioners from time to time will observe deposits such as keratic precipitates on the endothelial surface. These may be benign or may be associated with a broad range of uveal responses. In 1979 McMonnies and Zantos[1] described the appearance of endothelial deposits of uncertain origin in patients who were intolerant to contact lens wear (Figure 15.1). They de-

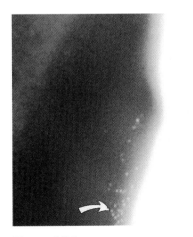

**Figure 15.1**
*Endothelial bedewing observed using marginal retro-illumination (arrow)*

scribed this condition as 'endothelial bedewing'. This condition was further discussed soon thereafter by Zantos and Holden;[2] however, since then, this topic has received little attention in the literature.

As will be discussed in this chapter it is not at all clear that endothelial bedewing is induced by contact lens wear; however, there appears to be an association between lens wear and endothelial bedewing. This association is worth considering because specific management strategies need to be employed to solve the problem.

## Incidence

The appearance of deposits or pigment spots on the endothelium is commonly encountered during routine slit-lamp examination of all patients. Corneal and/or lenticular pigmentation rarely affects vision.[3] McMonnies and Zantos[1] reported seeing 25 patients with endothelial bedewing associated with contact lens intolerance over a 9-month period, suggesting that this condition is not uncommon.

However, it is important to recognise

that these observations were made over 20 years ago when the contact lens market was dominated by soft contact lenses which were replaced infrequently, made of materials (primarily HEMA) of relatively low oxygen transmissibility, and maintained using relatively unsophisticated lens care systems. At that time contact lenses in general were associated with a higher prevalence of adverse reactions compared with the present-day situation.

Recent extensive surveys of adverse responses to contact lenses have failed to document the prevalence of endothelial dysfunction of any kind.[4,5] It is therefore not possible to deduce the prevalence of contact lens-associated endothelial bedewing (CLEB) in modern contact lens practice.

## Signs and symptoms

Contact lens-associated endothelial bedewing is characterised by the appearance of small particles in the region of the inferior central cornea near to or immediately below the inferior pupil margin. The area of bedewing can vary in shape. For example, CLEB may appear as an oval cluster

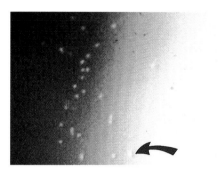

**Figure 15.2**
*Endothelial bedewing observed at high magnification, with individual cells displaying 'reversed illumination' (arrow)*

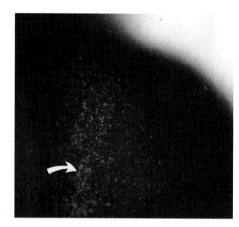

**Figure 15.3**
*Pigment dispersion observed using indirect retro-illumination (arrow)*

of particles or a less discrete dispersed formation. The condition is usually bilateral.[1]

The preferred slit-lamp observation technique is marginal retro-illumination, where the attention of the observer is directed to the region of the cornea in front of the border between the brightly illuminated iris and the dark pupil. Using this technique, the cells appear as small, discrete, circular, optically translucent entities. The cells invariably display an optical phenomenon known as 'reversed illumination', whereby the distribution of light within the cell is the opposite of the background distribution of light (Figure 15.2). This is optically identical to the 'reversed illumination' characteristic displayed by epithelial microcysts, although the underlying pathology is different from that of CLEB (see 'Pathology'). The optical basis for this appearance of 'reversed illumination' has been discussed in Chapter 10.

When viewed in direct illumination, CLEB can appear as fine white precipitates or as an orange/brown dusting of cells. The colour of the particles can give a clue to the length of time they have been present. Newly deposited cells are often whitish in colour, but these become pigmented over time.

Figure 15.3 is a slit-lamp photograph taken of the right eye of a 35-year-old male referred for assessment of suitability for contact lenses to correct myopia. An extensive 'dusting' of brown pigment can be observed in a spindle shape characteristic of pigment dispersion syndrome (the so-called 'Krukenberg spindle').

There appears to be no fixed pattern of associated signs. Among their detailed case reports of three patients, McMonnies and Zantos[1] noted these signs (in addition to

bedewing): conjunctival injection, epithelial erosion, epithelial oedema and reduced corneal transparency. There were no cases of flare in the anterior chamber.

The main associated feature of endothelial bedewing is either total or partial intolerance to lens wear. Some patients may present after having recently abandoned lens wear. Patients may also complain of 'fogging' of vision or stinging. It should be noted, however, that the association between bedewing and lens intolerance is not obligatory; McMonnies and Zantos[1] observed two cases of endothelial bedewing in successful lens wearers.

Mackie[6] describes a condition which he named 'total endothelial bedewing'. According to Mackie, this is an acute phenomenon that occurs in soft lens wearers. Patients usually present complaining of blurred vision. The condition resolves rapidly (within two days of lens removal) and does not recur. It is unclear whether Mackie was observing the same phenomenon as that reported by McMonnies and Zantos.[1]

## Pathology

McMonnies and Zantos[1] originally surmised that the bedewing particles were either droplets of clear fluid (oedema) within the endothelial cells or inflammatory cells such as leucocytes or macrophages resting on the posterior surface of the endothelium.

In view of the 'reversed illumination' optical appearance of bedewing, the more

likely explanation is that bedewing represents the presence of inflammatory cells. The reason for this is that 'reversed illumination' indicates the presence of material of higher refractive index within the entity displaying this appearance compared with the refractive index of the medium surrounding that entity.

The material of higher refractive index acts as a converging refractor causing a crossing over of the light rays. The cytoplasm, organelles and nucleus of an inflammatory cell resting on the endothelium would be of a higher refractive index than the surrounding clear aqueous humor, thus giving rise to reversed illumination.

Fluid droplets within the endothelium would be of a lower refractive index than the surrounding cytoplasm, organelles and nucleus of an endothelial cell and would therefore be expected to display 'unreversed illumination', whereby the distribution of light within the particles is the same as the background distribution of light. Since CLEB characteristically takes on a 'reversed illumination' appearance, it is more likely that the bedewing represents inflammatory cells rather than intracellular endothelial oedema.

Bergmanson and Weissman[7] have described an additional feature of endothelial bedewing – that inflammatory cells on the endothelial surface eventually become subsumed or engulfed by the endothelium and end up residing between adjacent endothelial cells and sealed off from the anterior chamber by zonula occludens.

These authors have produced convincing electron micrographs to support this hypothesis. Such engulfed inflammatory cells would be expected to produce a less pronounced appearance of reversed illumination because of the lower refractive index difference between the contents of the engulfed cell and the surrounding endothelial cells. It is likely that inflammatory cells observed in CLEB lie on the endothelium in the first instance, and some may become subsumed into the endothelium later.

Whatever the position of the inflammatory cells (on or within the endothelium), the very fact that these are inflammatory cells suggests that CLEB may have an inflammatory basis (see 'Aetiology'). Figure 15.4 is a schematic representation of endothelial bedewing.

On the assumption that CLEB represents a mild inflammatory uveal response, the origin of the inflammatory cells is likely to

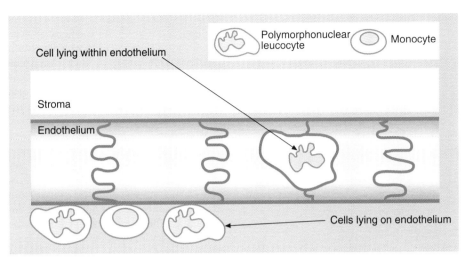

**Figure 15.4**
*Schematic representation of endothelial bedewing*

be the iris and/or ciliary body. During inflammation, vascular permeability is increased and inflammatory cells leave vessels in the iris and ciliary body and float around in the aqueous until they come to rest on the endothelial surface. One would therefore expect to occasionally observe mild aqueous flare in patients with CLEB, but this does not appear to have been reported.

## Aetiology

The appearance and characteristic distribution of endothelial bedewing, and the associated signs and symptoms of eye redness, stinging and blurred vision (aside from lens intolerance), strongly suggest that the syndrome of CLEB represents a mild anterior uveal inflammation. Although it is clear that contact lenses can induce a variety of inflammatory responses of the ocular surface tissues, it is less certain that contact lenses can induce a uveal inflammation.

Theoretically, contact lenses could induce a non-microbial inflammation. In most tissues, hypoxia can lead to the release of inflammatory mediators such as prostaglandins, which can cause inflammation. One possible mechanism is depicted in Figure 15.5. In this model, hypoxia induces the release of prostaglandins from corneal tissue which diffuse into the aqueous humor and eventually enter iris tissue. A mild inflammation is initiated and inflammatory cells are released into the aqueous; these eventually come to rest on the endothelial surface.

Efron *et al*[8] examined whether contact lens-induced corneal oedema was at least part inflammatory by measuring the level of oedema in response to contact lens wear in a group of human subjects who took prostaglandin inhibitor drugs prior to lens wear. There was no difference between the level of oedema in this group of subjects versus that in a control group who did not take prostaglandin inhibitor drugs, leading to a rejection of the hypothesis that contact lens-induced corneal oedema has an inflammatory component.

Nevertheless, a sequelae of events similar to that depicted in Figure 15.5 and described above is possible, perhaps with a family of inflammatory mediators other than prostaglandins.

It may well be the case that, instead of contact lenses inducing a mild uveal response of which endothelial bedewing is a sign, the converse is true. That is, a patient may develop a mild anterior uveal response for reasons unrelated to lens wear, but the mild inflammatory status of the eye causes lens intolerance. Indeed, the latter explanation is the more likely scenario. Whatever the causation, it is important that clinicians are aware of the association so that appropriate management strategies can be put in place.

## Patient management

As alluded to above, patients suffering from CLEB will have already devised strategies for alleviating the symptoms before they present to the clinic – namely, reducing wearing time or ceasing lens wear. Simply put, this is a condition that is managed by symptomatology rather than signs. Wearing time should be reduced to a level that represents the balance between the needs of the patient to wear lenses for a desired

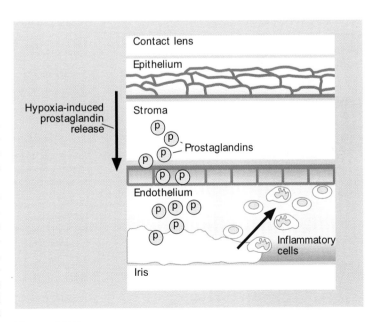

**Figure 15.5**
*Possible aetiology of endothelial bedewing*

length of time each day versus the level of discomfort that can be tolerated.

The presence of inflammatory cells on the endothelial surface should be viewed with great caution by clinicians, who need to consider a variety of possible causes. Certainly, all forms of uveitis should be considered as a possibility and tests should be conducted to exclude such possibilities (see 'Differential diagnosis').

In all cases of CLEB, intraocular pressures should be measured as there is a possibility that some inflammatory cells may have migrated into the anterior angle, creating a blockage of aqueous outflow. Gonioscopy is also indicated, especially if intraocular pressure is elevated.

## Prognosis

The pattern of recovery from CLEB is variable. McMonnies and Zantos[1] reported that in some cases the bedewing completely disappeared within four months, and in other cases it changed little over many months. These authors also reported that lens intolerance persisted for many months in some patients even after the bedewing had disappeared.

## Differential diagnosis

Various anomalies of the endothelium can potentially be confused with CLEB. Corneal guttata are focal accumulations of collagen on the posterior surface of Descemet's membrane which lead to localised bulging of the endothelial surface. This in turn

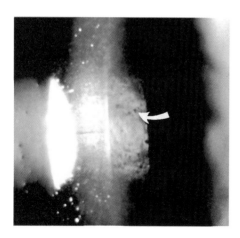

**Figure 15.6**
*Contact lens-induced endothelial blebs (arrow)*

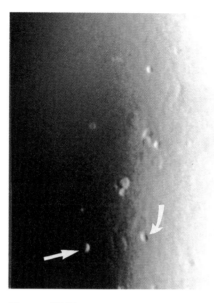

**Figure 15.7**
*Contact lens-induced epithelial microcysts (curved arrow; displaying reversed illumination) and fluid vacuoles (straight arrow; displaying unreversed illumination)*

leads to the appearance of dark spots in the endothelial mosaic when viewed using specular reflection.

Contact lens-induced endothelial blebs,

which are due to localised endothelial cell oedema, can take on an identical appearance to guttata (Figure 15.6). Differential diagnosis is effected by viewing the cornea using marginal retroillumination, thus confirming the presence of the reversed illumination appearance of bedewing. Guttata and blebs do not display this optical phenomenon.

When the cornea is viewed using marginal retro-illumination, endothelial bedewing takes on an appearance that is identical to epithelial microcysts (Figure 15.7). The procedure for differentiating between these two conditions is to view the cornea using a fine optical section at high magnification. If the endothelial bedewing is of the form whereby the cells are resting on the surface of the endothelium, then these will be observed as fine spots on the posterior corneal surface. If the bedewing cells have been engulfed into the endothelium, they may not be visible. Similarly, epithelial microcysts will not be observed in optic section. Thus, the appearance of spots on the endothelium when observed in optic section confirms the diagnosis of CLEB, whereas the absence of spots does not assist in differential diagnosis.

The associated signs will assist in the dif-

| Table 15.1 | Comparison of contact lens-associated endothelial bedewing and Fuch's heterochromatic cyclitis | |
|---|---|---|
| *Feature* | *Contact lens-associated endothelial bedewing* | *Fuch's heterochromatic cyclitis* |
| Age of onset | Any age | < 45 years |
| Sex | No preference | No preference |
| Associated factors | Contact lens wear | Vitreous opacities<br>Smudging of iris crypts<br>Iris pigment loss<br>Iris atrophy |
| Symptoms | Intolerance to lens wear<br>'Fogging' of vision<br>Stinging | Blurred vision |
| Signs | Conjunctival injection<br>Epithelial erosion<br>Epithelial oedema<br>Reduced corneal transparency | Feint anterior chamber flare |
| Cells | White or pigmented precipitates<br>Form at inferior cornea | Only white precipitates<br>Scattered diffusely over cornea |
| Laterality | Usually bilateral | Usually unilateral |
| Secondary complications | Glaucoma | Glaucoma<br>Cataract |

ferential diagnosis of CLEB versus epithelial microcysts. The latter is typically associated with extended lens wear and symptoms are minimal or absent. On the other hand, CLEB is associated with stinging, eye redness, corneal clouding and lens intolerance.

The possibility that the patient is suffering from a form of uveitis that has occurred coincidentally with lens wear must be considered as a distinct possibility. The signs and symptoms associated with CLEB can closely mimic some of the mild manifestations of uveitis, such as Fuch's heterochromatic cyclitis. Table 15.1 compares the signs and symptoms of CLEB and Fuch's heterochromatic cyclitis as a guide to differential diagnosis.

If a uveitis of any sort is suspected – including an intractable case of CLEB associated with indicators of active pathology such as a red irritable eye and/or anterior chamber flare – the patient must be referred for medical evaluation. Medical treatment may include the prescription of corticosteroids to dampen the inflammatory response, mydriatics to prevent the formation of posterior synechiae, and analgesics to reduce the pain. If uveitis is confirmed in a contact lens wearer, then lens wear should be ceased until the condition has fully resolved.

## REFERENCES

1 McMonnies CW, Zantos SG (1979) Endothelial bedewing of the cornea in association with contact lens wear. *Br J Ophthalmol* **63**: 478.

2 Zantos SG, Holden BA (1981) Guttate endothelial changes with anterior eye inflammation. *Br J Ophthalmol* **65**: 101.

3 Efron N, Collin HB (1979) Epicapsular stars with visual loss. *Am J Optom Physiol Opt* **56**: 441.

4 Stapleton F, Dart J, Minassian D (1992) Nonulcerative complications of contact lens wear. *Arch Ophthalmol* **110**: 1601.

5 Hamano H, Watanabe K, Hamano T (1994) A study of the complications induced by conventional and disposable contact lenses. *Contact Lens Assoc Ophthalmol J* **20**: 103.

6 Mackie IA (1993) Adverse reactions to soft contact lenses. In: *Medical Contact Lens Practice – A Systematic Approach.* Butterworth–Heinemann, Oxford, ch. 13.

7 Bergmanson JPG, Weissman BA (1992) Hypoxic changes in corneal endothelium. In: *Complications of Contact Lens Wear* (ed. A Tomlinson). Mosby Year Book, St Louis, p. 52.

8 Efron N, Holden BA, Vannas A (1984) Effect of the prostaglandin inhibitor naproxen on the corneal swelling response to hydrogel contact lens wear. *Acta Ophthalmol* **62**: 746.

# 16
# Blebs

Prevalence
Signs and symptoms
Pathology
Aetiology
Observation and grading
Management and prognosis
Differential diagnosis

Prior to 1977, it was thought that contact lenses could only affect the cornea by direct mechanical influence or oxygen deprivation. Because the endothelium is located on the posterior surface of the cornea and is known to obtain all of its required oxygen from that dissolved in the aqueous humor,[1] this tissue layer was thought to be immune from the effects of contact lenses.

The first clue that contact lenses could alter the corneal endothelium came from Zantos and Holden,[2] who noted that the endothelial mosaic undergoes a dramatic alteration in appearance within minutes of inserting a contact lens. Specifically, they reported observing a number of black, non-reflecting areas in the endothelial mosaic – which they called blebs – and an apparent increase in the separation between cells. These changes can be observed under high magnification (×40) using the slit-lamp biomicroscope (Figure 16.1).

The contact lens fraternity remained sceptical for some time, and it was not until the appearance of blebs was verified independently[3] and reports of contact lens-induced endothelial polymegethism were published by Schoessler and Woloschak in the early 1980s,[4,5] that serious research

commenced into understanding the endothelial response to lens wear.

## Prevalence

The prevalence of endothelial blebs is thought to be essentially 100 per cent among contact lens wearers.[2] That is, blebs can be observed in all patients within 10 minutes of lens insertion. There is a large variation in the intensity of the response between patients.[2]

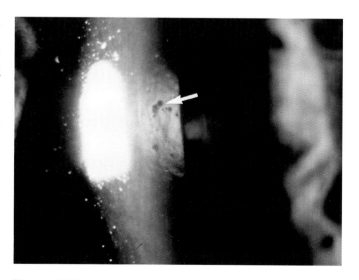

**Figure 16.1**
*Contact lens-induced blebs (arrow) in the endothelial mosaic*

## Signs and symptoms

The black, non-reflecting areas observed in the endothelial mosaic correspond with the position of individual cells or groups of cells. The initial impression one gains is that cells have 'fallen off' the posterior surface of the cornea, leaving behind gaps or black holes.[2] In corneas displaying a marked blebbing response, it also appears as if all endothelial cells throughout the field of view have become more separated and the endothelial surface takes on a more textured and three-dimensional appearance.[2]

The 'bleb response' displays a characteristic time course (Figure 16.2). Blebs can be observed within 10 minutes of lens insertion. The number of blebs peaks in 20–30 minutes, then subsides to a low level after about 45–60 minutes. A low-level bleb response can be observed throughout the remainder of the wearing period.[2]

Hydrogel lenses cause a greater bleb response than well fitting rigid lenses, and hydrogel lenses of greater average thickness also induce a greater response than thinner lenses. However, the design and fit of hydrogel lenses have little effect on the bleb response.[6]

Williams and Holden[7] observed two additional phenomena in patients wearing soft lenses on an extended wear basis. First, there appears to be an increase in the number of blebs in the late evening, prior to going to sleep. Second, the overall magnitude of the bleb response can be seen to decrease over the initial eight days of extended wear. Furthermore, Bruce and

Brennan[8] noted that the overall bleb response was reduced by approximately 50 per cent after 4 months of soft lens extended wear compared with baseline values. These observations suggest that some form of short-term[7] and long-term adaptation of the endothelium is taking place.[7,8]

Despite their stunning clinical appearance, blebs are asymptomatic and thought to be of little clinical significance. They are, however, of great interest to physiologists who are endeavouring to understand the workings of the cornea.

## Pathology

Histological studies of the endothelial bleb response were conducted by Vannas et al[9] using corneas from eyes that were enucleated (because of melanomas) and corneas of beating-heart, brain-death cadavers. The 'blebbed' endothelium displayed oedema of the nuclear area of cells, intracellular fluid vacuoles and fluid spaces between cells. Thus, endothelial blebs appear to be the result of a local oedema phenomenon, where the posterior surface of the 'blebbed' endothelial cell is bulged towards the aqueous. The endothelial cell bulges in the posterior direction as this represents the path of least resistance; that is, the posterior stromal surface (Descemet's membrane) offers much greater resistance to endothelial cell swelling than the aqueous humor.

A simple optical model can now be constructed to explain the appearance of blebs (Figure 16.3). When the endothelium is viewed using specular reflection, light

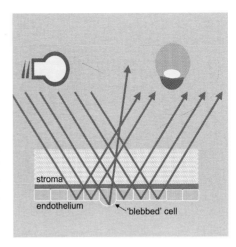

**Figure 16.3**
*Optical theory explaining the appearance of contact lens-induced endothelial blebs*

rays reflect from the tissue plane corresponding to the interface between the posterior surface of the endothelium and the aqueous humor. This interface acts as the reflective surface because it represents a significant change in tissue refractive index. The light rays that are reflected from this interface give rise to an observed image of an essentially flat (or slightly undulating) and featureless endothelial cell mosaic.

Light rays which strike 'blebbed' endothelial cells will be deflected away from the observation path, leaving a corresponding area of darkness. Thus, an endothelial bleb is simply an individual endothelial cell (or group of adjacent cells) that has become swollen and bulged in the direction of the aqueous humor, giving rise to the compelling optical illusion that the cell (or cells) has disappeared.

## Aetiology

The aetiology of endothelial blebs has been explained by Holden et al.[10] These authors attempted to induce blebs using a variety of stimulus conditions, and concluded that one physiological factor common to all successful attempts to form blebs was a local acidic pH change at the endothelium.

Two separate factors induce an acidic shift in the cornea during contact lens wear:

- An increase in carbonic acid due to retardation of carbon dioxide efflux (hypercapnia)[11] by a contact lens.

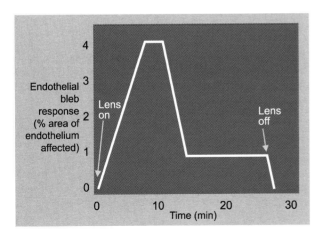

**Figure 16.2**
*Time course of appearance and resolution of contact lens-induced endothelial blebs*

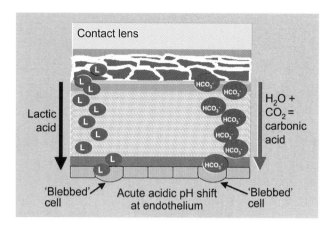

**Figure 16.4**
*Aetiology of contact lens-induced endothelial blebs*

- Increased levels of lactic acid as a result of lens-induced oxygen deprivation (hypoxia)[11] and the consequent increase in anaerobic metabolism (Figure 16.4).

When silicone elastomer contact lenses are worn, such metabolic changes do not take place because of the extremely high oxygen permeability of such lenses.

Bonnano and Polse[12] have confirmed by direct measurement that contact lens-induced hypoxia and hypercapnia result in an acidic shift in the cornea and these authors noted that the extent of acidosis that they measured is in the range where endothelial function may be affected. Furthermore, the time course of the appearance of blebs following lens insertion, and resolution following lens removal, is consistent with the time course of corneal pH change as measured by Bonnano and Polse.[12]

The cornea becomes hypoxic and hypercapnic during sleep so it would be expected that the consequent acidic changes would induce blebs. Various authors have indeed confirmed that there is a diurnal variation in the endothelial bleb response, whereby more blebs can be observed immediately upon awakening.[7,13]

The question arises as to the precise mechanism by which acidosis causes endothelial cells to swell. All cells in the human body function optimally when surrounded by extracellular fluid that is maintained within an acceptable range of pH, temperature, tonicity, ion balance etc. The carbonic acid and lactic acid may alter the physiological status of the environment surrounding the endothelial cells by shifting pH in the acidic direction. This may induce changes in membrane permeability and/or membrane pump activity, resulting in a net movement of water into endothelial cells. The resultant cellular oedema is observed as 'blebbing'.

## Observation and grading

The corneal endothelium can be viewed by specular reflection using a slit-lamp biomicroscope at ×40 magnification. In order to observe the endothelium using this technique, the angle between the illumination and observation systems must be symmetrical about a plane extending normally from the cornea, and will typically be between 75° and 90°. The endothelial mosaic can be seen adjacent to a bright reflex from the corneal surface (Figure 16.1). Using this technique, only the mid-peripheral nasal or temporal endothelium are viewed; this does not pose a problem because changes in these regions are representative of changes elsewhere in the cornea.[6]

Although individual endothelial cells can only just be resolved at ×40 magnification, blebs have a stark appearance and are easily recognisable. A variety of sophisticated automated cameras specifically designed for viewing the endothelium have become available in recent times;[14] these instruments offer higher magnification and superior resolution compared with slit-lamp observation. Automated endothelial cameras are invaluable as research tools when it is necessary to quantify endothelial changes; however, a general appraisal of the endothelial bleb response can be obtained satisfactorily with a good quality, high-magnification slit lamp.

The extent of endothelial bleb formation can be graded using the concept of a standard clinical severity scale extending from zero (normal) to four (severe);[15] however, the usual connotation that is associated with contact lens grading scales concerning the urgency for clinical action does not apply here because contact lens-induced endothelial blebs are thought to be innocuous, irrespective of the level of severity of blebbing. The 0 to 4 scale of the bleb response can be considered as being approximately linear. High-magnification slit-lamp photographs of endothelial blebbing of grades 0 (normal), 2 (slight) and 4 (severe) are shown in Figure 16.5.

## Management and prognosis

While the phenomenon of endothelial blebs is of immense interest from a physiological standpoint, there are no readily apparent clinical ramifications. The bleb response occurs to a greater or lesser degree in most patients, and displays a characteristic time course. It is not known whether a propensity for the endothelium of a patient to exhibit blebbing is a positive or negative attribute. Williams surmises that the severity of an endothelial bleb response is reduced in patients displaying increased levels of endothelial polymegethism, which could partially explain the apparent long-term adaptation of the bleb response.[6] Specifically, a low-level bleb response has been interpreted as an indication that the endothelium has lost its capacity to respond to changes in its immediate environment; that is, the endothelium has become 'exhausted'.

Theoretically, the bleb response can be used as a relative measure of the combined impact of contact lens-induced hypoxia and hypercapnia on the cornea of a given patient. That is to say, in a given patient, a lens with lower average oxygen transmissibility will induce a more severe bleb response.[6] Thus, a comparison of the severity of the bleb response could be used to help select a lens of optimal gas transmission characteristics. However, such applications have not been reported and further research is needed to ascertain whether the bleb response holds any information that could assist clinicians in evaluating the ocular response to lens wear.

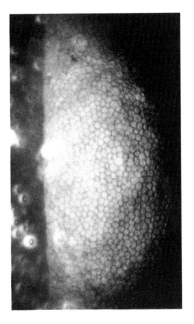 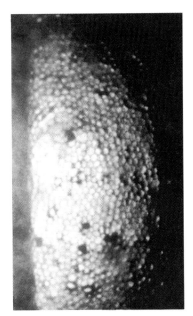 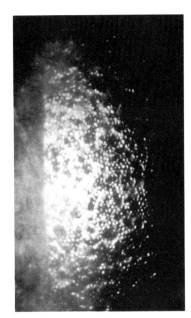

**Figure 16.5**
*High-magnification slit-lamp photographs of contact lens-induced endothelial blebs. Left, grade 0; centre, grade 2; and right, grade 4*

The prognosis for recovery from endothelial blebs is excellent. After removal of a contact lens, blebs disappear within minutes.[2]

## Differential diagnosis

Primary chronic corneal disorders such as Fuch's endothelial dystrophy are often characterised by the presence of guttata, which appear as small shallow depressions in the endothelial mosaic in the early stages of the disease process and as distinct black holes in advanced cases.[16] In the case of guttae due to dystrophy, extensive confluent areas of blebbing may be apparent (Figure 16.6); such confluence is not observed in contact lens-induced blebbing. The key distinction between guttae related to corneal dystrophy and contact lens-induced blebs is the permanence of guttae and the transience of blebs.

Interestingly, transient phenomena that closely resemble endothelial blebs have been observed in patients with acute superficial eye disorders. Specifically, Zantos and Holden[17] noted such transient changes in cases of acute 'red eye' associated with extended contact lens wear; these formations have exactly the same appearance as contact lens-induced blebs, but are different in that they persisted for many days following

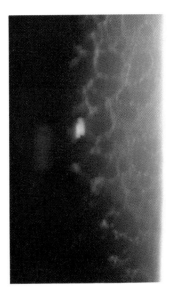

**Figure 16.6**
*Corneal dystrophy depicting severe guttate changes*

cessation of lens wear. Brooks *et al*[18] described transient 'subendothelial blebs' in patients with superficial keratopathy of various aetiology; however, these changes have a different appearance from contact lens-induced blebs in that the areas of darkness are more diffuse and there is no apparent separation of cells throughout the field.

## REFERENCES

1 Fatt I, Beiber MT (1968) The steady state distribution of oxygen and carbon dioxide in the *in vivo* human cornea. The open eye in air and the closed eye. *Exp Eye Res* **7**: 103.

2 Zantos SG, Holden BA (1977) Transient endothelial changes soon after wearing soft contact lenses. *Am J Optom Physiol Opt* **54**: 856.

3 Vannas A, Makitie J, Sulonen J (1981) Contact lens-induced transient changes in corneal endothelium. *Acta Ophthalmol* **59**: 552.

4 Schoessler JP, Woloschak MJ (1981) Corneal endothelium in veteran PMMA contact lens wearers. *Int Contact Lens Clin* **8**: 19.

5 Schoessler JP (1983) Corneal endothelial polymegethism associated with extended wear. *Int Contact Lens Clin* **10**: 144.

6 Williams L (1986) Transient endothelial changes in the *in vivo* human cornea. PhD Thesis, University of New South Wales.

7 Williams L, Holden BA (1986) The bleb response of the endothelium decreases with extended wear of contact lenses. *Clin Exp Optom* **69**: 90.

8 Bruce AS, Brennan NA (1993) Epithelial, stromal and endothelial responses

to hydrogel extended wear. *Contact Lens Assoc Ophthalmol J* **19**: 211.

9 Vannas A, Holden BA, Makitie J (1984) The ultrastructure of contact lens-induced changes in the human corneal endothelium. *Acta Ophthalmol* **62**: 320.

10 Holden BA, Williams L, Zantos SG (1985) The etiology of transient endothelial changes in the human cornea. *Invest Ophthalmol Vis Sci* **26**: 1354.

11 Efron N, Ang JHB (1990) Corneal hypoxia and hypercapnia during contact lens wear. *Optom Vis Sci* **67**: 512.

12 Bonanno JA, Polse KA (1987) Corneal acidosis during contact lens wear: effects of hypoxia and $CO_2$. *Invest Ophthalmol Vis Sci* **28**: 1514.

13 Khodadoust AA, Hirst LW (1984) Diurnal variation in corneal endothelial morphology. *Ophthalmol* **91**: 1125.

14 Stevenson RWW (1994) Non-contact specular microscopy of the corneal endothelium. *Optician* **208**: 22.

15 Woods R (1989) Quantitative slit-lamp observations in contact lens practice. *J Br Contact Lens Assoc (Scientific Meetings)*: 42–5.

16 Feeney ML, Garron LK (1961) Descemet's membrane in the peripheral cornea. In: *The Structure of the Eye* (GK Smelser, ed.). Academic Press, London.

17 Zantos SG, Holden BA (1981) Guttate endothelial changes with anterior eye inflammation. *Br J Ophthalmol* **65**: 101.

18 Brooks AMV, Grant G, Gillies WE (1989) The influence of superficial epithelial keratopathy on the corneal endothelium. *Ophthalmol* **96**: 704.

# 17
# Polymegethism

The normal endothelium
Defining endothelial changes
Contact lens effects
Prevalence
Signs and symptoms
Pathology
Aetiology
Observation and grading
Management
Prognosis
Differential diagnosis

As explained in Chapter 16, the observation by Zantos and Holden[1] in 1977 of acute transient changes ('blebs') in the corneal endothelium associated with contact lens wear provided the first clue to researchers and clinicians that the corneal endothelium was susceptible to alterations in the physiological environment at the ocular surface. Attention quickly turned to the possibility that contact lenses could induce chronic alterations to endothelial morphology in the same way that such changes were induced by other ocular and systemic disease processes; subsequent research confirmed these changes to occur.[2–6]

Concern that contact lenses may be adversely affecting the corneal endothelium has resulted in endothelial examination becoming a routine procedure during biomicroscopic examination of the cornea of contact lens wearers. Whether observable changes such as endothelial polymegethism are of immediate clinical significance is being debated; nevertheless, practitioners ought to be able to examine and assess the integrity of the endothelium, and should be prepared to interpret any changes observed in the context of current controversies concerning corneal endothelial structure and function.

## The normal endothelium

The corneal endothelium is a monolayer of about half a million cells (at birth) which constitutes the posterior corneal surface. Anteriorly, the endothelium is in apposition with a basement membrane which is formed by secretions from the endothelium itself. The basement membrane is known as the posterior limiting lamina (or Descemet's membrane). The anterior surface of the endothelial cell is known as the basal surface. The posterior (apical) surface of the endothelium is in direct contact with the aqueous humor.

On examination of the endothelium using specular reflection, the apparent size and shape of the component cells can be identified. In the normal endothelium of an infant, all cells are approximately the same size and have a characteristic hexagonal shape. These features can only just be resolved using a good quality slit-lamp biomicroscope at the highest magnification ($\times40$) (Figure 17.1).

## Defining endothelial changes

The conventional way of denoting cell size is in terms of the endothelial cell density, expressed as the number of cells per square millimetre (Figure 17.2). The variation in apparent size of cells is expressed as the coefficient of variation of cell size (COV); this dimensionless ratio is calculated by dividing the standard deviation of the cell areas in a defined field by the arithmetic mean area of all cells in that field.

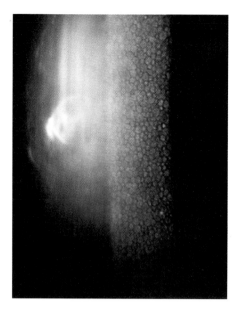

**Figure 17.1**

*High-magnification slit-lamp biomicroscope photograph of a corneal endothelium displaying extensive contact lens-induced polymegethism*

The COV is a measure of the degree of endothelial polymegethism. ('Polymegethism is derived from the Greek word *megethos* meaning 'size'; *poly* means 'many'.) The term endothelial polymorphism (or pleo-morphism) refers to a variation in cell shape (i.e. cells with four, five, six or seven sides, as distinct from the classical uniform six-sided endothelial cell appearance).

In the normal eye, endothelial cell density decreases from about 4400 cells/mm$^2$ at birth to 2200 cells/mm$^2$ at age 80.[7] In addition, the COV increases throughout life. Obviously, any changes thought to be attributed to contact lens wear must be considered in the context of these normal age changes.

Consequently, the term endothelial polymegethism, when discussed in this paper in the context of an induced change, should generally be taken to mean a degree of change in excess of that expected for a given age.

## Contact lens effects

Reports of contact lens-induced endothelial polymegethism were first published by Schoessler and Woloschak in the early 1980s.[2,3] These authors provided a convincing anecdotal demonstration of endothelial polymegethism in 10 patients who had worn PMMA lenses for at least five years. Subsequent research by Hirst *et al*,[4] Holden *et al*[5] and MacRae *et al*[6] provided statistical validation of this phenomenon.

Figure 17.3 is a compelling illustration of the effect of contact lens wear on the corneal endothelium; illustrated is a pair of endothelial photomicrographs of a patient who wore an extended wear lens for 5 years in one eye only because of uniocular myopia. The bottom frame is the endothelium of the lens wearing eye and the top frame is that of the fellow non-lens wearing eye. A greater variation in endothelial cell size (polymegethism) is clearly evident in the lens-wearing eye.

Hirst *et al*[4] also reported a substantially lower percentage of hexagonal cells in patients wearing PMMA contact lenses compared with matched non-lens wearing control eyes. Such polymorphic changes are generally associated with changes in polymegethism.

Until recently, researchers had been unable to provide evidence for a contact lens-induced reduction in endothelial cell density. However, McMahon *et al*[8] reported that a group of 16 long-term PMMA lens wearers had an endothelial cell density (2147 cells/mm$^2$) that was statistically significantly less than that of a matched control group of non-lens wearers (2865 cells/mm$^2$).

The question as to whether endothelial polymegethism is always accompanied by endothelial cell loss is a critical issue because, as will be explained later in this chapter, the answer will impact the development of models of the aetiopathology of age-related versus contact lens-induced polymegethism. In age-related polymegethism, it is assumed that cell loss results in a three-dimensional redistribution and spreading out of the cytoplasmic mass of existing cells to ensure full endothelial cell coverage of the posterior corneal surface.

This redistribution theory may also apply to contact lens-induced endothelial polymegethism if one accepts the data of McMahon *et al* that contact lenses induce endothelial cell loss;[8] however, if it is the case that contact lenses do not cause a loss of endothelial cells, then an alternative explanation of contact lens-induced polymegethism (that does not require redistribution of the cytoplasmic mass of existing cells) will need to be sought.

## Prevalence

Endothelial polymegethism is a natural age change that occurs in all humans. Contact

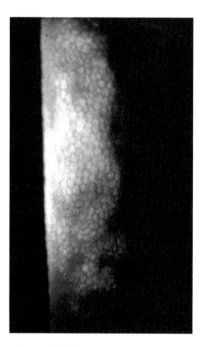 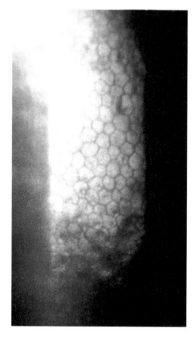

**Figure 17.2**

*Very high-magnification slit-lamp biomicroscope photographs of high (left) and low (right) contact lens-induced corneal endothelial cell density*

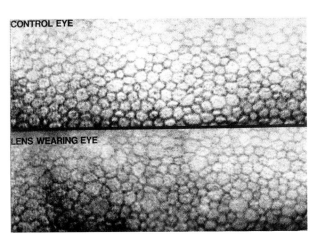

CONTROL EYE

LENS WEARING EYE

**Figure 17.3**
*Polymegethous corneal endothelium of the eye of a patient who wore an extended wear lens in one eye only (bottom frame) for five years because of uniocular myopia. The endothelium of the fellow non-lens wearing control eye is shown in the top frame*

lenses essentially have the effect of accelerating such changes. Although such accelerated changes are not observed when lenses of extremely high oxygen transmissibility are worn (such as silicone elastomer lenses),[9] virtually all other lens types that induce some measure of chronic hypoxic stress will induce a degree of endothelial polymegethism and polymorphism.

Because it has only recently been discovered that contact lenses can cause a reduction in cell density,[8] it is too early to speculate as to the prevalence of this particular complication in lens wearers generally.

## Signs and symptoms

The endothelium of a newborn baby has a very regular and uniform appearance, with all cells being almost exactly the same size and displaying classical hexagonality. In, say, a 25-year-old – an age when contact lens wear might begin – the endothelium will typically display a low degree of polymegethism. The ratio of the diameter of the smallest cell to the largest cell that can be seen could be 1 : 5.

In advanced cases of polymegethism, the ratio of smallest to largest cell can be as great as 1 : 20 (Figure 17.4). While it is possible to make a qualitative assessment of the extent of polymegethism based on observation of the endothelial mosaic, it is not possible for clinicians to make such an assessment concerning endothelial cell density. Techniques for measuring endothelial polymegethism and cell density are described under 'Observation and grading'.

Sweeney[10] has drawn an anecdotal association between endothelial polymegethism and a condition which she termed 'corneal exhaustion syndrome'. This is a condition in which patients who have worn contact lenses for many years suddenly develop a severe intolerance to lens wear characterised by ocular discomfort, reduced vision, photophobia and an excessive oedema response. These patients also display a distorted endothelial mosaic and moderate to severe polymegethism.

Although the link between endothelial polymegethism and corneal exhaustion syndrome is not proven, it is plausible that chronic lens-induced hypoxia has induced a number of pathological tissue changes (endothelial polymegethism being one of these) that can result in intolerance to lens wear.

Aside from the possibility of corneal exhaustion syndrome, no other symptoms are associated with endothelial polymegethism.

## Pathology

To understand precisely what happens to endothelial cells when polymegethism develops, it is important to understand how the classical appearance of the endothelium as viewed by specular reflection relates to the overall three-dimensional structure of endothelial cells.

When the endothelium is viewed using specular reflection, light rays reflect from

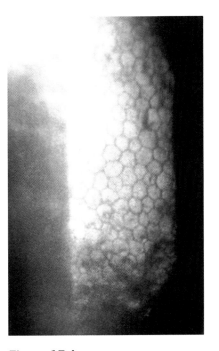
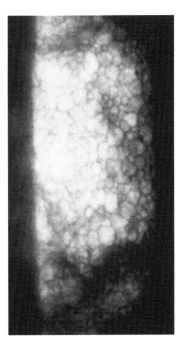

**Figure 17.4**
*Very high-magnification slit-lamp biomicroscope photographs of low grade (left) and high grade (right) contact lens-induced corneal endothelial polymegethism*

the tissue plane corresponding to the interface between the apical surface of the endothelium and the aqueous humor.

This interface acts as the main reflective surface because it represents a significant change in tissue refractive index; that is, the difference in refractive index between the apical surface of the endothelial cell and the aqueous humor is greater than that between the basal surface of the endothelial cell and posterior limiting lamina of the stroma.

The light rays that are reflected from the apical endothelium–aqueous interface give rise to an observed image of the endothelial mosaic. Light rays which strike the junction between endothelial cells are deflected away from the observation path, leaving corresponding dark lines which are observed as cell borders.

Assuming no change in endothelial cell density, the specular appearance of polymegethism would suggest that some cells are becoming smaller and some are becoming larger. If, on the other hand, a reduction in endothelial cell density is assumed, then the appearance of polymegethism would suggest that some cells are remaining the same size and some are becoming larger.

Irrespective of the assumption one makes concerning changes in cell density, a disparity in cell size is apparent. However, this disparity is evident only at the apical endothelium–aqueous interface, and does not necessarily relate to volumetric changes in the cytoplasmic mass of endothelial cells anterior to this interface. A true appreciation of the morphological changes that constitute polymegethism can be gained by considering the theoretical analysis of Bergmanson,[11] who conducted an ultrastructural study of the corneas of six long-term contact lens wearers. He observed that the lateral cell walls, which are normally extremely interdigitated but essentially oriented normal to the endothelial surface, had straightened out and oriented obliquely.

The interpretation of this observation in terms of the three-dimensional structure of the endothelium is that endothelial cells have changed shape but the volume of each cell has remained constant. Thus, by observing only the apical surface of the endothelium on specular reflection, one is presented with the compelling illusion that a disparity in cell size has developed. In reality, the cells have merely become

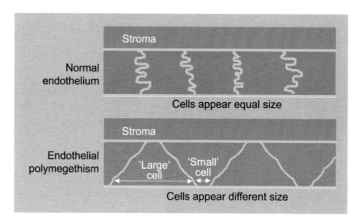

**Figure 17.5**
*Theory of Bergmanson explaining the pathogenesis and biomicroscopic appearance of corneal endothelial polymegethism (adapted from Bergmanson[11])*

reoriented in three-dimensional space (Figure 17.5).

A further observation of Bergmanson[11] of equal significance is that, although the endothelium of contact lens wearers showed some inter- and intra-cellular oedema, the cells were otherwise of a healthy appearance containing normal, undamaged organelles. This raises the interesting and controversial possibility that, rather than representing an adverse effect, endothelial polymegethism is a non-problematic adaptation to chronic metabolic stress.

The suggestion that endothelial polymegethism is a benign tissue change has been challenged by researchers who have demonstrated a link between endothelial polymegethism and corneal hydration control.[8,12] In these studies, the effect of contact lens wear on corneal hydration control was measured by inducing corneal oedema and then recording the exponential rate of corneal deswelling.

Recovery from oedema is significantly slower in the corneas of contact lens wearers (versus matched controls) and this deficit is dose-related (i.e. the effect is more pronounced the longer lenses have been worn). Figure 17.6 is a re-representation of the data of McMahon *et al*[8] demonstrating that corneal deswelling following induced oedema in PMMA lens wearers is considerably slower than that in non-lens wearers.

Such observations must be considered in the context of a loss of corneal hydration control being a normal age-related change in the human population; typically, the cornea of a 65-year-old person will take 10

per cent longer to recover from stromal swelling compared with that of a 20-year-old person.[13]

An unfortunate conundrum in science is that correlation does not prove causation. Thus, it cannot be concluded with absolute certainty that the loss of corneal hydration control in contact lens wearers is caused by lens-induced endothelial polymegethism. However, it is not unreasonable to postulate such a causal relationship in view of the critical role of the endothelium in corneal hydration control.

The corneal hydration control process – known as the 'pump-leak' mechanism[14] –

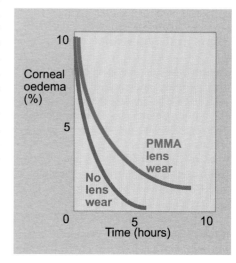

**Figure 17.6**
*Corneal deswelling following induced oedema in PMMA lens wearers vs non-lens wearers (adapted from McMahon et al[8])*

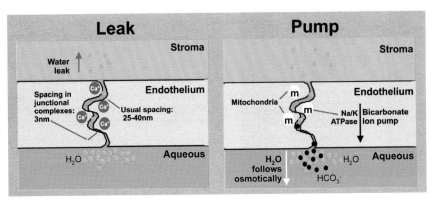

**Figure 17.7**
*The pump–leak process of corneal hydration control encompasses a 'leaky' endothelium (left) and an endothelial bicarbonate pump (right)*

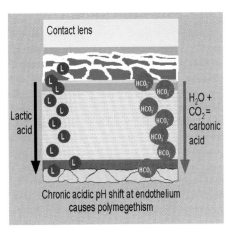

**Figure 17.8**
*Aetiology of contact lens-induced corneal endothelial polymegethism*

comprises, as the name suggests, two critical components, both of which are located in the endothelium. The leak refers to the constant tendency for water to move from the aqueous humor into the stroma through gaps between endothelial cells, and the pump refers to an active mechanism whereby endothelial cells pump bicarbonate ions into the aqueous, creating an osmotic force that draws water out of the stroma (Figure 17.7).[15]

These counter-acting forces are metabolically controlled so as to maintain a constant level of stromal hydration, while at the same time affording a mechanism of nutrient and waste exchange between the cornea and aqueous humor.

The suggestion that contact lens-induced endothelial damage results in either an increased leak or a reduction in pump efficiency, or both, is confounded by the failure of Bergmanson[11] to detect such damage upon ultrastructural examination of the organelles of endothelial cells of long-term contact lens wearers.

## Aetiology

It is likely that the aetiology of endothelial polymegethism is precisely the same as the aetiology of endothelial blebs, whereby the former represents a chronic response and the latter represents an acute response to the same stimuli.

The aetiology of endothelial blebs – or acute localised endothelial oedema – was considered in Chapter 16. The key evidence comes from Holden *et al*,[16] who attempted to induce blebs using a variety of stimulus conditions, and concluded that one physio-

logical factor common to all successful attempts to form blebs was a local acidic pH change at the endothelium. It is suggested here that polymegethism in contact lens wearers is also due to lens-induced endothelial acidosis, for the simple reason that the extent of polymegethism is apparently governed by the same dosed hypoxic response as blebs, albeit on a different time scale. This theory was originally proposed by Efron and Holden[17] over a decade ago and was restated by Clements in 1990.[18]

Two separate factors induce an acidic shift in the cornea during contact lens wear:

- An increase in carbonic acid due to retardation of carbon dioxide efflux (hypercapnia)[19] by a contact lens.
- Increased levels of lactic acid as a result of lens-induced oxygen deprivation (hypoxia)[19] and the consequent increase in anaerobic metabolism (Figure 17.8).

When silicone elastomer contact lenses are worn, such metabolic changes do not take place because of the extremely high oxygen permeability of such lenses. No evidence of endothelial polymegethism could be found by Schoessler *et al*[9] in the corneas of patients wearing silicone elastomer lenses.

Bonnano and Polse[20] have confirmed by direct measurement that contact lens-induced hypoxia and hypercapnia result in an acidic shift in the cornea and these authors noted that the extent of acidosis that they measured is in the range where endothelial function may be affected.

The cornea becomes hypoxic and hypercapnic during sleep so it would be expected that the consequent acidic changes would

induce endothelial polymegethism, which is known to be age-related.[7] Schoessler and Orsborn[21] published a case report of extreme endothelial polymegethism in the right eye (compared with the left eye) of a 23-year-old female following four years of unilateral ptosis in the right eye.

Consideration needs to be given to the mechanism by which acidosis causes changes to the three-dimensional shape of endothelial cells, which in turn gives rise to the appearance of polymegethism when viewed by specular reflection. All cells in the human body function optimally when surrounded by extracellular fluid that is maintained within an acceptable range of pH, temperature, tonicity, ion balance etc. The carbonic acid and lactic acid may cause an acidic pH shift in the extracellular fluid surrounding endothelial cells.

This may induce changes in membrane permeability and/or membrane pump activity, resulting in water movement that acts to elongate endothelial cell walls.[11] A reconfiguration of cell shape then occurs in order to preserve cell volume, resulting in the appearance of polymegethism at the apical surface of the endothelium.

## Observation and grading

The corneal endothelium can be viewed by specular reflection using a variety of instruments, such as contact or non-contact specular microscopes, confocal microscopes or slit-lamp biomicroscopes. To observe the endothelium using the slit-lamp biomicroscope, a magnification of at least ×40 must be used and the angle between the illumination and observation systems should be symmetrical about a plane extending normally from the cornea, and will typically be between 75° and 90°. The endothelial mosaic can be seen adjacent to a bright reflex from the corneal surface. Using this technique, only the mid-peripheral nasal or temporal endothelium are viewed; this does not pose a problem if the same approximate area is observed each time for comparative purposes (e.g. assessing changes in a patient over time).

Figure 17.1 is an enlarged view of the slit-lamp biomicroscopic appearance of the endothelium of a young female who had been wearing a soft lens of low oxygen transmissibility (38 per cent water content HEMA) for 10 years. Considerable variation in the size of individual endothelial cells (polymegethism) is clearly evident.

The observation of individual endothelial cells is at the very limit of resolution when using a slit-lamp biomicroscope at ×40 magnification. Even with the assistance of a graduated eyepiece graticule or a reference grading scale, endothelial cell density and degree of polymegethism are difficult to estimate, and often impossible with normal involuntary micronystagmoid and vibratory eye movement.

Sophisticated automated cameras specifically designed for viewing the endothelium, which incorporate digital video image-capture and computer image-analysis technology, have only become available relatively recently.[22] These instruments offer higher magnification and superior resolution compared with slit-lamp observation, and are essential if endothelial morphology is to be graded.

For example, the Topcon specular microscope SP1000 provides a photographic print-out of the endothelium which includes a five-point scale for grading endothelial cell density within the range 1000 to 3000 cells/mm² (Figure 17.9). Hume[23] demonstrated that a given observer can make consistent gradings. The extent of endothelial polymegethism can also be graded (see Appendix A).

Another automated instrument – the Keeler Konan Nocon Robo non-contact specular microscope – provides a printout (Figure 17.10) that contains an image of endothelial mosaic as well as detailed results of a morphometric analysis, including the number of cells analysed (NUM), aver-

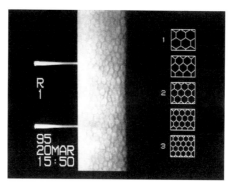

**Figure 17.9**
*Printout from Topcon specular microscope SP1000, showing corneal endothelial mosaic and cell density grading scale*

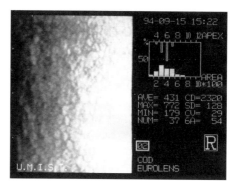

**Figure 17.10**
*Printout from the Keeler Konan Nocon Robo non-contact specular microscope, showing corneal endothelial mosaic and the results of a detailed morphometric analysis*

age (AVE), maximum (MAX) and minimum (MIN) cell areas, cell density (CD), standard deviation of mean cell area (SD), percen-

tage co-efficient of variation of cell size (CV) and the percentage of cells that are hexagonal (6A). The distribution of cell area and number of cell sides is also plotted in bar graph form.

Doughty[24] has outlined the following limitations with respect to quantification of the degree of polymegethism in terms of the COV:

- The co-efficient is valid only for the individual from whom it was obtained, and so cannot be used for intersubject comparison.
- The COV can be ambiguous in that it does not indicate whether there is an overall increase or decrease in mean cell area (the COV can be the same in either case).
- The error associated with calculation of COV, typically by measuring up to 200 cells, is too great (analysis of 3000 cells is required for good accuracy, which is generally precluded because of time and cost constraints).

Despite this critical analysis, evaluation of the degree of endothelial polymegethism against grading scales is a valuable technique upon which clinically relevant differences can be detected and management decisions can be based.

## Management

Figure 17.11 is a construction of the approximate relationship between COV and oxygen transmissibility, which indicates that lenses of lower oxygen performance will induce higher levels of polymegethism.

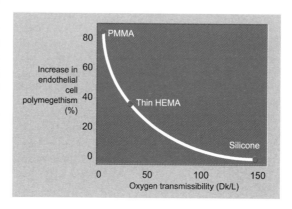

**Figure 17.11**
*Relation between percentage increase in co-efficient of variation (COV) of endothelial cell size (polymegethism) vs lens oxygen transmissibility (Dk/L). Units of Dk/L are '×10⁻⁹ (cm×mlO₂)/(sec×ml×mmHg)'*

Although this relationship provides a clear indication as to how to minimise or prevent contact lens-induced polymegethism, it is unclear whether there is a need to take any measures to reverse or prevent this process because of the uncertainty as to whether endothelial polymegethism is an unwanted pathological change or a harmless physiological adaptation.

Whether or not one would wish to reverse or prevent endothelial polymegethism from the perspective of the health of the endothelium itself is an interesting but secondary consideration. What is certain is that endothelial polymegethism provides an indication that the cornea has been subjected to prolonged metabolic stress.

The source of this stress is probably chronic tissue acidosis, which in turn has been caused by chronic contact lens-induced hypoxia and hypercapnia. Clinicians have long recognised the importance of minimising lens-induced hypoxia and hypercapnia because these changes are known to induce a wide variety of adverse effects in all layers of the cornea and conjunctiva.[5]

Thus, from a clinical perspective, it is essential to take note of the presence of significant endothelial polymegethism and to take action to minimise the metabolic stress to the cornea, known to be associated with this change. Strategies for alleviating contact lens-induced hypoxia and hypercapnia include the following:

- Fitting soft lenses made from higher oxygen permeable materials.
- Fitting rigid lenses made from materials of higher oxygen permeability.
- Reducing lens thickness.
- Sleeping in extended lenses less frequently.
- Changing from extended lens wear to daily lens wear.
- Reducing lens wearing time.
- Fitting rigid lenses with more movement and edge lift (to enhance oxygen-enriching tear exchange).

The real battle against contact lens-induced endothelial polymegethism and indeed all chronic lens-induced changes is being fought in the polymer laboratories and lens design studios of the major contact lens manufacturers. Although practitioners will always have a choice to make concerning the best lens for a given patient, such decisions can only be made within an

envelope of available lens designs and materials. As time goes on, this envelope will shift to encompass more and more sophisticated and highly permeable polymers which will be capable of being manufactured in thin designs. The natural outcome will be an overall lowering of the degree of polymegethism and related chronic tissue changes in the world-wide population of lens wearers.

## Prognosis

The prognosis for recovery from endothelial polymegethism is poor. After removal and cessation of wear of high water content contact lenses that had been worn on an extended wear basis for an average of 5 years, Holden *et al*[25] were unable to detect a recovery from endothelial polymegethism during an observation period of 6 months (Figure 17.12).

Furthermore, McLaughlin and Schoessler[26] were unable to demonstrate a significant improvement in endothelial morphology 4 months after re-fitting patients who had been wearing PMMA lenses with rigid lenses of high oxygen transmissibility. Thus, all available evidence suggests that contact lens-induced endothelial polymegethism is essentially a permanent change; if there is any recovery back to age-related normality, this would be likely to take many years.

The prognosis for overall corneal health based upon action taken as a result of observed endothelial polymegethism may be excellent, despite the fact that the endothelium may remain polymegethous for a considerable period of time or perhaps forever.

The reason for this is that many other changes induced by chronic hypoxia and hypercapnia, such as reduced epithelial thickness, reduced oxygen consumption, epithelial microcysts and stromal oedema,[5] will dissipate in a matter of weeks or months following cessation of lens wear.[5,25] These changes can subsequently be minimised by adopting strategies for optimising corneal oxygen availability during lens wear, such as those outlined above (in 'Management').

Notwithstanding the good prognosis for *corneal health* described above, it has been suggested that the existence of endothelial polymegethism in itself may represent a continuing liability in view of the finding of Rao *et al*[27] that corneal oedema induced by cataract surgery takes a lot longer to recover in patients displaying preoperative corneal endothelial polymegethism.

Although this observation has subsequently been challenged,[28] the possibility that endothelial polymegethism may compromise corneal health if surgical intervention of the eye is required later in life should not be discounted.

## Differential diagnosis

A variety of degenerative (acquired) and dystrophic (hereditary) changes in the endothelium have been described, but a detailed account of these is beyond the scope of this chapter. Such conditions are characterised by opacities, lesions or bleb-like formations (as in the case of Fuch's endothelial dystrophy), which generally cannot be confused with endothelial polymegethism.

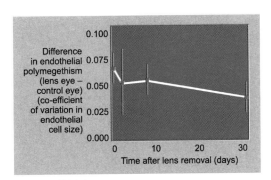

**Figure 17.12**
*Degree of polymegethism plotted for 30 days following cessation of lens wear (relative to non-lens wearing control eyes). The apparent trend towards recovery is not statistically significant (adapted from Holden et al[5])*

What is more important in the context of differential diagnosis is the capacity to distinguish between the aetiologies of any observed endothelial changes. As well as being a natural age change,[7] endothelial polymegethism can occur as a result of, or in association with, both ocular insult (such as injury,[29] chronic solar radiation,[30] ptosis,[21] endothelial guttata,[31] intraocular surgery[32] and keratoconus[33]) and systemic disease (diabetes mellitus and cystic fibrosis[34]).

Practitioners should therefore be alert to the fact that endothelial polymegethism observed in the eyes of contact lens patients may have been caused by factors or conditions other than contact lens wear.

## REFERENCES

1 Zantos SG, Holden BA (1977) Transient endothelial changes soon after wearing soft contact lenses. *Am J Optom Physiol Opt* **54**: 856.

2 Schoessler JP, Woloschak MJ (1981) Corneal endothelium in veteran PMMA contact lens wearers. *Int Contact Lens Clin* **8**: 19.

3 Schoessler JP (1983) Corneal endothelial polymegethism associated with extended wear. *Int Contact Lens Clin* **10**: 144.

4 Hirst LW, Aver C, Cohn J (1984) Specular microscopy of hard lens wearers. *Ophthalmology* **91**: 1147.

5 Holden BA, Sweeney DF, Vannas A (1985) Effects of long-term extended contact lens wear on the human cornea. *Invest Ophthalmol Vis Sci* **26**: 1489.

6 MacRae SM, Matsuda M, Shellans S (1986) The effects of hard and soft contact lenses on the corneal endothelium. *Am J Ophthalmol* **102**: 50.

7 Yee RW, Matsuda M, Schultz RO (1985) Changes in normal corneal endothelial cellular pattern as a function of age. *Curr Eye Res* **4**: 671.

8 McMahon TT, Polse KA, McNamara N (1996) Recovery from induced corneal edema and endothelial morphology after long-term PMMA contact lens wear. *Optom Vis Sci* **73**: 184.

9 Schoessler JP, Barr JT, Fresen DR (1984) Corneal endothelial observations of silicone elastomer contact lens wearers. *Int Contact Lens Clin* **11**: 337.

10 Sweeney DF (1992) Corneal exhaustion syndrome with long-term wear of contact lenses. *Optom Vis Sci* **69**: 601.

11 Bergmanson JPG (1992) Histopathological analysis of corneal endothelial polymegethism. *Cornea* **11**: 133.

12 Nieuwendaal CP, Odenthal MTP, Kok JHC (1994) Morphology and function of the corneal endothelium after long-term contact lens wear. *Invest Ophthalmol Vis Sci* **35**: 3071.

13 O'Neal MR, Polse KA (1986) Decreased endothelial pump function with ageing. *Invest Ophthalmol Vis Sci* **27**: 457.

14 Maurice DM (1972) The location of the fluid pump in the cornea. *J Physiol* **221**: 43.

15 Hodson S, Miller F (1976) The bicarbonate ion pump in the endothelium which regulates the hydration of rabbit cornea. *J Physiol* **263**: 563.

16 Holden BA, Williams L, Zantos SG (1985) The etiology of transient endothelial changes in the human cornea. *Invest Ophthalmol Vis Sci* **26**: 1354.

17 Efron N, Holden BA (1986) A review of some common contact lens complications. II. The corneal endothelium and conjunctiva. *Optician* **192**: 17.

18 Clements LD (1990) Corneal acidosis, blebs and endothelial polymegethism. *Contact Lens Forum* March: 39.

19 Efron N, Ang JHB (1990) Corneal hypoxia and hypercapnia during contact lens wear. *Optom Vis Sci* **67**: 512.

20 Bonanno JA, Polse KA (1987) Corneal acidosis during contact lens wear: effects of hypoxia and $CO_2$. *Invest Ophthalmol Vis Sci* **28**: 1514.

21 Schoessler JP, Orsborn GN (1987) A theory of corneal endothelial polymegethism and aging. *Curr Eye Res* **6**: 301.

22 Stevenson RWW (1994) Non-contact specular microscopy of the corneal endothelium. *Optician* **208**: 22.

23 Hume DE (1994) Evaluation of endothelial assessment using the Topcon specular microscope SP1000 in clinical practice. MSc Dissertation, UMIST.

24 Doughty MJ (1990) The ambiguous coefficient of variation: polymegethism of the corneal endothelium and central corneal thickness. *Int Contact Lens Clin* **17**: 240.

25 Holden BA, Vannas A, Nilsson KT (1985) Epithelial and endothelial effects from the extended wear of contact lenses. *Curr Eye Res* **4**: 7392.

26 McLaughlin R, Schoessler J (1990) Corneal endothelial response to refitting polymethyl methacrylate wearers with rigid gas-permeable lenses. *Optom Vis Sci* **67**: 346.

27 Rao GN, Aquavella JV, Goldberg SH (1984) Pseudophakic bullous keratopathy: relationship to pre-operative corneal endothelial status. *Ophthalmology* **91**: 1135.

28 Bates AK, Cheng H (1988) Bullous keratopathy: a study of endothelial cell morphology in patients undergoing cataract surgery. *Br J Ophthalmol* **72**: 409.

29 Ling T, Vannas A, Holden BA (1988) Long-term changes in corneal morphology following wounding in the cat. *Invest Ophthalmol Vis Sci* **29**: 1407.

30 Good GW, Schoessler JP (1988) Chronic solar radiation exposure and endothelial polymegethism. *Curr Eye Res* **7**: 157.

31 Burns RR, Bourne WM, Brubaker RF (1981) Endothelial function in patients with corneal guttata. *Invest Ophthalmol Vis Sci* **20**: 77.

32 Matsuda M, Suda T, Manabe R (1984) Serial alterations in endothelial cell shape and pattern after intraocular surgery. *Am J Ophthalmol* **98**: 313.

33 Matsuda M, Suda T, Manabe R (1984) Quantitative analysis of the endothelial mosaic pattern changes in anterior keratoconus. *Am J Ophthalmol* **98**: 43.

34 Lass JH, Spurney RV, Dutt RM (1985) A morphologic and fluorophotometric analysis of the corneal endothelium in Type I diabetes mellitus and cystic fibrosis. *Am J Ophthalmol* **100**: 783.

# Part VII
# Corneal Topography

# 18
# Corneal shape change

Incidence
Signs and symptoms
Pathology
Aetiology
Patient management
Prognosis
Differential diagnosis
Intentional corneal moulding

Because contact lenses are in direct contact with the eye, it stands to reason that physical forces can act to change the shape of both the lens and the eye. Indeed, both types of change have been documented and both can have important clinical sequelae. This chapter will concentrate on changes in ocular shape induced by contact lens wear. Primary consideration will be given to corneal shape changes because these are critical to vision and lens fitting techniques. However, it is true that contact lenses can also alter the surface topography of the conjunctiva (indentation rings) and the form of the upper lid (rigid lens-induced ptosis).

Consideration will be given to the various manifestations of contact lens-induced changes in corneal topography. The term 'change in topography' is chosen deliberately because it covers all possible deviations in surface shape from normality. A myriad of terms have been coined by various authors to describe different phenomena; these include deformation, distortion, warpage, indentation, steepening, flattening, sphericalisation, imprinting and wrinkling. These terms are generally self-explanatory and will be used when discussing specific forms of corneal shape change. A severe case of corneal warpage is shown in Figure 18.1.

While most contact lens-induced shape changes are unintentional, it must not be overlooked that some clinicians have fitted lenses with the deliberate intention of inducing shape change; the two best-known practices, which have attracted consider-

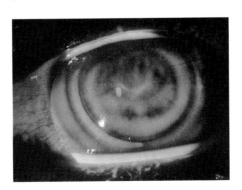

**Figure 18.1**
*Severe case of corneal warpage in a keratoconic eye seen here wth the aid of fluorescein after removal of an ill-fitting hybrid rigid centre-soft surround lens*

able controversy, are apical bearing in keratoconus (with the aim of flattening the cone to halt or slow its progression), and orthokeratology (with the aim of flattening the cornea to reduce myopia). These concepts will also be reviewed briefly.

## Incidence

The incidence of corneal shape change due to various categories of lens wear is well known. Finnemore and Korb[1] reported that 98 per cent of PMMA lens wearers develop central corneal clouding, which will inevitably cause some degree of corneal steepening. More generalised distortion, or 'warpage', was noted in 30 per cent of PMMA lens wearers by Rengstorff.[2]

When assessed using conventional keratometric techniques, current generation rigid lenses of high oxygen transmissibility (Dk/L) induce little or no change in overall corneal shape during daily wear or extended wear.[3,4] Similarly, keratometry fails to highlight significant corneal shape changes in daily[5] and extended[6] wear of soft lenses.

Modern videokeratographic corneal mapping techniques reveal that all forms of contact lens wear are capable of inducing small but statistically significant changes in corneal topography. Ruiz-Montenegro *et al*[7] reported the prevalence of abnormalities in corneal shape to be 8 per cent in a control group of non-contact lens wearers versus 75 per cent in PMMA lens wear, 57 per cent in daily RGP lens wearer, 31 per cent in daily soft lens wear, and 23 per cent in extended soft lens wear. These authors attached some clinical significance to their findings because:

- Decreases in best spectacle-corrected visual acuities of up to one line of Snellen acuity were noted in many of the PMMA and RGP lens wearers, and
- Correlations were noted between lens decentration and corneal shape change.

Lens binding is known to occur with daily and extended wear of rigid lenses, the clinical evidence of which is an indentation of the cornea that can be seen in white light and with the aid of fluorescein. Based on subject reports, lens binding occurred in 29 per cent of daily wear and 50 per cent of extended wear RGP patients, respectively.[3]

Most other forms of lens-induced corneal shape change, such as corneal wrinkling, are either rare or are known to be associated with specific types of poorly designed or ill-fitting lenses; thus, it is not possible to assign incidence figures to such phenomena.

## Signs and symptoms

The clinical presentation of lens-induced corneal shape change – characterised by time course and precise topographical alterations – can manifest in a variety of forms and will depend primarily upon the material, design and fit of the lens. The signs and symptoms of shape change will be considered in the context of the various forms of topographical alterations that have been described.

### Change in overall curvature
Much of the earlier literature concentrates on overall changes in curvature; that is, steepening or flattening of the anterior corneal surface as measured by keratometry. Results have been expressed as changes in either corneal curvature (millimetres), surface corneal power (dioptres) or refraction (dioptres).

Central corneal clouding often occurred during the initial period of adaptation to PMMA lens wear and was generally associated with a myopic shift (see 'Aetiology' below). Thus, newly fit PMMA patients would complain of hazy vision due to the excess oedema and resultant reduced vision upon removing their lenses and putting on spectacles. Some patients would complain of mild ocular discomfort, but this probably related more to the underlying cause (excessive oedema) rather than the actual change in corneal shape.

This problem of blurred vision with spectacles following contact lens wear was termed 'spectacle blur', which posed a significant clinical problem because many patients could only wear PMMA lenses for a limited period of time and needed to wear spectacles at the end of the wearing period.

As the patient adapted and the central corneal oedema subsided, there was a reversal of the induced myopia and the corneal curvature and refraction returned to pre-fitting levels. After 12 months of PMMA lens wear, the cornea often displayed central flattening, resulting in a hyperopic creep, or reduction in myopia.

RGP lenses can also induce changes in overall curvature, whereby the extent of change is inversely proportional to the Dk/L and flexibility of the lens. The higher the Dk/L and the more flexible the lens, the less likelihood there is of lens-induced changes, assuming a well-fitting lens. Changes of corneal curvature of more than 0.25D are rare with flexible, high Dk/L RGP lenses and hydrogel lenses.

Clinical evaluation of corneal curvature has traditionally been achieved using the optical keratometer. This instrument is still invaluable and can generally be relied upon to detect overall compromise to corneal shape. The difficulty arises when attempting to assess asymmetric or localised regions of corneal distortion, because most keratometers are based upon an optical configuration that relies upon corneal reflections emanating from a 3 mm diameter circle on the corneal surface. Thus, localised swelling within, outside or partially covering this 'circle' will either go undetected or be misinterpreted.

### Change in corneal symmetry
Numerous videokeratoscopes are currently available and all have computerised algorithms for quantifying the degree of irregularity of corneal surface shape. The

Topographic Modelling System (TMS-1, Computed Anatomy, New York) used by Ruiz-Montenegro *et al*[7] computes a function known as the Surface Asymmetry Index (SAI). Specifically, the SAI provides a quantitative measure of the radial symmetry of the four central videokeratoscope mires surrounding the vertex of the cornea. The higher the degree of central corneal symmetry, the lower the SAI. A high degree of central radial symmetry is characteristic of normal corneas.

Ruiz-Montenegro *et al*[7] reported SAI mean values (± standard error of mean) associated with the following forms of lens wear: non-lens wearing controls $0.35 \pm 0.03$; PMMA $0.86 \pm 0.22$; daily wear RGP $0.48 \pm 0.09$; daily wear soft $0.48 \pm 0.11$; extended wear soft $0.46 \pm 0.08$. The SAI was statistically significantly greater than the control group for all forms of lens wear except for daily wear soft.

The clinical significance of this finding was highlighted by the fact that the authors observed a correlation between the nature of corneal deformation and the fit of the lens. For example, a superior riding rigid lens was associated with superior flattening, thus explaining the increase in SAI in that case. Such correlations were only observed in PMMA and RGP lens wearers, and an example is depicted in Figures 18.2 and 18.3.

Obvious corneal asymmetry can be detected using a keratometer, whereby the mires will not be perfectly circular; that is, they may take on an elliptical, pear or egg-shaped appearance.

### Change in corneal regularity
In addition to SAI, the TMS-1 also computes a function known as the Surface Regularity Index (SRI). The SRI is a quantitative measure of central and paracentral corneal irregularity derived from the summation of fluctuations in corneal power that occur along semi-meridians of the 10 central videokeratoscope mires. The more regular the anterior surface of the central cornea the lower the SRI. The SRI is highly correlated with best spectacle-corrected visual acuity.

Ruiz-Montenegro *et al*[7] reported SRI mean values (± standard error of mean) associated with the following forms of lens wear: non-lens wearing controls $0.41 \pm 0.04$; PMMA $1.17 \pm 0.34$; daily wear RGP $0.93 \pm 0.18$; daily wear soft $0.52 \pm 0.08$; extended wear soft $0.51 \pm 0.06$. The SRI was statistically

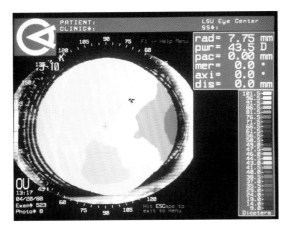

**Figure 18.2**
*Videokeratogram of cornea immediately following removal of a high-riding PMMA lens. Note superior corneal flattening*

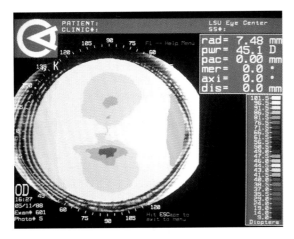

**Figure 18.3**
*Same cornea depicted in Figure 18.2 above, 3 weeks following lens removal. The cornea has recovered normal with-the-rule astigmatism*

significantly greater than the control group for PMMA and daily RGP lens wear but not for daily or extended soft lens wear.

The clinical significance of changes in SRI was confirmed by the observation of the authors of an association in PMMA and RGP lens wearers whereby a decrease in best spectacle corrected visual acuity occurred in patients displaying an increased SRI. The patients did not suffer significant discomfort.

A keratometer can detect gross corneal irregularity in the form of lack of clarity of the mires; that is, various sections of the mires will appear to be more in focus than others, and the circular mire lines may not appear to be perfectly smooth.

Of course, such an assessment will only relate to the 3 mm diameter ring of corneal surface that a keratometer samples optically. Other inexpensive instruments such as the Placido disc and Klein keratoscope can provide a similar assessment to that offered by the keratometer, but over a wider expanse of cornea. Needless to say, modern videokeratoscopes offer disinct advantages over traditional instruments in terms of the extent of corneal coverage, sensitivity, accuracy, objectivity, computational power and data presentation.

**Corneal wrinkling**
Corneal wrinkling is a rare but severe ocular complication of contact lens wear. Described originally by Quinn[8] and later more fully by Lowe and Brennan[9] this con-

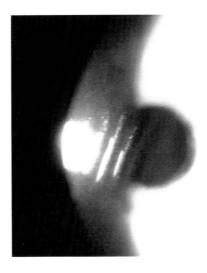

**Figure 18.4**
*Wrinkling of the central cornea following removal of 42.5 per cent water content lens of 0.035 mm centre thickness*

dition is characterised by the appearance of a series of deep parallel grooves in the cornea giving the impression of a 'wrinkled' cornea (Figure 18.4). The case described by Lowe and Brennan[9] took the form of two linear wave patterns of fluorescein pooling across the cornea and intersecting at an angle of 70°. Several discrete spots were observed at the points of intersection of the two wave patterns.

This condition is observed in patients wearing highly elastic, ultra-thin mid-water content lenses. In the two cases described in the literature,[8,9] the lenses that induced corneal wrinkling were either specifically designed by the practitioner or were experimental; that is, they were apparently not standard commercial products.

As one would expect with such a severe distortion of the cornea, vision loss is dramatic. Indeed, vision dropped to less than 6/60 within five minutes of lens insertion.[8,9] The condition is also extremely painful.

Clinical evaluation of corneal wrinkling is best achieved by slit–lamp examination under white light and with fluorescein under cobalt blue light. Computerised videokeratoscopy can provide useful supplementary information by viewing the unprocessed image of the reflected mires.

**Corneal indentation**
Rigid lenses can adhere to the cornea

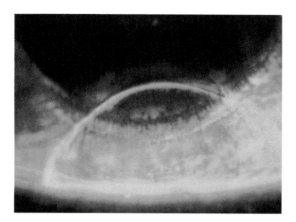

**Figure 18.5**
*Corneal and conjunctival imprint of an inferiorly mislocated bound RGP lens viewed with fluorescein immediately following lens removal*

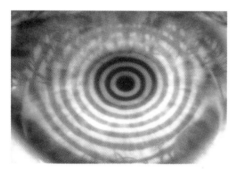

**Figure 18.6**
*Superior arcuate imprint observed in unprocessed mires of videokeratoscope following lens removal*

during open-eye[3] or closed-eye[3,10] wear. Adherence can occur at any time of the day in open-eye wear, but is characteristically noticed immediately upon eye opening following overnight wear. In the latter case, the lens usually begins to move freely after a few blinks; persistent binding for more than a few minutes is considered to be problematic.

Upon removal of a bound lens, an impression of the lens edge is usually evident on the cornea. Slit-lamp examination with fluorescein reveals the presence of an annular indentation in the cornea (Figure 18.5), mild punctate keratitis primarily outside the lens edge and dense corneal desiccation inside the lens edge. An imprint from the bound edge following lens removal is clearly visible in Figure 18.6, which is an unprocessed image of videokeratoscope

rings. Lens binding is usually asymptomatic but can be mildly uncomfortable.

## Pathology

All known forms of contact lens-induced changes to corneal topography can be explained in terms of three underlying pathological mechanisms:

- Physical pressure on the cornea exerted either by the lens and/or eyelids.
- Contact lens-induced oedema.
- Mucus binding beneath rigid lenses.

The contributions of these factors vary with the type of topographical alteration.

### Change in overall curvature
A comprehensive explanation of corneal shape change during PMMA lens wear has been provided by the classic analysis of Carney[11] – an analysis that can be extrapolated from PMMA lens wear to explain virtually all cases of overall corneal shape change with rigid and soft lens wear.

Carney[11] observed corneal shape changes induced by PMMA lenses in normal atmospheric conditions (21 per cent oxygen) and in artificial conditions ranging from 0 per cent oxygen (anoxia) to 100 per cent oxygen. He demonstrated convincingly that corneal shape change during PMMA lens wear could be attributed to a combination of lens-induced oedema due to hypoxia and physical pressure from the lens. The distribution of these two influences can explain the various forms of

topographical changes observed with all forms of lens wear (see 'Aetiology', below).

### Change in SAI and SRI
The precise pathological processes that explain corneal shape changes characterised by SAI and SRI are difficult to derive because research has not been conducted to differentiate mechanisms that underlie changes in corneal symmetry and regularity. In the absence of other explanatory mechanisms, one can only conclude that surface asymmetry and irregularity are caused by differing contributions of the two key factors identified earlier – physical pressure by the lens/lids and lens-induced hypoxia.

It may also be true that individual differences in corneal rigidity may be a governing factor. Ruiz-Montenegro *et al*[7] noted that much of the variance in their data could be attributed to a small number of patients displaying large alterations in SAI and SRI. The implication here is that some patients with 'softer' or more pliable corneas will be more susceptible to lens-induced shape changes, and that such patients will be slower to recover.

### Corneal wrinkling
Lowe and Brennan[9] argue that corneal wrinkling involves the epithelium and anterior stroma. This view is based upon their observations of the extreme variance in intensity of fluorescence across the ridges of a wrinkled cornea (Figure 18.7), implying deep furrows, and the extreme distortion of photokeratometric mires reflected off a wrinkled cornea (Figure 18.8). The intensity of the wrinkling pattern increased with time following a blink, indicating fluorescein pooling within deep troughs.

### Corneal indentation
Indentation associated with lens binding appears to be more related to physical pressure and less to the effects of hypoxia. In the case of overnight wear, mucus accumulation beneath the lens is a feature of lens binding (Figure 18.9), the aetiological significance of which will be considered below.[12]

## Aetiology

Theoretical and experimental analyses have been undertaken to explain the aetiology of lens-induced corneal shape changes.

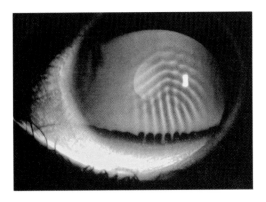

**Figure 18.7**
*Extreme corneal wrinkling as revealed by fluorescein*

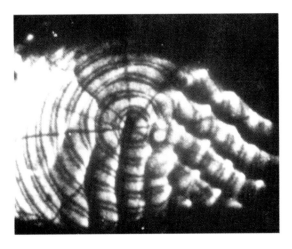

**Figure 18.8**
*Photokeratogram of cornea displaying extreme wrinkling*

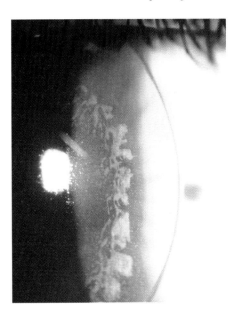

**Figure 18.9**
*Build-up of mucus and debris beneath a bound RGP lens, pictured here two and a half hours after waking*

to explain lens-induced corneal shape change:

- Local lens-induced hypoxia causing localised oedema, corneal swelling and myopic shift.
- Overall lens bearing causing corneal flattening and a hyperopic shift.

A less likely influence is a steep lens moulding the cornea into a more curved shape, thereby inducing myopia.

It can be presumed that rigid lenses of higher oxygen performance will influence corneal shape more by way of physical bearing than hypoxic oedema. Certainly, there will be an inceasing shift in favour of physical bearing and against hypoxic oedema, as aetiological factors in lens-induced shape change, as RGP lens Dk/L increases.

Because modern-generation soft lenses have relatively high Dk/L values and contribute little direct tangential physical force to the cornea, soft lens-induced shape changes are rarely observed. Soft lenses of lower Dk/L can induce low to moderate levels of oedema across the cornea. An optical analysis of this phenomenon leads to the conclusion that there will be virtually no refractive shift in association with a

These will be considered with respect to the various forms of shape changes described earlier.

### Change in overall curvature

The typical pattern of refractive change during PMMA lens wear – an initial myopic shift during adaptation followed by a recovery over 3–6 months and subsequent myopia reduction – can be explained using the model of Carney.[11] A centrally fitting PMMA lens will induce hypoxia beneath the lens, resulting in oedema in the corresponding central region of the cornea. This phenomenon, known as central corneal clouding (CCC), is characterised by an increased curvature of the central cornea as the stroma in that region thickens, resulting in a myopic shift. Baron[13] calculated

that a moderate increase in corneal thickness of 2 per cent over a 4 mm wide central zone would increase corneal surface power (and thus myopia) by 1.78D.

Following the initial adaptation (subsequent to possible lens refits to provide more movement), the hypoxia will be alleviated and the cornea may return to its original shape. Another influence would be occurring concurrently – a progressive overall flattening of the cornea due to the constant bearing of the lens against the corneal apex. This flattening would lead to a hyperopic shift in refraction, which would presumably have been masked by the initial marked apical steepening due to hypoxia during the adaptive phase described above.

While the explanation provided above cannot be considered to be definitive, the following general principles can be applied

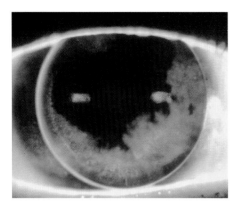

**Figure 18.10**
*Gradual penetration of fluorescein beneath a bound lens as the mucus adhesion breaks down*

uniform area of oedema greater than 8 mm in diameter.[13]

### Change in SAI and SRI

The data of Ruiz-Montenegro *et al*[7] provide quantitative proof that RGP lenses disturb corneal symmetry and regularity less than PMMA lenses, and that soft lenses least affect SAI and SRI. This can only be presumed to be attributed to less physical deformation by softer lenses and less lens-induced hypoxic oedema with RGP and soft lenses.

A likely cause of increased SAI in RGP lens wearers could be physical pressure from a lens that is constantly tending to decentre in a predictable manner. Ruiz-Montenegro *et al*[7] noted a correlation between lens decentration and corneal topographic change. The precise cause of increased SRI cannot be easily explained in terms of improper lens fitting.

Further experimentation along the lines of the studies of Carney[11] would be required to provide a full explanation of the specific aetiology of lens-induced changes to SAI and SRI.

### Corneal wrinkling

It is interesting to observe that in both reports of corneal wrinkling,[8,9] the lenses that caused the problem were ultra-thin mid-water content lenses. Excessive elastic forces are thought to draw corneal tissue inwards from the limbus, causing the corneal tissue to collapse in a concertina-like action, creating a wrinkled appearance.

The force could be derived from an intrinsic elastic force created when a relatively steep lens is compressed against the eye (the lens used by Lowe and Brennan[9] had a fairly steep base curve of 8.20 mm); in an attempt to return to its original shape, an inward force would be created.

If the lens also displayed a high propensity for dehydration, lens dehydration (and associated base curve steepening) and lens diameter reduction would provide an additional inward force. However, the lens reported by Lowe and Brennan[9] was made of a vinyl pyrrolidone methyl methacrylate (VP-MMA) co-polymer and thus would be categorised using the FDA system as Group II (high water content, non-ionic). Such lenses are chacteristically dehydration-resistant.

Bruce and Brennan[13] have suggested that corneal wrinkling may have an osmotic aetiology in view of the observation of Dixon[14] that complete evaporation of the tear film in normal humans can cause an almost identical corneal wrinkling and vision loss to lens-induced wrinkling.

### Corneal indentation

Binding of RGP lenses to the cornea during overnight wear has been explained by Swarbrick.[12] Thinning of the post-lens tear film during sleep leaves a very thin, highly viscous layer of mucus-rich tears between the lens and cornea which acts as a form of glue to bind the lens to the cornea. This tear film thinning is due to constant lid pressure against the lens during eye closure.

On eye opening the shear force imparted by the eyelid may be insufficient to initiate lens movement, and the lens will remain bound until the mucus film is diluted and thickened by the gradual penetration of aqueous tears. Evidence for this theory comes from clinical observations of fluorescein movement under RGP lenses as the lens becomes unstuck (Figure 18.10).[12]

RGP lens binding during open-eye lens wear occurs less frequently, and may be partially explained by mucus-mediated adhesion. Another possibility is that, in the course of moving around the cornea and being intermittently compressed by the lids, an RGP lens may assume a position whereby a slight negative pressure is created beneath the lens. This could create a mild suction that temporarily holds the lens in place and results in corneal indentation due to the mild pressure of a static lens edge.

## Patient management

Because PMMA lenses are rarely fitted today, the difficult fitting problems encountered with such lenses are only of historical interest. However, as has been revealed above, RGP lenses can induce clinically significant changes in corneal topography, which may be especially evident in patients with higher prescriptions requiring thicker lenses. Such lenses will impart greater physical and hypoxic stress on the cornea compared with thinner lenses made of the same material.

Of course, in any case of contact lens-induced corneal shape change, refitting into soft lenses will usually provide a cure because soft lenses are known to have little or no effect on corneal topography. The following discussion will therefore be based on the assumption that, for clinical reasons, refitting with another form of rigid lens is required.

### Change in overall curvature

Refractive instability in an RGP patient is a possible sign of lens-induced corneal shape change. One must rule out other possible causes of refractive instability such as unstable diabetes or advancing keratoconus. Once other possibilities have been ruled out, the direction of refractive change may provide a clue as to the likely cause. A myopic shift suggests increased corneal curvature which could be due to a steeply fitting lens or central hypoxic oedema. A hyperopic shift suggests a flat lens fit and excessive central lens bearing.

Although it is not always possible to determine the precise cause of a shift in refraction, a solution to the problem can be based upon the principle that a well-fitting lens of high oxygen performance will induce minimum corneal shape change.

If the clinical decision has been made that the present lens is unacceptable, then a new lens must be fitted. Three basic approaches have been suggested for refitting RGP patients suffering from corneal shape changes. These are:

- *Sudden discontinuation* – the patient is advised to cease lens wear for an extended period of time (perhaps many weeks). The theory behind this approach is that the cornea is allowed to recover completely in the total absence of the influence of lenses.[5]
- *De-adaptation* – the patient is advised to

continue wearing lenses but wearing time is gradually reduced to zero. The cornea is then monitored and lenses are refitted when stability has been reached.[6]

- *Immediate refit* – the patient is immediately refitted with lenses of superior design and higher Dk/L, so that recovery will occur more gradually during wear of the replacement lenses.[15,17]

Sudden discontinuation is not considered to be a viable technique for two reasons. First, patients who discontinue in this way, especially following PMMA lens wear, show excessive and unpredictable fluctuations in refractive state and corneal curvature.[18] In addition, permanent corneal distortion has been noted in some patients following sudden discontinuation of PMMA lens wear.[19] Second, this procedure is disconcerting to patients who must endure the wild refractive changes and suffer the inconvenience of not wearing lenses for some time.

De-adaptation is a compromise between the patient management techniques of 'sudden discontinuation' and 'immediate refit'. The preferred technique is 'immediate refit'.[15,17,20] The aim is to refit the patient with a lens of better fit and higher Dk/L. It is beyond the scope of this chapter to provide a full set of guidelines for achieving a superior RGP lens fit – suffice it to say that a thin, large diameter, aspheric back surface alignment fit often gives the best results.

During RGP lens wear, the tear layer will mask any deleterious effects on vision arising from corneal distortion. Thus, patients will be satisfied because they can continue to wear lenses, and vision will be adequate.

Patients should be advised that their new lenses will be more flexible and less scratch-resistant, and that greater caution will be required when cleaning and handling lenses.

If supplementary spectacles are to be prescribed; it is obviously preferable to delay this until there has been a stabilisation of corneal shape. This could take three weeks following the lens refit, although a longer period should be allowed if the corneal distortion that prompted the refit was particularly severe.[15]

### Change in SAI and SRI
Gross changes in corneal asymmetry may be attributed to rigid lens decentration, with corneal flattening in the region of the decentered lens. Refitting a lens with good centration should solve the problem; this may involve fitting a larger diameter lens and avoiding excessive central bearing.

The exact cause of excessive lens-induced corneal surface irregularity may be difficult to ascertain. If vision has dropped by more than one line of Snellen acuity, then refitting with a large diameter lens of high Dk/L may allow the cornea to recover to a more normal topographic form.

Ruiz-Montenegro *et al*[7] stated that they do not routinely discontinue contact lens wear in patients who are asymptomatic and have mild alterations to SAI and/or SRI, even if the changes are associated with a small decrease in best spectacle-corrected visual acuity.

### Corneal wrinkling
The treatment protocol for a patient experiencing corneal wrinkling is to immediately cease lens wear. Patients suffering from this condition may be alarmed at the extreme discomfort and loss of vision; it is therefore important to reassure patients that this is only a transient problem and that the cornea will recover fully within 24 hours.

Although the appearance of wrinkling will indeed have disappeared within 24 hours, the patient should not wear lenses for one week as a precaution to allow possible sub-clinical compromise to resolve. The patient should then be refitted with a soft lens that is devoid of inherently high elastic forces. Specifically, ultra-thin mid-water content FDA Type II lenses should be avoided, but if such lenses are to be fitted, the lens centre thickness should be at least 0.08 mm and the base curve should be as flat as possible. Alternatively, rigid lenses can be fitted because corneal wrinkling does not occur with such lenses.

### Corneal indentation
Although there is little doubt that mucus adhesion is the principle mechanism of binding of a rigid lens to the cornea,[12] the literature is full of ambiguous and often contradictory opinions as to lens fitting strategies for avoiding this problem. A review of the pertinent literature by Woods and Efron[21] produced a list of the various opinions that have been suggested: flatten base curve, steepen base curve, increase centre thickness, reduce centre thickness, reduce back optical zone diameter, reduce total diameter, increase axial edge lift, increase edge band width, use an aspheric design and prescribe lubricants.

It has recently been suggested that rigid lens binding may be in some way related to long-term deposit formation and lens surface modification. This theory is derived from research which shows that the incidence of rigid lens binding in extended-wear patients can be reduced by regular lens replacement.[21] Interestingly, lens binding was not alleviated in daily wear RGP patients by regularly replacing lenses.[21]

Swarbrick and Holden[22] observed that RGP lens binding is a patient-dependent phenomenon. Their analysis did not reveal patient attributes that would allow a clinician to predict whether a given patient is likely to display binding. Nevertheless, the observation of patient dependence is useful as it serves to alert clinicians to the fact that binding is likely to recur in a given patient unless some remedial action is taken.

Significant changes to lens design could be attempted to alleviate further occurrences of binding in a given patient, although it must be recognised that this can only be effected using a systematic 'trial-and-error' approach in the absence of definitive guidelines in the literature.

Because lens binding is a problem that relates specifically to rigid lenses, refitting with soft lenses is an obvious solution to this problem.

## Prognosis

The prognosis for recovery of normal corneal topography is highly variable and dependent upon the magnitude and duration of the lens-induced deformation forces. While the time course of recovery from physical forces on the cornea may be difficult to predict, recovery from chronic lens-induced oedema is known to occur within 7 days of cessation of lens wear.[25]

### Change in overall curvature
Dramatic changes in corneal curvature following cessation of long-term PMMA lens wear have been documented by Rengstorff.[18] There is an initial reduction in myopia over the first 3 days, averaging 1.32D, followed by a gradual return to baseline over the next 3 weeks. The extent of these changes correlates with the length of time that the PMMA lenses are worn. In

general, the refractive changes occur in parallel with corneal shape changes.

Bennett and Tomlinson[15] observed that the pattern of corneal recovery following PMMA lens wear is the same irrespective of whether a 'sudden discontinuation' or 'immediate refit' strategy is adopted. Because vision is better and more stable when adopting the 'immediate refit' strategy, this procedure is favoured by the authors.

The prognosis of recovery from severe corneal warpage is not good. Hartstein[19] reported 12 cases of contact lens-induced corneal warpage deemed permanent. Morgan[23] reported that in 74 cases of severe PMMA-induced corneal warpage, only half of the corneas displayed satisfactory resolution within 3 months of cessation of lens wear. Willson *et al*[24] advise that rigid lens-induced corneal warpage can take between 5 and 8 months to recover fully.

### Change in SAI and SRI

The patterns of recovery of corneas that have been rendered asymmetric or irregular as detected by videokeratoscopy are likely to be similar to those described above relating to changes in overall curvature. Assuming that soft lens-induced changes in corneal topography are due primarily to the effects of oedema, recovery of SAI and SRI would be expected to occur within 7 days.[25]

### Corneal wrinkling

The time course of recovery of corneal wrinkling has been shown to be related to the period of wear of the lens that induced the changes. Lowe and Brennan[9] noted that corneal wrinkling took 3, 90 and 240 minutes to recover after 5, 90 and 300 minutes of lens wear, respectively.

### Corneal indentation

In relation to a specific binding episode (with associated corneal indentation), prognosis for recovery is good. Swarbrick and Holden[22] reported that 25 per cent of all lenses bound on eye opening were mobile within 10 minutes and 50 per cent were mobile within 30 minutes; however, 40 per cent were still bound 60 minutes later. All lenses could eventually be freed by gentle manipulation of the lens through the lids. In almost two-thirds of cases where lenses had been assessed as bound on eye opening, clinical signs of binding were apparent 2 hours after eye opening.[22]

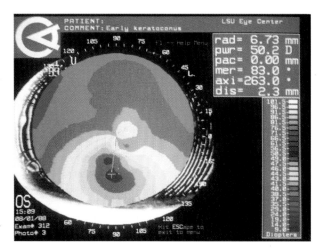

**Figure 18.11**
*Early keratoconus, which takes on a similar appearance to corneal warpage induced by a high-riding rigid lens (compare this image with Figure 18.2)*

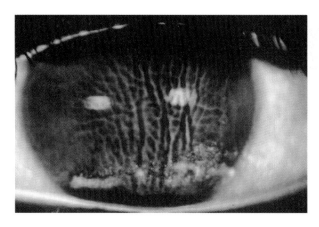

**Figure 18.12**
*Classic Fischer–Schweitzer polygonal mosaic following removal of a thick hydrogel lens, which takes on a similar appearance to corneal wrinkling (compare this image with Figure 18.7)*

All signs of binding disappear within 24 hours in the absence of lens wear.

The prognosis for avoiding future episodes of RGP lens binding is not good given that binding is a patient-dependent phenomenon. A satisfactory prognosis can only be effected if significant changes are made to lens design or type.

## Differential diagnosis

It is generally possible to differentiate vision loss due to corneal shape change from that due to other causes by reconciling refractive shifts with changes in corneal curvature. Although this relationship generally holds true, it is important to recognise that other factors such as localised oedema and changes to other refractive components of the eye can alter refractive status.

Contact lens-induced corneal warpage can take on a very similar clinical appearance to keratoconus (Figure 18.11). The key differentiating features of these two conditions are that patients with keratoconus often display corneal thinning, Vogt's striae, Fleischer's ring and progressive corneal steepening (cone development), whereas lens-induced corneal warpage recovers after cessation of lens wear and is not associated with clinically detectable corneal thinning, striae and ring pathology.

Suggestions that rigid lens wear can induce keratoconus[26] have been dismissed because of lack of sound evidence. Any as-

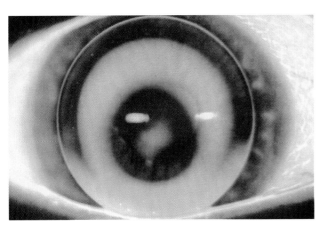

**Figure 18.13**
*Rigid lens fitted to a keratoconic eye, with the fluorescein pattern indicating central and superior arcuate bearing*

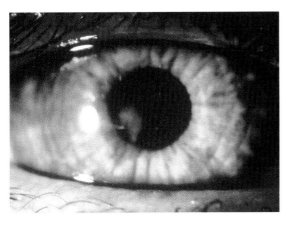

**Figure 18.14**
*Same eye as depicted in Figure 18.13, pictured here in white light and revealing central corneal scarring induced by the apical lens bearing*

socation between keratoconus and rigid lens wear is almost certainly coincidental rather than causative.

Corneal wrinkling should not be confused with epithelial wrinkling – the latter being a reversible phenomenon associated with PMMA lens wear. Epithelial wrinkles have been described as minute branching lines or furrows in the epithelial surface that are revealed with fluorescein, and are thought to be caused by physical bearing of the lens. They may be localised or cover the whole corneal surface and recover rapidly following lens removal.[14]

Another clinical phenomenon that appears remarkably similar to corneal wrinkling is the Fischer–Schweitzer polygonal mosaic, which can sometimes be observed following RGP extended wear, thick hydrogel lens wear or aggressive rub-

bing of the eyes through the closed eyelid (Figure 18.12).[27] This pattern is thought to be due to epithelial groove formation due to wrinkling of Bowman's membrane during physical deformation of the cornea. The Fischer–Schweitzer mosaic disappears within 10 minutes of removing the initiating corneal stress.

## Intentional corneal moulding

Brief mention needs to be made of two clinical approaches that attempt to utilise the known corneal moulding properties of rigid lenses for the purpose of reshaping the cornea.

### Cone compression
Confirmed cases of keratoconus are almost

always fitted with rigid lenses so as to neutralise corneal distortions and provide satisfactory vision. A variety of fitting philosophies can be adopted to fit the keratoconic eye, including apical bearing, apical clearance, three-point-touch and lid attachment procedures. The theory behind the first of these – apical bearing – is that constant bearing on the cone will arrest or slow the progression of the cone. Both scleral and rigid lenses have been used historically for this reason (Figure 18.13).

Korb *et al*[28] warned that an apical bearing lens fit can result in scarring of the apex of the cone (Figure 18.14). Furthermore, Ruben and Trodd[29] demonstrated that there was no difference in the rate of progression of keratoconus in lens-wearing versus non-lens wearing groups. Despite these observations, the apical bearing technique appears to have been favoured by 75 per cent of practitioners in a recent national US survey of 1579 keratoconic patients.[30]

### Orthokeratology
Orthokeratology is a term used to describe the clinical procedure of deliberately fitting rigid lenses in such a manner that the cornea is moulded into a new shape, with the aim of altering the refractive status of the eye. The typical approach is to prescribe flat-fitting lenses to myopic patients with the intention of reducing the degree of myopia.

Orthokeratology must be discounted as a viable clinical alternative mode of refractive error correction because the results of the treatment are variable, unreliable and largely inefficacious. Kerns[31] reported that a large number of orthokeratology patients gave poor results. Binder *et al*[32] reported an unsatisfactory outcome in 61 per cent of his orthokeratology patients. The procedure at best can only correct 1.00D to 1.50D of myopia, although the effect is largely reversible.[32,33] Thus, orthokeratology only has extremely limited application for low myopes.

A supposedly more sophisticated approach to orthokeratology has recently been advocated. This is known as 'modern orthokeratology' or 'accelerated orthokeratology', and uses 'reverse geometry lenses' to mould the cornea during either daily or overnight lens wear. Wai-on[34] recently conducted a rigorous controlled, masked and randomised study of the efficacy of accelerated orthokeratology and demonstrated that this procedure represents only a marginal improvement over previous approaches.

## REFERENCES

1 Finnemore VM, Korb JE (1980) Corneal edema with polymethylmethacrylate versus gas-permeable rigid polymer contact lenses of identical design. *J Am Optom Assoc* **51**: 271.

2 Rengstorff RH (1965) The Fort Dix report: longitudinal study of the effects of contact lenses. *Am J Optom Arch Am Acad Optom* **42**: 153.

3 Woods CA (1997) The Benefits of Planned Replacement of Rigid Contact Lenses. PhD Thesis, University of Manchester.

4 Polse KA, Rivera RK, Bonanno J (1988) Ocular effects of hard gas-permeable lens extended wear. *Am J Optom Physiol Opt* **65**: 358.

5 Baldone JA (1975) Corneal curvature changes secondary to the wearing of hydrophilic gel contact leases. *Contact Intraoc Lens Med J* **1**: 175.

6 Rengstorff RH, Nisson KT (1985) Long-term effects of extended-wear lenses: changes in refraction, corneal curvature and visual acuity. *Am J Optom Physiol Opt* **62**: 66.

7 Ruiz-Montenegro J, Mafra CH, Wilson SE (1993) Corneal topographic alterations in normal contact lens wearers. *Ophthalmology* **100**: 128.

8 Quinn TG (1982) Epithelial folds. *Int Contact Lens Clin* **9**: 365.

9 Lowe R, Brennan NA (1987) Corneal wrinkling caused by a thin medium water content lens. *Int Contact Lens Clin* **10**: 403.

10 Swarbrick HA, Holden BA (1987) Rigid gas-permeable lens binding: significance and contributing factors. *Am J Optom Physiol Opt* **64**: 815.

11 Carney LG (1975) The basis of corneal shape change during contact lens wear. *Am J Optom* **52**: 445.

12 Swarbrick HA (1988) A possible aetiology for RGP lens binding (adherence). *Int Contact Lens Clin* **15**: 13.

13 Bruce AS, Brennan NA (1990) Corneal pathophysiology with contact lens wear. *Surv Ophthalmol* **35**: 25.

14 Dixon J (1964) Ocular changes due to contact lenses. *Am J Ophthalmol* **58**: 424.

15 Bennett ES, Tomlinson A (1983) A controlled comparison of two techniques of refitting long-term PMMA contact lens wearers. *Am J Optom Physiol Opt* **60**: 139.

16 Arner RS (1977) Corneal deadaptation: the case against abrupt cessation of contact lens wear. *J Am Optom Assoc* **48**: 339.

17 Bennett ES (1983) Immediate refitting of gas permeable lenses. *J Am Optom Assoc* **54**: 239.

18 Rengstorff RH (1968) Variations in myopia measurements: an after-effect observed with habitual wearers of contact lenses. *J Am Optom Assoc* **39**: 262.

19 Hartstein J (1965) Corneal warping due to contact lenses: a report of 12 cases. *Am J Ophthalmol* **60**: 1103.

20 Rengstorff RH (1979) Refitting long-term wearers of hard contact lenses. *Rev Optom* **116**: 75.

21 Woods CA, Efron N (1996) Regular replacement of rigid contact lenses alleviates binding to the cornea. *Int Contact Lens Clin* **23**: 13.

22 Swarbrick HA, Holden BA (1989) Rigid gas-permeable lens adherence: a patient dependent phenomenon. *Optom Vis Sci* **66**: 269.

23 Morgan JF (1982) For keratoconus diagnosis: 'qualitative' ophthalmometry. *Ophthalmol Times* **7**: 33.

24 Wilson SE, Lin DTC, Klyce SD (1990) Topographic changes in contact lens-induced corneal warpage. *Ophthalmology* **97**: 734.

25 Holden BA, Sweeney DF, Vannas A (1985) Effects of long-term extended contact lens wear on the human cornea. *Invest Ophthalmol Vis Sci* **26**: 1489.

26 Gasset AR, Houde WL, Garcia-Bengochea M (1978) Hard contact lens wear as an environmental risk in keratoconus. *Am J Ophthalmol* **85**: 339.

27 Bron AJ, Tripathi RC (1969) Anterior corneal mosaic – further observations. *Br J Ophthalmol* **53**: 760.

28 Korb DR, Finnemore VM, Herman JP (1982) Apical changes and scarring in keratoconus as related to contact lens fitting techniques. *J Am Optom Assoc* **53**: 199.

29 Ruben M, Trodd C (1976) Scleral lenses in keratoconus. *Contact Intraoc Lens Med J* **2**: 18.

30 Edrington TB, Zadnik K, Barr JT (1991) Scarring and contact lens fit in keratoconus: results from the CLEK screening study. *Invest Ophthalmol Vis Sci* **32** (Suppl): 738.

31 Kerns RL (1978) Research on orthokeratology: part VIII. Results, conclusions and discussions of techniques. *J Am Optom Assoc* **49**: 308.

32 Binder PS, May CH, Grant SC (1980) An evaluation of orthokeratology. *J Am Acad Ophthalmol* **87**: 729.

33 Brand RJ, Polse KA, Schwalbe JS (1983) The Berkeley orthokeratology study, part II: Efficacy and duration. *Am J Optom Physiol Opt* **60**: 87.

34 Wai-on TL (1998) Orthokeratology on Chinese patients with low myopia: Efficacy, safety and corneal topographic changes. MPhil Dissertation, The Hong Kong Polytechnic University.

# Part VIII
# Grading and Classification

# 19
# Grading scales and morphs

Photographic vs painted scales
Painted grading scales
Explanation of illustrations
Method of grading
Interpretation of grading
Grading morphs
Tear film classification
Conclusions

In all health care disciplines, it is important to record as accurately as possible the clinical signs observed in patients. Classically, this has involved a discursive account of the condition being entered onto a record card. The severity of the condition would be recorded using wording that offered a general connotation of the level of severity, such as mild or severe. A potential problem with this approach is that these terms are somewhat general and have been used in the absence of any form of standardisation; that is, what appears to be 'mild' to one clinician may seem to be 'severe' to another.

As an aid to accurate record keeping, health care practitioners of all disciplines have, in more recent times, resorted to the use of standardised grading scales of various functions and qualities. A grading scale may be defined as: 'A tool that enables quantification of the severity of a condition with reference to a set of standardised descriptions or illustrations.'

Descriptive grading scales take the form of an agreed series of numbers or letters, each corresponding to a written account of the severity of a condition. The clinician makes a judgement of the severity of a con-

dition being observed with reference to the descriptive grading scale and records the appropriate number or letter.

Illustrative grading scales represent a more advanced form of denoting the severity of a clinical condition (Figure 19.1). A series of photographs, paintings or drawings depicting a given condition in various stages of severity offers the clinician a visual reference against which the severity of a condition can be assessed and future changes in severity may be judged. Indeed,

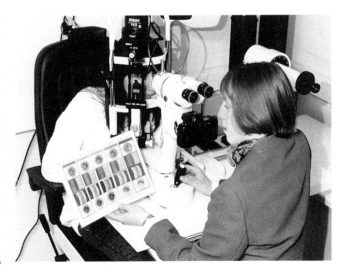

**Figure 19.1**
*Grading scales (A4 version) in use*

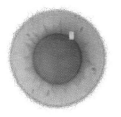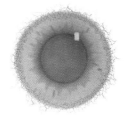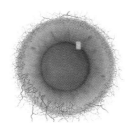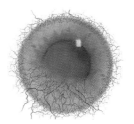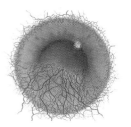

**Figure 19.2**
*Stromal neovascularisation from (l to r) grade 0 to 4*

the use of illustrative scales to grade the degree of severity or progression of a particular clinical sign is becoming increasingly popular. Grading scales also offer clinicians a 'common language' for describing clinical phenomena.

Such principles are of course relevant to the field of contact lenses. Patients can present with a variety of contact lens-induced complications of the anterior ocular structures. A standard set of grading scales for a representative range of the most frequently viewed and clinically relevant conditions would be an asset to contact lens practitioners, both as individuals and as part of an international community that shares its clinical experiences in trying to understand, manage and prevent adverse responses to lens wear.

This chapter describes the design and clinical application of a set of standardised illustrative grading scales for contact lens complications which are presented in Appendix A.

## Photographic vs painted scales

### Problems with photographic grading scales

The first important decision was whether to develop photographic or artist-rendered grading scales. The advantage of photographic grading scales is that real conditions are depicted. However, it was judged that there were too many disadvantages in developing a set of photographic grading scales. An immense slide library is required – but even if such a resource was available, a number of compromises would need to be made.

For example, a given condition such as neovascularisation can present in many different forms, and it is generally not possible to identify a series of photographs that

display precisely the same manifestation of that condition at various levels of severity.

A series of photographs of a given condition at varying levels of severity will also be confounded by the fact that the photographs are of different patients, and are taken from various angles, at different magnifications, with various illumination conditions, using different levels of staining etc.

The use of different types of photographic film and variations in photographic processing techniques will result in inconsistencies in colour rendering of sequential images. The precise level of severity of a condition may not be available from the slide library, leading to further compromise.

In addition, some complications such as epithelial microcysts or stromal striae and folds are extremely difficult to photograph; indeed, few photographs of such conditions exist. This artificially constrains the range of complications from which a series of graded photographic images can be compiled.

### Advantages of painted grading scales

The advantages of using artist-rendered (painted) versus photographic grading scales are as follows:

- The desired level of severity of a given condition can be depicted.
- Any chosen manifestation of a given condition can be depicted.
- The severity of the manifestation of a given condition can be systematically advanced.
- All images of a given complication can be painted using precisely the same colour scheme, and can be standardised with respect to angle of view, magnification, and associated ocular features (such as iris colour).
- Confounding artefacts unrelated to the complication being depicted (such as associated or secondary complications) can be avoided.

- Artistic licence can be adopted to embellish certain features or obscure others for clarity.
- Ancillary clues can be introduced to reinforce the notion of 'increasing severity' (such as increasing light scatter of the slit-lamp illumination reflex or increasing limbal hyperaemia).

Many of the design features described above can be seen in Figure 19.2, which is the grading scale sequence for stromal neovascularisation. The key pathological change is obvious – vessels of a given type (superficial plexus) progressively encroach onto the cornea from the 6 o'clock location. Associated subtle pathological signs are deliberately painted in to reinforce the notion of a worsening condition: the limbus becomes progressively more engorged, the corneal slit-lamp reflex progressively more diffuse, and the central cornea progressively more hazy. All other factors are kept constant: the full cornea is depicted from the same angle ('front on') in each case, iris size is constant, and the iris detailing and colouring is identical in each of the five frames. All these features combine to form a powerful, self-evident and unambiguous sequence of progressive stromal neovascularisation.

## Painted grading scales

In view of the arguments presented above, it was decided to develop a series of painted grading scales. The renowned British medical ophthalmic artist Terry Tarrant was commissioned to illustrate the complications. Mr Tarrant was provided with detailed specifications as to what was required; this comprised written instructions, colour sketches and colour photographs depicting the various conditions. The paintings were then generated and altered until the desired result was obtained.

## Principles of design

The primary design criterion was simplicity and ease of use by clinicians. Eight of the most important and interesting complications of contact lens wear were selected and categorised according to the tissue layer affected. Specifically, two complications from each of the corneal epithelium, corneal stroma, corneal endothelium and conjunctiva are depicted. The specific complications are given in Table 19.1.

A critical design feature of these grading scales is that only one series of illustrations is presented for each complication, requiring estimation of only a single grading score per complication. Other systems can be exceedingly complex because a given complication is sometimes depicted in numerous manifestations. This complexity can be further compounded by requiring individual gradings to be undertaken in a number of defined zones. While such grading schemes can have useful applications in certain research settings, the level of complexity is generally inappropriate for routine clinical use, where practitioners require a simple system that strikes a balance between accuracy and expediency.

Each complication is illustrated in five stages of increasing severity (from 0 to 4) (see Appendix A). The adoption of such a five-step grading scale has been advocated by Woods[1] as a concept that is widely used and certainly applicable to the field of contact lenses; indeed, the 0 to 4 scheme has been adopted by other authors of grading scales for contact lens complications.

An important conclusion drawn by Woods[1] is that, in clinical practice, assessment of the severity of an ocular reaction need not be restricted to those complica-

tions depicted in a given set of grading illustrations. This is because a universally applicable interpretation of clinical severity is assigned to each grading level. The grading scales described in this book were designed to cover the four key tissue types affected by contact lens wear so that estimation of the level of severity of tissue reactions not specifically depicted in these grading scales can be achieved by subjective extrapolation, albeit less accurately. That is, the procedure of estimating the level of severity will be easier to accomplish when this is performed with reference to an illustrated grading scale.

The depiction of each complication at each level of severity is based on an appraisal of accumulated evidence in the literature, and clinical experience. The maximum level of severity depicted (grade 4) is based upon the 'worst case scenario' likely to be seen in a contact lens clinic. 'Traffic light' colour banding from green (normal) to red (severe) denotes increasing severity; this feature will assist clinicians to instantly recognise a given grade.

### Image size

Each complication has been painted to an equivalent level of magnification that addresses the compromise between (a) being high enough to depict the key features of the tissue changes, and (b) being low enough to relate to what practitioners can observe with available clinical techniques. The approximate magnification of each of the eight complications (relative to a whole cornea depicted as ×1) is given in Table 19.1.

A consequence of these magnification levels is that, although epithelial microcysts and endothelial blebs can be detected and graded at ×40 magnification on a slit-lamp biomicroscope, they will not be viewed at the resolution depicted. Furthermore, endothelial polymegethism can only be assessed with the aid of an endothelial microscope. The other five complications can be viewed at the resolution depicted and are capable of being graded by direct observation and/or using a slit-lamp biomicroscope at up to ×40 magnification.

## Explanation of illustrations

Great attention has been paid to detail in the design and painting of the grading

scale sequences in order to make the images as realistic as possible. Below is a description of the essential features depicted in the painted images of each of the eight tissue complications. In each case, the painting corresponding to grade 4 (severe) is depicted because this image contains all elements of the pathological changes which have become manifest as the level of severity has increased.

### Epithelial staining

The whole cornea is illustrated in general diffuse illumination (Figure 19.3). A significant amount of limbal injection is depicted which intensifies throughout the grades to denote increasing severity. The bright green colour depicts staining with fluorescein. A combination of punctate, diffuse and coalescent staining is evident, along with a full-thickness epithelial erosion in the mid-peripheral cornea at 4 o'clock. The corneal slit-lamp reflex is blue because a cobalt blue light is used to induce fluorescence; the reflex becomes more diffuse throughout the grades due to an assumed generalised epithelial decompensation. Limbal hyperaemia increases with increasing grade.

### Epithelial microcysts

This image (depicted at ×100 magnification) is of a small section of cornea at the right-hand edge of the pupil (Figure 19.4). The microcysts are observed here in indirect retro-illumination, against an illuminated iris on the right and a dark pupil on the left. Over 100 microcysts can be observed, each displaying a characteristic reversed illumination; that is, a dark shadow is present on the right-hand side of each microcyst,

| Table 19.1 | Magnification at which complications are depicted |
| --- | --- |
| *Complication* | *Magnification* |
| Epithelial staining | ×1 |
| Epithelial microcysts | ×100 |
| Stromal oedema | ×40 |
| Stromal neovascularisation | ×1 |
| Endothelial polymegethism | ×600 |
| Endothelial blebs | ×200 |
| Conjunctival hyperaemia | ×2 |
| Papillary conjunctivitis | ×1 |

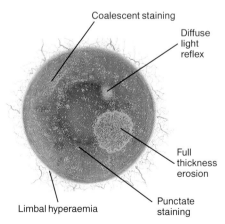

**Figure 19.3**
*Epithelial staining (grade 4)*

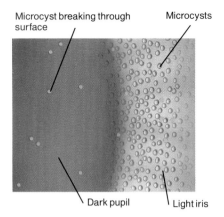

**Figure 19.4**
*Epithelial microcysts (grade 4)*

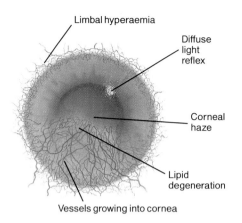

**Figure 19.6**
*Stromal neovascularisation (grade 4)*

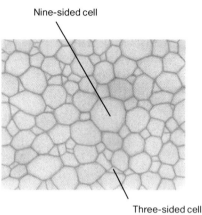

**Figure 19.7**
*Endothelial polymegethism (grade 4)*

which is the opposite dark/light orientation of the background. Microcysts to the extreme right of the field, and overlapping onto the pupil, are less visible because they are on the edge of the field of illumination. The bright green dots represent microcysts breaking through the epithelial surface and staining with fluorescein.

### Stromal oedema

The cornea is viewed here in optic section at ×40 magnification, with the epithelial surface to the right and the endothelium to the left (Figure 19.5). Artistic licence is adopted to depict the three classic signs of oedema in a single field of view. Vertical striae are visible in the posterior stroma; these typically represent at least 5 per cent oedema and are normally observed in optic section. Folds are seen in the endothelial mosaic; these usually indicate at least 8 per cent oedema and are normally observed in specular reflection. Bullous keratopathy is

observed in the epithelium; this usually suggests about 15 per cent oedema and is normally seen using diffuse illumination.

### Stromal neovascularisation

As with epithelial staining, the whole cornea is illustrated in general diffuse illumination (Figure 19.6). Limbal injection becomes more severe throughout the grades to denote increasing severity. A plexus of superficial vessels encroaches from the 6 o'clock area of the cornea into the central (pupillary) region. The cornea has suffered a considerable loss of transparency (depicted as a blue-green haze against a normally black pupil) and lipid degeneration is evident at the leading edge of the vessels. The corneal slit-lamp reflex becomes more diffuse throughout the grades due to epithelial compromise. (The full grading scale sequence relating to this condition is shown in Figure 19.2.)

### Endothelial polymegethism

The endothelial mosaic is shown in specular reflection at ×600 magnification (Figure 19.7). Severe endothelial polymegethism is depicted with the ratio of largest to smallest cell diameter being about 20 : 1. Considerable pleomorphism is also present, with a spectrum of shapes ranging from small three-sided to large nine-sided cells. It is not possible to grade the level of endothelial polymegethism using a conventional slit-lamp biomicroscope (which is typically limited to ×40 magnification), although it is possible to detect gross polymegethism (grade 4) because the larger cells can just be resolved. In general, endothelial polymegethism can only be graded with the aid of an endothelial microscope.

### Endothelial blebs

The endothelial mosaic is shown in specular reflection at ×200 magnification for clarity (Figure 19.8); however, it should be noted that it is possible to observe endothelial blebs at ×40 magnification using a slit-lamp biomicroscope. The 'blebs' are seen as black non-reflecting areas; these can be single cells or groups of adjacent cells. The separation between cells has grown with increasing severity.

### Conjunctival hyperaemia

The bulbar conjunctiva is viewed under general diffuse illumination, lateral to the 9 o'clock corneal location (Figure 19.9). The image is depicted at a magnification of about ×2. The superficial conjunctival vessels are grossly distended; a light reflex is depicted on the large horizontal vessel in the bottom third of the frame. Considerable underlying ciliary flush can be observed and the limbus is especially engorged.

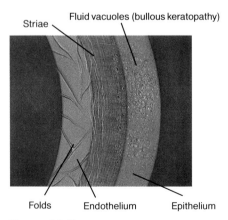

**Figure 19.5**
*Stromal oedema (grade 4)*

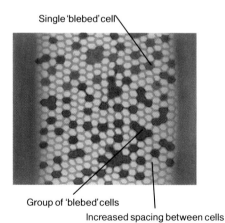

**Figure 19.8**
*Endothelial blebs (grade 4)*

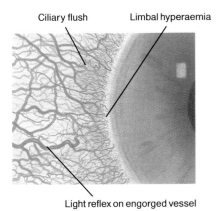

**Figure 19.9**
*Conjunctival hyperaemia (grade 4)*

## Papillary conjunctivitis

The upper eyelid has been everted to reveal the tarsal conjunctiva, which is viewed here without magnification under general diffuse illumination (Figure 19.10). The tarsal plate is covered with giant papillae, each of which displays a characteristic central vascular tuft. Numerous white reflexes emanating from the illumination source can be observed on the papillae. Mucus strands lie between papillae and on the corneal surface. The corneal slit-lamp reflex seen at the bottom of the frame becomes more diffuse and limbal hyperaemia increases throughout the grades due to generalised ocular decompensation.

## Method of grading

The tissue change of interest is observed using the slit-lamp biomicroscope under high and/or low magnification as required and the grading is estimated to the nearest 0.1 scale unit. For example, a tissue change that is judged to be considerably more severe than grade 2, but not quite as severe as grade 3, may be assigned a grade of 2.8 or 2.9. Although this procedure can sometimes be difficult, grading to the nearest 0.1 scale unit (rather than simply assigning a whole digit grade of 0, 1, 2, 3 or 4) accords much greater precision and increases the sensitivity of the grading scale for detecting real changes or differences in severity.[2]

Various grading scales are becoming available, so it is important that practitioners clearly designate on their record cards the grading system used and the specific tissue change being graded. For example, the following entry could be made on the record card:

'Epithelial staining – Efron 3.1'

A more expedient approach would be to print or stamp the eight tissue changes onto the record card, each with an accompanying box into which the assigned grade is entered. It may be necessary to add additional annotations to more fully describe the condition, such as (with respect to the example of epithelial staining above) superior, superficial, punctate etc.

An example of how a record card could be designed for use in association with the grading scales described here is given in Figure 19.11. The eight complications are listed in the same order as depicted on the grading scales in Appendix A. A data entry box is positioned on either side of each of the complications in which the numerical grade can be entered for each eye. It may be thought of as good practice to enter a grading for each of the eight complications listed (in most instances it will not be possible to enter a grading for endothelial polymegethism); however, it is not mandatory to do so. At 5–10 seconds per grading, it is estimated that a complete grading of both eyes (excluding endothelial polymegethism) would take about 2 minutes, which is thought to be commensurate with the time generally taken to perform a slit-lamp biomicroscope examination of a contact lens patient.

Additional spaces are provided below the eight specified complications so that other tissue changes and estimated gradings can be noted. A schematic outline of an everted eyelid and a cornea appear on each side of the list of complications for additional annotations and notes if required.

## Interpretation of grading

The 0 to 4 grading scale adopted here is based on a universally accepted concept that denotes increasing clinical severity as the numeric grade increases.[1] As described above, this schema can be applied to any tissue change – not only to those depicted. The interpretation of each grading step is given in Table 19.2. Perhaps the only exception with respect to these interpretations relates to the appearance of endothelial blebs, which require no clinical action even at grade 4. It must be recognised that this is only a general guide, and clinical action will be varied depending upon individual clinical opinion as well as other factors such as patient

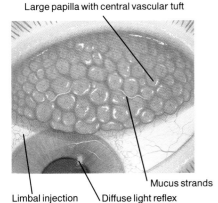

**Figure 19.10**
*Papillary conjunctivitis (grade 4)*

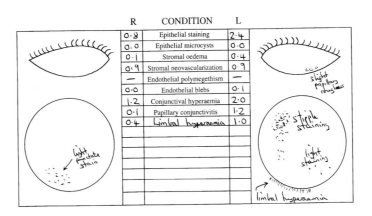

| R | CONDITION | L |
|---|---|---|
| 0·8 | Epithelial staining | 2·4 |
| 0·0 | Epithelial microcysts | 0·0 |
| 0·1 | Stromal oedema | 0·4 |
| 0·9 | Stromal neovascularization | 0·9 |
| — | Endothelial polymegethism | — |
| 0·0 | Endothelial blebs | 0·1 |
| 1·2 | Conjunctival hyperaemia | 2·0 |
| 0·1 | Papillary conjunctivitis | 1·2 |
| 0·4 | Limbal hyperaemia | 1·0 |

**Figure 19.11**
*Suggested design of record card for use in conjunction with Efron grading scales*

| Table 19.2 | Interpretation of grading levels |
| --- | --- |

| Grade | Interpretation |
| --- | --- |
| 0 | Normal – no tissue changes |
| 1 | Trace – clinical action not required |
| 2 | Mild – clinical action may be required |
| 3 | Moderate – clinical action usually required |
| 4 | Severe – clinical action urgently required |

symptomatology, the condition of the contact lenses, general health considerations etc.

In general, a grading of more than 2, or a change or difference in grading of more than 1.0 grading scale units,[3] is considered to be statistically and clinically significant.

## Grading morphs

As explained previously, accurate grading can be effected by interpolation to the nearest 0.1 grade unit. Most practitioners find the process of mental interpolation between two discrete grading steps to be quite difficult, notwithstanding the fact that this task becomes easier with practice. One way of partially overcoming this difficulty is to re-engineer the grading scales into a continuous movie sequence, progress through which can be controlled by the clinician attempting to decide upon a grade. Modern computer software technology is available to undertake such tasks; the process of merging discrete images into a continuous movie sequence is known as 'morphing'. The results of morphing will be familiar to many readers because this technique is used extensively in the visual arts to change the appearance of an object or person into another – for example, changing the face of a man into an ape.

Morphing is a technique that allows accurate interpolation of numerous progressively changing images between a 'start' and 'end' image, which are calculated pixel by pixel. When these images are presented one after the other in rapid succession, a movie or animation results, which allows one to observe the 'start' image being transformed into the 'end' image. The greater the number of interpolated images, the smoother will be the movie sequence. If the 'start' and 'end' images are not identical, the morphing technician can program the computer to link common elements in these images which are identified manually. The only limitation to the number of interpolated images is the amount of computer memory available, because a high-resolution image in many colours can be memory-intensive.

Morphing animation sequences have been developed for each of the complications depicted in Appendix A, and are incorporated into the accompanying CD-ROM. For each complication, it is possible to view the morph sequence as a continuous movie from grade 0 to grade 4, by manual adjustment (see Appendix C). Initial viewing of a continuous sequence is a useful exercise as it provides an overview of the extremes of severity of a condition and provides insights into the way in which a given condition worsens over time.

Chong *et al*[4] constructed morph sequences of three clinical conditions using clinical photographs – 3 and 9 o'clock staining, bulbar hyperaemia and palpebral conjunctival papillae. They compared the accuracy of grading using these morph sequences, versus that using a verbal descriptors scale and a discrete photographic scale. There was little difference between the three grading techniques with respect to the precision of grading, although the authors did suggest that bulbar hyperaemia and palpebral conjunctival papillae could be graded to a slightly higher degree of precision using morphs.

Whether or not increased precision using morphs can be definitively proven, it is clear that with computer-based management of administrative and clinical data becoming more commonplace, some practitioners will prefer to use morphs for convenience (and perhaps enjoyment) to grade the severity of contact lens-related ocular complications.

## Tear film classification

Classification and clinical interpretation of the appearance of the tear film was discussed in detail in Chapter 8. Particular attention was paid to the technique of viewing the tear film in specular reflection, which can be accomplished using a slit-lamp biomicroscope or a hand-held instrument such as the Tearscope (Keeler Limited, Windsor, UK).[5]

Photographs of the various forms of appearance of the lipid layer of the tear film as viewed with the Tearscope are presented in Appendix B. Five basic patterns that can be observed when examining the pre-ocular tear film are depicted for patients with light and dark eyes. The appearance of various degrees of lipid contamination due to the use of cosmetics, eye ointments and face creams, is also depicted.

Two image sequences show the appearance of the tear film on the surface of a soft lens and rigid lens over time as the eyelids are held open. In both cases, aqueous fringes begin to appear as the lipid and aqueous layers become thinner due to evaporation of the tear film.

It is important to note the essential difference between the grading scales in Appendix A and the tear film classification system in Appendix B. The grading scales are used to denote the level of severity of a given condition, whereas the tear film classification system facilitates categorisation of tear film types without necessarily inferring that one pattern is more or less severe than another, notwithstanding general trends of increasing or decreasing thickness of the component layers of the tear film. For example, a higher grading is always more severe than a lower grading when using the scales in Appendix A; however, a very thin or absent lipid layer (as indicated by an open meshwork pattern) may be just as problematic, for different reasons, as an excessive amount of lipid (as indicated by a globular, multi-coloured lipid pattern), determined using Appendix B. Certainly, both Appendix A and Appendix B can, in different ways, be of immense clinical value in conceptualising ocular complications of contact lens wear.

## Conclusions

Artist-rendered grading scales and a photographic-based tear film classification system have been devised as a clinical aid to accurate record keeping. These provide a practitioner-friendly means of recording adverse responses to contact lens wear and monitoring changes in severity over time and of accurately classifying various appearances of the tear film. The assignment of general guidelines relating to the necessity for clinical action with respect to each level of severity can be of assistance to clinicians in formulating a general framework for patient management. The grading scales will also nurture a common language that can assist practitioners to communicate clinical information within and beyond the confines of contact lens practice.

Clinicians are encouraged to use Appendices A and B as part of their routine contact lens practice so as to foster a disciplined and consistent approach to clinical decision making, which will ultimately be to the benefit of our patients.

## REFERENCES

1 Woods R (1989) Quantitative slit-lamp observations in contact lens practice. *J Br Contact Lens Assoc (Scientific Meetings)*: 42.
2 Bailey IL, Bullimore MA, Raash TW (1991) Clinical grading and the effects of scaling. *Invest Ophthalmol Vis Sci* **32**: 422.
3. Katsara SF (1998) Precision of grading contact lens complications. MSc Dissertation, University of Manchester.
4. Chong T, Simpson TL, Pritchard N (1996) Repeatability of discrete and continuous clinical grading scales. *Optom Vis Sci* **12s**: 232.
5. Guillon JP, Guillon M (1988) Tear film examination in the contact lens patient. *Contax* May: 14.

# Appendices

# Appendix A
# Grading scales for contact lens complications

# Epithelial staining

Grade 0

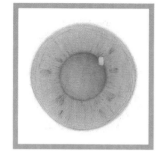

Whole view of cornea overlying dark pupil and grey iris (Referent: ×1 magnification)
Clear cornea with no evidence of staining
Note light blue reflex (indicating blue light in use to observe fluorescence) on upper right pupil border

Grade 1

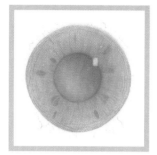

Trace amounts of punctate staining appear in the superior cornea
Trace conjunctival hyperaemia

Grade 2

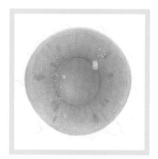

Mild punctate staining
Mild conjunctival hyperaemia

Grade 3

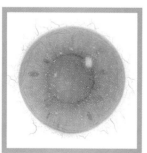

Moderate amount of diffuse punctate staining covering most of the cornea
Note that the light blue reflex on the upper right pupil border has become diffuse
Moderate conjunctival hyperaemia

Grade 4

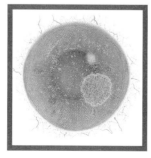

Severe diffuse punctate staining covering most of the cornea with full-thickness epithelial erosion to the lower right
Note that the light blue reflex on the upper right pupil border has become very diffuse
Marked conjunctival hyperaemia

# Epithelial microcysts

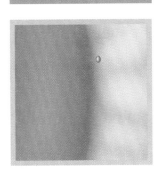

**Grade 0**

Very high-magnification view (×100) of cornea overlying slightly out-of-focus pupillary margin
The dark pupil is on the left and the yellow/brown iris is on the right
The cornea is clear

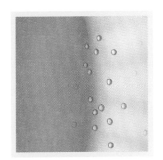

**Grade 1**

Trace response: a single microcyst appears in the superior field at the pupil–iris border
Note that the distribution of light within the microcyst (darker on the right and lighter on the left) is the opposite to the distribution of light in the background (lighter on the right and darker on the left)

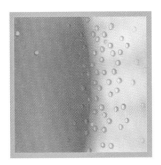

**Grade 2**

Mild response: approximately 20 microcysts are now visible
Some faint microcysts can be observed to the right of the field and over the dark pupil; these are newly formed microcysts which are deeper in the epithelium and thus less visible

**Grade 3**

Moderate response: approximately 70 microcysts are now visible
Some faint microcysts can still be observed
Bright green spots represent pits in the epithelial surface staining with fluorescein, at locations where the microcysts have broken through the epithelial surface

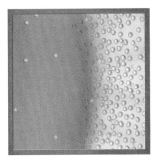

**Grade 4**

Severe microcyst response
Approximately 180 microcysts are now visible
Some faint microcysts can still be observed
More microcysts have broken through the epithelial surface and stain with fluorescein (depicted as green dots)

# Stromal oedema

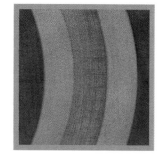

Grade 0

Thick (3 mm) optic section of normal cornea observed at ×40 magnification
*Left band*: endothelium in specular reflection
*Central band*: stroma with a slightly coarse texture
*Right band*: epithelium in direct illumination

Grade 1

Trace amount of oedema (4%)
A single, faint, white, vertical stria can be observed in the posterior stroma, slightly superiorly

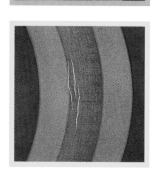

Grade 2

Mild amount of oedema (7%)
Three white, vertical striae can be observed in the posterior stroma, in the centre of the field

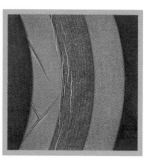

Grade 3

Moderate amount of oedema (11%)
Nine white, vertical striae can be observed in the posterior stroma
Two fold formations (one single fold and one Y-shaped fold) can be observed in the endothelium

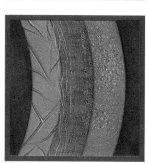

Grade 4

Severe amount of oedema (17%)
Approximately 16 white, vertical striae can be observed in the posterior stroma
Approximately 10 fold formations can be observed in the endothelium
The epithelium has become grossly oedematous and epithelial bullae can be observed

# Stromal neovascularisation

Grade 0

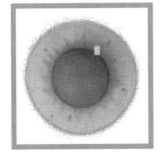

Whole view of cornea overlying dark pupil and light grey iris (×1 magnification)
Clear cornea with no evidence of neovascularisation
Note white reflex on upper right pupil border
Note prominent but normal limbal vasculature

Grade 1

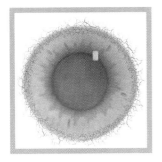

Trace amount of circumlimbal neovascularisation (<1 mm)
Cornea clear
Reflex sharp

Grade 2

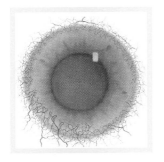

Mild amount of neovascularisation encroaching from the inferior right field
(2–3 mm)
Trace amount of background circumlimbal neovascularisation (<1 mm)
Mild limbal hyperaemia
Cornea clear
Reflex slightly speckled

Grade 3

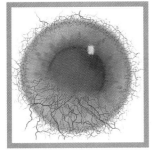

Moderate neovascularisation encroaching from the inferior right field (4–5 mm)
Trace amount of background circumlimbal neovascularisation (<1 mm)
Moderate limbal hyperaemia
Cornea slightly hazy
Reflex speckled

Grade 4

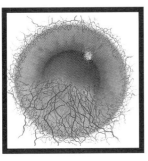

Severe neovascularisation encroaching from the inferior right field (6 mm)
Trace amount of background circumlimbal neovascularisation (<1 mm)
Intense limbal hyperaemia
Cornea very hazy
Reflex extremely diffuse

# Endothelial polymegethism

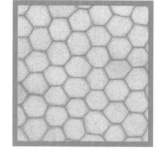

**Grade 0**

Extremely high-magnification view (×600) of the endothelium seen in specular reflection
Cells approximately all the same size
Co-efficient of variation: approximately 0.15
Normal endothelium of newborn baby
Cells primarily hexagonal in shape

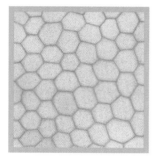

**Grade 1**

Trace variation in cell size
Co-efficient of variation: approximately 0.25
Normal endothelium of a 20-year-old
Cells primarily hexagonal in shape

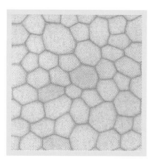

**Grade 2**

Mild variation in cell size
Co-efficient of variation: approximately 0.35
Normal endothelium of a 40-year-old
Cells primarily hexagonal in shape

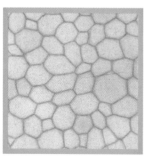

**Grade 3**

Moderate variation in cell size
Co-efficient of variation: approximately 0.45
Normal endothelium of a 60-year-old
Cells primarily hexagonal in shape, but some 4-, 5- and 7-sided cells

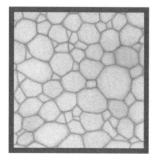

**Grade 4**

Severe variation in cell size
Co-efficient of variation: approximately 0.55
Normal endothelium of an 80-year-old
Cells primarily hexagonal in shape, but some 3-, 4-, 5-, 7-, 8-, and 9-sided cells

# Endothelial blebs

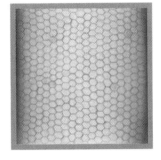

Grade 0

Very high-magnification view (×200) of the endothelium seen in specular reflection
No blebs visible
Cells primarily hexagonal in shape
Cells approximately all the same size

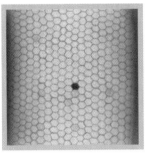

Grade 1

Trace bleb response
A single black bleb is visible
Cells primarily hexagonal in shape
Cells approximately all the same size

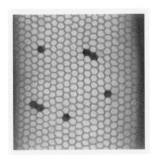

Grade 2

Mild bleb response
Severe black blebs are visible
Cells primarily hexagonal in shape
Cells approximately all the same size
Apparent increased separation of cells

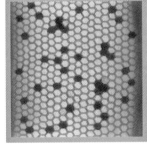

Grade 3

Moderate bleb response
Approximately 35 black blebs are visible, many joined in groups of 2 or 3
Cells primarily hexagonal in shape
Cells approximately all the same size
Further increase in cell separation

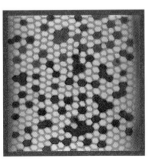

Grade 4

Severe bleb response
Approximately 80 black blebs are visible, many joined in groups of up to 6
Cells primarily hexagonal in shape
Cells approximately all the same size
Extensive cell separation

# Conjunctival hyperaemia

**Grade 0**

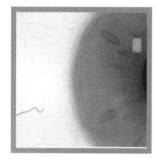

View of one-third of the cornea (*right*) and large field of conjunctiva (*left*) (×2 magnification)
Clear conjunctiva with one major vessel inferiorly
Limbus clear
Cornea clear

**Grade 1**

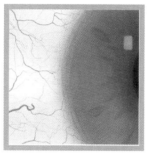

Trace conjunctival hyperaemia
Very slight increase in conjunctival redness
Very slight increase in limbal redness
Cornea clear

**Grade 2**

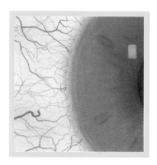

Mild conjunctival hyperaemia
Further increase in conjunctival redness
Further increase in limbal redness
Slight ciliary flush
Cornea clear

**Grade 3**

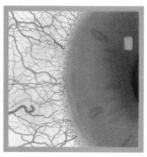

Moderate conjunctival hyperaemia
Conjunctiva quite red
Moderate limbal engorgement
Moderate ciliary flush
Cornea clear

**Grade 4**

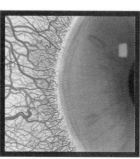

Severe conjunctival hyperaemia
Conjunctiva extremely red
Intense limbal engorgement
Intense ciliary flush
Cornea clear

# Papillary conjunctivitis

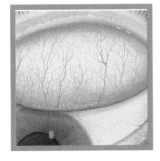

**Grade 0**

View of superior third of the cornea and everted superior eyelid revealing the upper tarsal conjunctiva (×1 magnification)
Hyperaemic tarsal conjunctiva with slight roughness at inferior tarsal fold (both normal)
Limbus and bulbar conjunctiva clear
Cornea clear

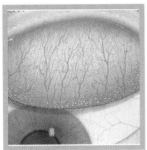

**Grade 1**

Trace papillary conjunctivitis
Increased hyperaemia of tarsal conjunctiva with increased roughness at inferior tarsal fold
Trace hyperaemia of limbus and bulbar conjunctiva
Cornea clear

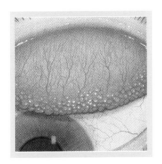

**Grade 2**

Mild papillary conjunctivitis
Mild hyperaemia of tarsal conjunctiva with roughness and papillae near inferior tarsal fold
Mild hyperaemia of limbus and bulbar conjunctiva
Corneal reflex slightly hazy

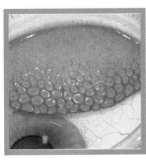

**Grade 3**

Moderate papillary conjunctivitis
Moderate hyperaemia of tarsal conjunctiva with large papillae covering the inferior two-thirds of the tarsal conjunctiva
Mild hyperaemia of limbus and bulbar conjunctiva
Corneal reflex hazy
Fine mucus strands on cornea and tarsus

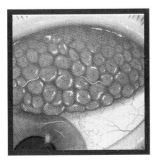

**Grade 4**

Severe papillary conjunctivitis
Severe hyperaemia of tarsal conjunctiva with very large papillae covering all of the tarsal conjunctiva
Mild hyperaemia of limbus and bulbar conjunctiva
Corneal reflex very hazy
More fine mucus strands on cornea and tarsus

# Appendix B
# Guillon–Keeler tear film classification system

All the pre-ocular and pre-lens tear film patterns depicted in this Appendix were imaged and captured photographically using the Tear-scope Plus. All tear film lipid patterns should be assessed before any other examination and should be judged two seconds after the blink when the upward motion of the tear film (a viscosity characteristic) has stopped.

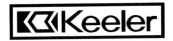

# Pre-ocular tear film lipid patterns

| | **Dark eye** | **Light eye** | |
|---|---|---|---|
| Open meshwork (marmorial) | 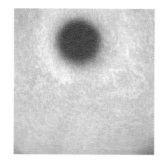 | 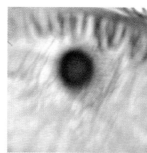 | Observed in 21% of population<br>13–50 nm thickness<br>Grey appearance of low reflectivity<br>Sparse, open meshwork pattern faintly visible following the blink<br>In the lower thickness range it may not be visible at low magnification<br>Thought to represent a deficient lipid layer |
| Closed meshwork (marmorial) | 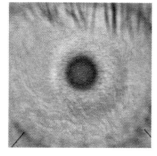 | 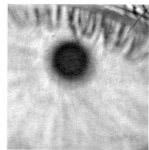 | Observed in 10% of population<br>30–50 nm thickness<br>Grey appearance of average reflectivity<br>More compact meshwork pattern<br>Thought to represent a normal lipid layer |
| Wave (flow) | 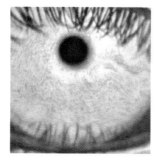 | 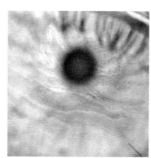 | Observed in 23% of population<br>50–80 nm thickness<br>Pattern of vertical or horizontal grey waves of good visibility between blinks<br>Most common lipid layer |
| Amorphous | 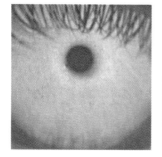 | 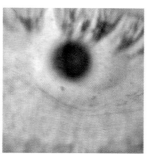 | Observed in 24% of population<br>80–90 nm thickness<br>Even pattern with whitish highly reflective surface<br>Thought to represent an ideal, well-mixed lipid layer |
| 1st order colour fringes | 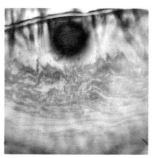 | 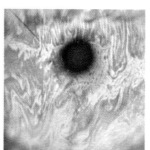 | Observed in 10% of population<br>90–140 nm thickness<br>Discrete brown and blue well-spread lipid layer interference fringes superimposed on a whitish background<br>Thought to represent a regular, very full lipid layer |

# Excessive and contaminated lipids

**2nd order colour fringes**

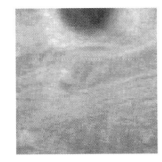

Observed in 5% of population
140–180 nm thickness
Discrete green and red tightly packed lipid layer interference fringes superimposed on a whitish background
Thought to represent an abnormal lipid layer of increased thickness in the coloured areas

**Globular lipid with multiple colours**

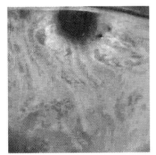

Observed in 7% of population
> 180 nm thickness
Highly variable colours, but typically combinations of brown, blue, green and red, irregularly spread
Sometimes globules of intense colour appear
Thought to represent an extremely heavy and irregular lipid layer, often associated with oversecretion, blepharitis or lipid contamination

**Lipid break-up and cosmetics**

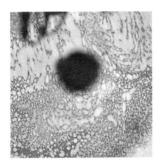

Abnormal lipid pattern
Seen when cosmetic products invade the tear film and break the lipid layer. The area devoid of lipid coverage appears dark grey as the light is specularly reflected from the bare aqueous phase. The area covered by lipid is highly reflective and can be confined to form isolated circular islands.

**Eye ointments**

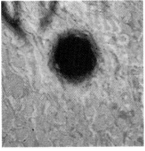

Abnormal appearance
Ointments destroy the normal tear film structure
Heavy striated fringes of yellow, brown, blue, green and purple, which are often irregularly distributed, indicating the variable thickness of the ointment

**Face cream**

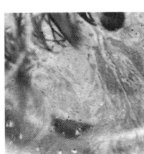

Lipid break-up observed when moisturisers or face creams invade and break the lipid layer
Coloured fringes on grey background

# Pre-soft lens tear film

The following sequence of images can be taken to represent an ideal pre-lens tear film going through the process of thinning due to drainage and evaporation. Initially, the presence of a superficial lipid layer reduces evaporation and the thick aqueous phase ensures the separation of the lipid and mucus phases. Following thinning of the aqueous phase, some lipid components migrate posteriorly and come into contact with the mucus phase and lens surface, producing non-wetting patches.

An alternative interpretation of this sequence of images is that they represent different tear film structures as they would appear immediately following eye opening. In this case, the images are arranged from 'best' to 'worst' and can be used to grade the quality of the pre-lens tear film.

Meshwork lipid coverage

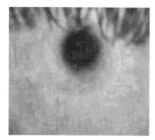

Appearance of a good tear film on the surface of a soft contact lens immediately after eye opening
Thin lipid layer present
Aqueous layer fringes not visible denote an aqueous phase of $> 3.5\ \mu m$ thick

Lipid with aqueous fringes

Appearance of tear film on the surface of a soft contact lens 4 seconds after eye opening
Very thin lipid layer of low visibility
Blue, green, yellow, and red aqueous interference fringes faintly visible under the lipid layer
Aqueous layer $2–3.5\ \mu m$ thick

Aqueous fringes

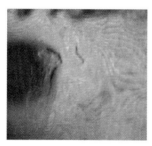

Appearance of tear film on the surface of a soft contact lens 8 seconds after eye opening
Lipid layer virtually absent
Narrow green and red aqueous interference fringes are easily visible
Aqueous layer $2\ \mu m$ thick

Dry area

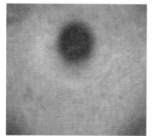

Appearance of tear film on the surface of a soft contact lens 12 seconds after eye opening
Lipid layer absent
Widely spaced, bright green and red aqueous interference fringes visible
Aqueous layer $< 1\ \mu m$ thick
Edge of the mucus layer visible
Lens surface visible at the centre of the dry spot

Lipid contamination

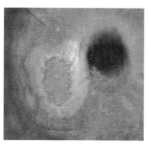

Appearance of tear film on the surface of a soft contact lens contaminated with lipid
Oval non-wetting patch occurring immediately after eye opening
Contaminating lipids highly visible
Blue, green, yellow and red interference fringes visible in a thin aqueous phase

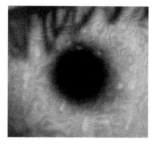

# Pre-RGP lens tear film

As for the pre-soft lens tear film, the following sequence of images of the pre-RGP lens tear film can be taken to represent either (a) an ideal pre-lens tear film going through the process of thinning, or (b) different tear film structures immediately following eye opening ranked from 'best' to 'worst'.

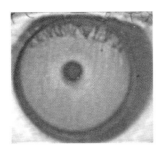

Complete lipid cover

Appearance of an ideal tear film on the surface of an RGP lens immediately after eye opening
Seen in only 5% of cases
Thin and complete lipid cover
Blue, green, yellow and red aqueous layer interference fringes faintly visible

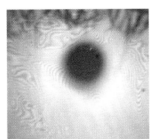

Thick aqueous layer

Appearance of tear film on the surface of an RGP lens 4 seconds after eye opening
Very thin lipid layer
Narrow aqueous layer interference fringes denote a thick aqueous phase
Aqueous layer > 2 μm thick

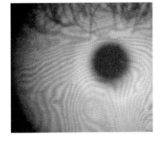

Medium aqueous layer

Appearance of tear film on the surface of an RGP lens 8 seconds after eye opening
Lipid layer absent
Well-defined aqueous layer interference fringes
Thinning of aqueous phase superiorly may be induced by the upper tear meniscus
Aqueous layer 1–2 μm thick

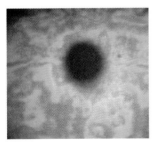

Thin aqueous layer

Appearance of tear film on the surface of an RGP lens 12 seconds after eye opening
Lipid layer absent
Broad, bright red and green aqueous layer interference fringes
Aqueous layer < 1 μm thick

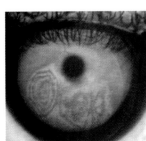

Drying

Appearance of tear film on the surface of an RGP lens 16 seconds after eye opening
Lipid layer absent
Irregular broad, bright red and green aqueous layer interference fringes visible, some in a circular pattern, formed by the evaporating tear film
Aqueous layer < 0.5 μm thick inferiorly and absent superiorly

# Appendix C
# Instructions for use of grading morphs on CD-ROM

## System requirements

This software will operate on either IBM compatible PC or Apple Macintosh platforms. The system requirements for operation of this software on an IBM compatible PC are as follows:

- 486 processor or better
- Windows 95 operating system
- 8 MB available RAM
- Monitor capable of displaying 16 bit colour ('thousands of colours')
- CD-ROM drive for installation
- 20 MB hard disk space (if transferring the program to your hard disk)

The system requirements for operation of this software on an Apple Macintosh computer are as follows:

- 68040 or PowerPC processor
- MacOS 7.6 or higher
- 8 MB available RAM
- Monitor capable of displaying 16 bit colour ('thousands of colours')
- CD-ROM drive for installation
- 20 MB hard disk space (if transferring the program to your hard disk)

This software may also operate on other computer configurations; full testing has only been performed on the above configurations.

## Installation of the CD-ROM

The software can be run directly from the CD-ROM but better performance will be achieved if the software is copied on to your hard disk. If you are operating the software directly from the CD-ROM, locate and open the 'Morphs CD' icon using Explorer or My Computer (Win 95) or on your Desktop (Mac). Now open the folder 'Morphs', and you are ready to begin.

Preferably, copy the folder 'Morphs' to your hard disk. Now, locate and open the folder 'Morphs' on your hard disk, and you are ready to begin.

## How to begin

After you have opened the folder 'Morphs', locate and start the application 'Go Morphs'.

Following the appearance of an introductory screen, you are presented with the following four options:

- Grading Morphs
- Information about Butterworth-Heinemann
- Information about *Optician*
- Exit

By selecting 'Grading Morphs', you will open this program (see below).

By selecting 'Information about Butterworth-Heinemann', you can find out about current and forthcoming titles from this publishing house.

By selecting 'Information about *Optician*', you can access information concerning this journal. Selecting 'Exit' will allow you to quit the application.

## How to use the program 'Grading Morphs'

When 'Grading Morphs' is selected, the grading morphs program will begin to run, and a title page appears with an instruction to 'View Morphs'.

Click on 'View Morphs'; a second window appears, from which you can choose any one of the eight available grading morphs shown in the menu along the top of the window.

A particular grading morph can be selected by clicking on the relevant picture in the menu bar along the top of the window. When this is done, the selected grading morph will be displayed in the right hand frame. The slide bar beneath the grading morph frame can be adjusted by clicking and holding the small black rectangular slide bar control handle and moving it in the appropriate direction. When the slide bar control handle is moved to the right, the grading morph advances and the level of severity increases. Moving the slide bar control handle to the left will reverse the grading morph to a lower level of severity. The slide bar control handle can be moved

back and forth in this way until the desired level of severity is achieved.

The numeric grading indicating the level of severity of the condition is indicated in the left hand frame as the grading morph is adjusted. This numeric grading is indicated to the nearest 0.1 grading scale unit, within the range from 0.0 (normal) to 4.0 (severe). The slide bar control handle can be released, re-engaged and moved as many times as required, before either selecting an alternative grading morph or quitting.

A different grading morph can be selected by clicking on the picture relating to any one of the other seven available grading morphs shown in the menu bar along the top of the window. The operating procedure as described above is identical for all eight grading morphs.

Clicking the 'Help' button on the lower blue menu bar opens a separate window which pictorially indicates how the program should be used. In this view, clicking on the red box in the lower left corner entitled 'Return to morph movies' will reopen the main window platform from which any of the eight grading morphs can again be selected.

The program can be restarted by clicking the 'Restart' button on the lower blue menu bar. Pressing this button returns the user back to the very beginning.

Clicking the 'Quit' button on the lower blue menu bar returns the user to the original four options on the introductory screen.

## In the event of problems

There is no technical support available for this CD-ROM. If you experience any problems, please make sure that your system meets the requirements detailed above. If problems persist, then in the first instance write to:

Butterworth-Heinemann
Linacre House
Jordan Hill
Oxford
OX2 8DP
UK

# Index

*Acanthamoeba* keratitis, 36, 118, 120, 121, 123, 124
Acidic shift
  bulbar hyperaemia, 35
  chemically induced, 35
  endothelial blebs, 135–6
  metabolically induced, 35
  polymegethism, 143, 145
Acute red eye syndrome, 36
*see also* CLARE (contact lens-induced acute red eye)
Acute spastic entropion, 15
Aging changes
  aponeurogenic ptosis, 14
  endothelial polymegethism, 140–1, 142, 143
  involutional ectropion, 14
  involutional entropion, 15
  meibomian gland dysfunction, 21
Alcian blue, 75
Allergic reactions
  atopic individuals, 44
  bulbar hyperaemia, 35
  papillary conjunctivitis, 43–4
  staining, 78–9, 80
Angiogenic inhibitors, 102
Antibiotics
  meibomian gland dysfunction, 22
  microbial infiltrative keratitis, 122
  staphylococcal anterior blepharitis, 25
Aponeurogenic ptosis, 11–12, 13, 14
Arcuate stains, 76
Artificial tears, 22, 25
Atopy, 44

Bacterial adherence, 37, 46, 120, 121, 122
Bandage lenses
  dry eye problems, 69
  microbial infiltrative keratitis, 122
  superior limbic keratoconjunctivitis, 56
Bedewing, 129–33
  aetiology, 131
  differential diagnosis, 132–3
  incidence, 129

  management, 131–2
  pathology, 130–1
  prognosis, 132
  signs/symptoms, 129–30
Benzalkonium chloride hypersensitivity, 78, 80
Blebs, 134–7
  aetiology, 135–6, 143
  differential diagnosis, 137
  grading, 136, 164, 177
  management, 136–7
  pathology, 135
  prevalence, 134
  signs/symptoms, 135
Blepharitis, 19
  seborrhoeic anterior, 25
  staphylococcal anterior, 24–5
Blepharospasm, 12, 14
Blindness, 116
Blink
  complete, 4
  forced, 4
  incomplete, 4
  inter-blink period, 4, 5
  pattern, 4, 5
  rate, 4, 5
  training, 8
  twitch, 4
Blinking, 3–8
  mechanism, 3–4
  purpose, 4–5
  spontaneous, 3–5
  types, 4
Blinking abnormalities, 5–8
  contact lens-induced ptosis, 12
  differential diagnosis, 8
  management, 8
Blurred vision
  meibomian gland dysfunction, 19, 20, 22
  total endothelial bedewing, 130
Bromhexine, 69
Bulbar hyperaemia, 33–9
  aetiology, 35–6
  definition, 33, 34

  differential diagnosis, 38–9
  grading, 34, 36–7, 164–5, 178
  pathology, 35
  prevalence, 34
  prognosis, 38
  signs/symptoms, 34–5
  treatment, 37–8

Care systems
  allergic reactions, 43
  bulbar hyperaemia, 35, 37
  disinfection efficacy, 120
  dry eye problems, 68
  microbial infiltrative keratitis, 120, 122–3
  papillary conjunctivitis, 43, 46
  staining, 78–9, 80
  sterile infiltrative keratitis, 112, 113
  superior limbic keratoconjunctivitis, 50, 51
  thimerosal-containing, 55
Central corneal clouding, 91–2
Chalazion (meibomian cyst), 8, 19, 22
  ptosis, 14
Chlamydial conjunctivitis, 47
Chlorhexidine, 78, 120
  allergic reaction, 78–9, 80
  dry eye problems, 68
  toxic reaction, 112, 113
Cicatricial ectropion, 14
Cicatricial entropion, 15
CLARE (contact lens-induced acute red eye), 109, 110
  bacterial aetiology, 111
  lens deposits, 112
  management, 112, 113
  prognosis, 113
Climate, warm, 121, 122
Cold compresses, 113
Collagen shield, 122
Complete blink, 4
Congenital ectropion, 14
Congenital entropion, 15
Conjunctival follicles, 47
Conjunctival haemorrhage, 39

Conjunctival hyperaemia *see* Bulbar hyperaemia
Conjunctival irrigation, 37, 46
Conjunctival papillae, 41, 47
Corneal exhaustion syndrome, 141
Corneal guttata, 132, 137, 146
Corneal hydration control, 142–3
Corneal infection, 79, 80
Corneal shape change, 149–57
  aetiology, 152–3
  curvature, 150, 152, 153–5, 156
  differential diagnosis, 156–7
  incidence, 149–50
  indentation, 151–2, 154, 155, 156
  keratoconus treatment, 149, 157
  management, 154–5
  orthokeratology, 149, 157
  pathology, 152
  prognosis, 155–6
  regularity, 150–1
  signs/symptoms, 150–2
  symmetry, 150, 152, 154, 155, 156
  wrinkling, 150, 151, 152, 154, 155, 156
Corneal surgery, 56
Corneal ulcer, 116, 117, 118
  hypoxia-induced oedema, 121
  overnight lens wear, 6
  *see also* Microbial infiltrative keratitis
Cotton thread test, 22, 62–3
Cromolyn sodium, 46, 47
Cryotherapy, 29
Culture-negative peripheral ulcer, 109, 110, 111
  management, 112
  prognosis, 113
Cyclosporin A, 69
Cystic fibrosis, 146

Debridement, 122
Delayed hypersensitivity, 43–4
*Demodex brevis*, 27
*Demodex folliculorum*, 27
Demodicosis, 26
Dermatochalasis, 14
Diabetes mellitus, 121, 146
Dimple stains, 76
Dimple veiling, 86
Disinfection efficacy, 120
Distichiasis, 29
Distortion *see* Corneal shape change
Dry eyes, 4, 66
  differential diagnosis, 22, 70
  meibomian gland dysfunction, 19, 22
  subtypes, 70
  tear ferning test, 67
  treatment, 68–70
  *see also* Tear film dysfunction

Ectropion, 14
  cicatricial, 14
  congenital, 14
  involutional, 14
  paralytic, 14
Electrolysis, 29
Eledoisis, 69
Embedded lens, 14–15
  ptosis, 14
Endothelium, 139
  contact lens-induced changes, 140
  size change definition, 139–40
Endotoxins, 111
Entropion, 15
  acute spastic, 15
  cicatricial, 15
  congenital, 15
  involutional, 15
  pseudo-entropion, 15
Ephedrine, 38
Epidemic keratoconjunctivitis, 114, 119
Epilation, 29
Epithelial desiccation, 5
'Epithelial plug', 76, 77
'Epithelial splitting' (superior epithelial arcuate lesion), 76, 77
Epithelial wrinkling, 156–7
Exposure keratitis, 78
  management, 79–80
Extended wear *see* Overnight wear
External hordeolum (stye), 22, 24
Eyelash disorders, 24–9
Eyelash parasitic infestations, 25–8
Eyelid
  absent, 16
  surgery, 13

Facial palsy, 14
Fischer–Schweitzer polygonal mosaic, 156, 157
Fluorescein, 75
  sequential staining, 76
  staining complications *see* Staining
  tear film assessment, 64–5
  use, 75–6
Flurbiprofen, 104
Folds, 92, 93
  differential diagnosis, 97
  pathology, 93
Foreign body tracks, 78
Fuch's endothelial dystrophy, 97, 137, 145
Fuch's heterochromatic cyclitis, 132, 133
Fungal keratitis, 119

Ghost vessels, 104, 105
  differential diagnosis, 105
Giant papillary conjunctivitis *see* Papillary conjunctivitis
Grading morphs, 166

Grading scales, 161–6, 167, 172–9
  conjunctival hyperaemia, 34, 164–5, 178
  design principles, 163
  endothelial blebs, 136, 164, 177
  endothelial polymegethism, 143–4, 164, 176
  epithelial microcysts, 85, 163–4, 173
  epithelial staining, 79, 163, 172
  image size, 163
  interpretation, 165–6
  methods of use, 165
  painted, 161–3
  papillary conjunctivitis, 45, 165, 179
  photographic, 161
  stromal neovascularisation, 103, 161, 164, 175
  stromal oedema, 95, 164, 174
Grave's disease, 8
Grey line, 24
Guillon–Keeler tear film classification system, 180–4

Haze, 92–3
  microbial infiltrative keratitis, 117
  pathology, 93
  sterile infiltrative keratitis, 109, 111
Herpes simplex keratitis, 119, 124
Histamine, 36
Horner's syndrome, 14
Humidification, 69
Hypercapnia, 6–7
  bulbar hyperaemia, 35
  endothelial blebs, 135, 136
  polymegethism, 143, 145
  staining, 78, 80
  *see also* Metabolic stress
Hypopyon, 116, 118
Hypoxia, 6–7
  alleviation strategies, 96
  bulbar hyperaemia, 35
  corneal shape change, 153, 154
  endothelial bedewing, 131
  endothelial blebs, 136
  microbial infiltrative keratitis, 120–1
  neovascularisation, 102
  oedema, 94, 95–6, 121, 131
  polymegethism, 143, 145
  prostaglandin-mediated vasodilatation, 36, 37
  staining, 78, 80
  sterile infiltrative keratitis, 111–12, 113
  superior limbic keratoconjunctivitis, 54–5
  *see also* Metabolic stress

Immediate hypersensitivity, 43
Immune system compromise, 25
Incomplete blink, 4
Infectious corneal ulcer, 79

Infectious keratitis, 108, 117
  *see also* Microbial infiltrative keratitis
Inferior epithelial arcuate lesion ('smile
  stain'), 76
Infiltrates, 108
  asymptomatic, 110–11
  intra-epithelial, 108
  sterile keratitis, 109–10
  stromal, 109
  sub-epithelial, 108–9
Infiltrative keratitis, 108
  classification, 109
  *see also* Microbial infiltrative keratitis;
    Sterile infiltrative keratitis
Inflammation, 36
Infra-red ocular thermography, 67
Injection, 33, 34
Insect entrapment, 28
Internal hordeolum, 22–3
Intrapalpebral fit, 8, 16
Involutional ectropion, 14
Involutional entropion, 15
3-Isobutyl-1-methylxanthine, 69

Keratitis *see Acanthamoeba* keratitis;
    Microbial infiltrative keratitis;
    *Pseudomonas* keratitis; Sterile infiltrative
    keratitis; Ulcerative keratitis
Keratoconus, 146, 156
  apical bearing, 149
  cone compression treatment, 157
Keratometry, 151
Krukenberg spindle, 130

Lacrimal gland function tests, 22
Lactic acid
  endothelial blebs, 136
  neovascularisation, 102
  oedema, 94
  polymegethism, 143
Lactoplate test, 22
Lagophthalmos, 15
Lens surface drying, 5
Lens binding, 150, 152, 154, 155
Lens deposits, 5, 37
  allergic reactions, 43
  calcium carbonate, 65
  'jelly bumps', 65
  microbial adherence, 37, 46, 121, 122
  papillary conjunctivitis, 43, 45
  protein deposits, 37, 43, 45–6, 54
  sterile infiltrative keratitis, 112
  superior limbic keratoconjunctivitis, 54
  tear-derived components, 65-6
Lens design, 8
  bulbar hyperaemia, 37
  dry eye problems, 68
  hypoxia alleviation strategies, 96, 123

microbial infiltrative keratitis, 122
  neovascularisation prevention, 104
  papillary conjunctivitis, 45–6
  polymegethism, 144–5
Lens fit, 8
  corneal shape change, 154–5
  staining, 77–8
  sterile infiltrative keratitis, 111, 113
Lens hygiene
  compliance, 121, 122–3
  microbial infiltrative keratitis, 121, 123
  sterile infiltrative keratitis, 112, 113
Lens movement, 16
  post-lens tear stagnation prevention, 6, 16
Lens positioning functions of lids, 16
Lens removal methods, 12, 14
Levator aponeurosis changes, 11–12, 13
Lice infestation, 27–8
  treatment, 28
Lid attachment fit, 8, 16
Lid hygiene
  bulbar hyperaemia, 37
  microbial infiltrative keratitis, 121
  papillary conjunctivitis, 46
  staphylococcal anterior blepharitis, 25
Lid scrubs
  meibomian gland dysfunction, 21–2
  mite infestation, 27
  papillary conjunctivitis, 46
Limbal hyperaemia, 99
Linear abrasions, 76
Loteprednol, 47
Lysozyme, 120

Marcus Gunn sign, 14
Marginal blepharitis, 24–5
Mast cell degranulation, 36
Mechanical trauma
  aponeurogenic ptosis, 14
  bulbar hyperaemia, 36
  microbial adherence, 121, 122
  microcysts, 85
  papillary conjunctivitis, 43
  shed eyelashes in eye, 29
  sterile infiltrative keratitis, 112, 113
  superior limbic keratoconjunctivitis, 54
Meibomian cyst *see* Chalazion
Meibomian gland dysfunction, 18–23
  aetiology, 20–1
  differential diagnosis, 22
  dry eye problems, 69
  grading system, 20
  management, 21–2
  papillary conjunctivitis, 44
  pathology, 20
  prevalence, 19
  prognosis, 22
  signs/symptoms, 19
Meibomian glands, 18

mechanical expression, 22
mechanical stimulation, 21
Meibomitis, 19
Metabolic stress
  bulbar hyperaemia, 35
  management options, 85–6
  microcysts, 84, 85
Microbial infiltrative keratitis, 108, 116–24
  aetiology, 120–2
  climatic factors, 121, 122
  definition, 116–17
  differential diagnosis, 123–4
  disposable lenses, 121–2
  incidence, 117
  management, 122–3
  microbial agents, 118–19
  pathology, 118–20
  prognosis, 123
  relative risk, 117
  signs/symptoms, 117–18
  time course, 118
Microcysts, 82–6, 132
  aetiology, 84–5
  differential diagnosis, 86
  grading, 85, 163–4, 173
  management, 85–6
  optical effects, 83–4
  pathology, 84
  prevalence, 82, 83
  prognosis, 86
  slit-lamp biomicroscope appearance, 82–3
  time course of onset, 84
Micropunctate staining, 76
Mite infestation, 25
  treatment, 27–8
Mucus balls, 86
Muscular dystrophy, 14
Myasthenia gravis, 14
Mydriatics, 122
Myogenic disease, 14
Myopia, 149
  orthokeratology, 157
Myopic shift, 153

Naphazoline, 38
Neovascularisation, 99–106
  aetiology, 102–3
  deep stromal, 101
  differential diagnosis, 105
  grading, 103, 161, 164, 175
  management, 103–4
  pathology, 101
  prevalence, 99–100
  prognosis, 104–5
  signs/symptoms, 100–1
  superficial, 100
  terminology, 99
  vascular pannus, 101

Neural control of vascular response, 102
Nits, 27
Non-steroidal anti-inflammatory drugs, 96, 122
Nutritional supplements, 69

Ocular decongestants, 37–8, 39
Ocular hygiene
  bulbar hyperaemia, 37
  papillary conjunctivitis, 46
Oedema, 91–7
  aetiology, 94–5
  central corneal clouding (CCC) criterion, 91–2
  contact lens-induced ptosis, 11, 12, 13
  corneal shape change, 153, 154
  definition, 91
  differential diagnosis, 97
  grading, 95, 164, 174
  hypoxia, 121, 131
  management, 95–6, 98
  neovascularisation, 102
  pathology, 93
  polymegethism, 142
  prevalence, 92
  prognosis, 97
  ptosis, 14
  signs/symptoms, 92–3
  stromal thinning, 93, 94–5, 102
Optic atrophy, 116
Oral contraceptives, 4
Orbicularis spasm, 15
Orthokeratology, 149, 157
Osmolarity changes
  bulbar hyperaemia, 35
  chemically induced, 35
  corneal wrinkling, 154
  metabolically induced, 35
Overnight wear
  microbial infiltrative keratitis, 120, 122, 123
  oedema management, 96
  post-lens tear stagnation prevention, 6
  sterile infiltrative keratitis, 111
Oxytetracycline, 56

Palpebral aperture size increase, 14
Papillary conjunctivitis, 40–8
  aetiology, 43–4
  classification, 41
  contact lens-induced ptosis, 12, 13
  differential diagnosis, 47–8
  grading, 45, 165, 179
  meibomian gland dysfunction, 44
  observation, 44–5
  pathology, 42–3
  prevalence, 40–1
  prognosis, 47
  ptosis, 14

signs/symptoms, 41–2
  treatment, 45–7
Parkinson's disease, 8
Pediculosis, 27
*Pediculus humanus capitis*, 27
*Pediculus humanus corpus*, 27
Phenylephrine, 38
Phthiriasis, 27–8
  treatment, 28
*Phthirus pubis*, 24, 27–8
Pilocarpine, 69
Polymegethism, 136, 139–46
  aetiology, 143
  definition, 139–40
  differential diagnosis, 145–6
  grading, 143–4, 164, 176
  management, 144–5
  pathology, 141–2
  prevalence, 140–1
  prognosis, 145
  signs/symptoms, 141
Polysorbate 80, 47
Post-lens tear stagnation, 5–6, 7
Posterior blepharitis, 18
Potassium metabolism, 35
Pre-corneal tear film, 5, 61–2
  lipid patterns, 2, 181
  maintenance, 4
Pre-lens tear film, 5
  RGP lens, 184
  soft lens, 183
Preservative-free care solutions, 37, 46
Pressure patching, 56
Prostaglandins
  endothelial bedewing, 131
  vasodilatation mediation, 36, 37
*Pseudomonas* keratitis, 118, 119–20, 121, 123, 124
Pseudotrichiasis, 15
Ptosis, 8, 10–16, 146
  aetiology, 12
  differential diagnosis, 14
  management, 13–14
  measurement, 11
  pathology, 11–12
  prevalence, 11
  prognosis, 14
  signs, 10–11
  symptoms, 11
  time course of onset, 11
Ptosis crutch/lugs, 13–14
'Pump-leak' mechanism, 143
Punctal plugs, 69
Punctate staining, 76

Red eye, 33
  acute red eye syndrome, 36
  contact lens-induced acute (CLARE), 109, 110

definition, 33–4
  differential diagnosis, 38–9
  *see also* Bulbar hyperaemia
Re-wetting drops, 68–9
Rigid lens 'bridging', 15–16
Rose bengal, 75
  mechanism of staining, 77
  use, 76

Schirmer test, 22, 62
Scleral lens, 13–14
Sebaceous gland carcinoma, 23
Secretory IgA, 67
Shed eyelashes in eye, 28–9
'Smile stain' (inferior epithelial arcuate lesion), 76
Smoking, 121
Soaking soft lenses, 69
Solar radiation, 146
Staining, 75–80
  aetiology, 77–9
  differential diagnosis, 80
  grading, 79, 163, 172
  management, 79–80
  microbial infiltrative keratitis, 117
  ocular discomfort, 77
  pathology, 77
  prevalence, 75
  prognosis, 80
  signs, 75–7
  slit-lamp biomicroscope appearance, 76
Sterile infiltrative keratitis, 108–14
  differential diagnosis, 114, 123
  management, 112–13
  pathology, 111
  prevalence, 109
  prognosis, 113–14
  signs/symptoms, 109–10
  terminology, 108–9
Sterile keratitis, 108
  *see also* Sterile infiltrative keratitis
Striae, 92
  differential diagnosis, 97
  pathology, 93
Stromal infiltrates, 114
Stromal thinning, 93, 94–5
  neovascularisation, 102
Superficial punctate erosion, 76
Superficial punctate keratitis, 76
Superior epithelial arcuate lesion ('epithelial splitting'), 76, 77
Superior limbic keratoconjunctivitis, 50–6, 101
  aetiology, 52–5
  differential diagnosis, 56
  pathology, 52
  prevalence, 50–1
  prognosis, 56
  signs/symptoms, 51–2

treatment, 55–6
Suprofen, 47
Surface Asymmetry Index, 150, 151, 152
Surfactant lens cleaning, 22
Sympathetic innervation, 35–6

Tap water, 121, 123
Tarsal conjunctiva, 41
Tear break-up mechanism, 67
Tear break-up time, 4, 5, 62, 67
    measurement, 64, 65
    tear film dysfunction, 64
Tear evaporation rate, 5
Tear exchange, 4
Tear ferning, 67
    meibomian gland dysfunction, 20
Tear film
    composition, 66–7
    function during contact lens wear, 62
    lipid patterns, 63–4, 181, 182
    meibomian gland function, 18
    structure, 61–2
    temperature, 67
    turnover, 67
Tear film classification, 166
    Guillon–Keeler system, 180–4
Tear film dysfunction, 61–70
    differential diagnosis, 70
    lens deposits, 65–6
    observations, 62
    ocular surface staining, 64
    pathology, 66–8
    post-lens tear film thinning, 66
    prognosis, 70
    signs, 62–6
    symptoms, 66
    tear film stability, 64
    tear film structure, 63–4
    tear volume assessment, 62–3
    treatment, 68–70

*see also* Dry eyes
Tear mixing, 7
Tear pH, 66
Tear stimulants, 69
Tear tonicity, 66
Tear volume assessment, 62–3
    meibomian gland dysfunction, 22
Tearscope, 63, 64, 166
Tetrahydrozaline, 38
Theodore's superior limbic
    keratoconjunctivitis, 50, 52, 56
Thimerosal
    contact lens solutions, 55
    dry eye problems, 68
    hypersensitivity, 43, 52, 53–4, 78–9, 80
    keratoconjunctivitis/keratopathy, 50, 51
    papillary conjunctivitis, 43
    toxic reaction, 54, 112, 113
Third nerve palsy, 14
Three and nine o'clock staining, 7–8, 15–16,
    64, 68, 78
Tissue adhesives, 122
Topical steroids
    neovascularisation prevention, 104
    papillary conjunctivitis, 47
    staphylococcal anterior blepharitis, 25
    sterile infiltrative keratitis, 113
    superior limbic keratoconjunctivitis, 56
Topographic changes *see* Corneal shape
    change
Topographic Modelling System, 150
Toxic reactions
    bulbar hyperaemia, 35
    care solutions *see* Care systems
    staining, 78, 80
Trapped debris, 5, 6, 7
Trichiasis, 29
Tumours
    blinking abnormalities, 8
    ptosis, 14

Ulcerative keratitis, 108, 117
Uveitis, 132, 133

Vascular pannus, 101
Vascular response, 99
    abnormal, 100–1
    normal, 100
Vascularisation, 99
Vascularised limbal keratitis, 105
Vascularity, 33, 34
Vasoproliferation, 99
Vasostimulatory factors, 102
Vernal conjunctivitis, 47, 48
    ptosis, 14
Vessel penetration, 99
Videokeratography, 150, 151
Viral conjunctivitis, 47
Vision loss, 108
    corneal shape change, 156
    corneal wrinkling, 151, 155
    microbial infiltrative keratitis, 116
    microcysts, 84
    neovascularisation, 101, 104
    staining, 76–7
Vitamin A therapy, 47

Warm compresses
    meibomian gland dysfunction, 21
    papillary conjunctivitis, 46
Warpage *see* Corneal shape change
Wear time reduction
    dry eye problems, 69–70
    endothelial bedewing, 131–2
    neovascularisation prevention, 104
    oedema management, 96
    sterile infiltrative keratitis, 112–13

Yellow mercuric oxide ointment, 27, 28

# Subscribe to Optician

## And receive your own personal copy every week

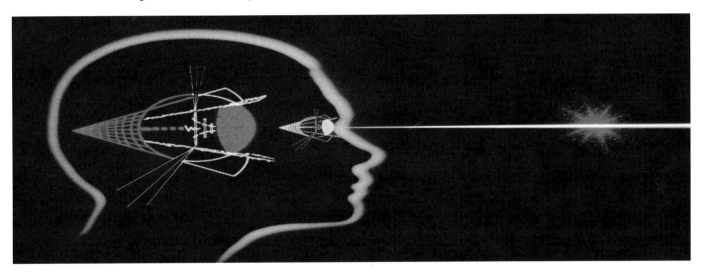

- ■ exclusive news coverage
- ■ latest job vacancies
- ■ fashion trends
- ■ approved continuing education
- ■ college approved CET
- ■ clinical and technical features

- ■ business management information
  AND a range of supplements throughout the year:
- ● eyestyle
- ● instrument insight
- ● optical technician
- ● recruitment
- ● optical yearbook
- ● wallplanner

For current subscription rates simply telephone 01444 475634 or fax 01444 445447
Quote code 124.

Or fill in the coupon below and return it to: Optician Subscriptions, FREEPOST RCC2619, HAYWARDS HEATH, RH16 3BR
(please affix stamp if posted outside the UK)

- - - - - - - - - - - - - - - - - - - - - - - - - - - - - - - - - - - - - - - - - - - - - - - - - - - - - - -

☐ Please send me the current subscription rates for Optician

Title       Initial      Surname

Job title

Address    ☐ home    ☐ practice

Postcode            Telephone               Code 124